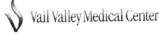
This Material Graciously Donated By the
Community Cancer Coalition

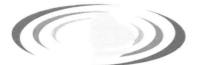

SHAW REGIONAL
CANCER CENTER

Toward the Elimination of Cancer Disparities

Howard K. Koh, MD, MPH
Editor

Toward the Elimination of Cancer Disparities

Clinical and Public Health Perspectives

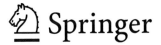 Springer

Editor

Howard K. Koh, MD, MPH
Department of Health Policy
  and Management
Division of Public Health Practice
Harvard School of Public Health
677 Huntington Ave.
Boston, MA 02115
USA

MassCONECT Publication Credit:

This publication was supported in part by MassCONECT funded under Grant Number 5 U01
CA114644 from the National Cancer Institute. Its contents are solely the responsibility of the
authors and do not necessarily represent the official views of the National Cancer Institute's
Center to Reduce Cancer Health Disparities.

ISBN 978-0-387-89442-3   e-ISBN 978-0-387-89443-0
DOI 10.1007/978-0-387-89443-0
Springer Dordrecht Heidelberg London New York

Library of Congress Control Number: 2009920396

Printed on acid-free paper

Springer is part of Springer Science+Business Media (www.springer.com)

Preface

The societal burden of cancer is one of the major public health challenges of our time. Yet that burden is not equally shared by all. Troubling disparities have been documented not only by racial/ethnic group but also by social class, insurance status, geography, and a host of other dimensions. Furthermore, such disparities represent the end result of a constellation of forces stemming from inside and outside the health care system. Many cancer disparities should be preventable.

Few have attempted to capture the breadth and depth of the dimensions of cancer disparities from both clinical as well as public health perspectives. To address this need, we present this volume to:

- broaden concepts of disparities beyond traditional discussions of race/ethnicity to explore how, where, and why they occur;
- focus on cancer disparities in the US, while citing some major examples from abroad;
- analyze certain major cancers with respect to disparities, with emphasis on socioeconomic position;
- examine the sources of disparities from both inside and outside the health care system;
- identify initial interventions that attempt to reduce and eliminate these disparities; and
- identify issues that deserve attention with respect to future research.

Our monograph addresses cancer disparities across the continuum (from prevention to mortality and by the domains of social inequality). We begin by exploring broad dimension such as definitions of disparities, data systems, the role of genes and environment, and the role of work and occupation in cancer disparities. Then we move into specific challenges in cancer disparities such as tobacco use and lung cancer, breast cancer, colorectal cancer, prostate cancer, cervical cancer, melanoma, and hepatocellular carcinoma. We then conclude with some avenues to address cancer disparities, including policy and advocacy, health communication, overcoming barriers to cancer care, and community-based approaches. Our efforts are far from exhaustive, but they represent one of the first attempts to address cancer disparities from such a comprehensive perspective.

This volume reflects the work of a number of national experts in cancer disparities. Many are members of the Executive Committee of the Cancer Disparities Program-in-Development of the Dana-Farber/Harvard Cancer Center. Still others are also investigators in the National Cancer Institute Community Network Program MassCONECT (Massachusetts Community Networks to Eliminate Cancer Disparities through Education, Research and Training). Also, this volume updates and expands a earlier 2005 monograph on the topic published in the journal *Cancer Causes and Control*. All authors are dedicated to the goal of eliminating cancer disparities and I am indebted to them.

I am particularly grateful to Rachel Warren, Terra Zipoyrn Snider, and Dr. Claudia Arrigg for their unending encouragement and support. It is my hope that this monograph represents another contribution toward helping all people enjoy their highest attainable standard of health.

Boston, MA   Howard K. Koh, MD, MPH

Contents

Contributors

Christopher A. Aoki Division of Gastroenterology and Hepatology, Department of Internal Medicine, School of Medicine, University of California, Davis, CA

Otis W. Brawley American Cancer Society and Emory University, Atlanta, GA

Marcela del Carmen Division of Gynecologic Oncology, Massachusetts General Hospital, Harvard Medical School, Boston, MA

Moon S. Chen Division of Hematology and Oncology, Department of Internal Medicine, School of Medicine, University of California, Davis, CA

Dexter Cooper Behavioral Research Center, American Cancer Society, National Home Office, Atlanta, GA

Teresa Diaz-Montez Division of Gynecologic Oncology, The Johns Hopkins Medical Institutions, Baltimore, MD

Karen Donelan MGH Cancer Center, Massachusetts General Hospital, Boston, MA

Loris Elqura Division of Public Health Practice, Harvard School of Public Health, Boston, MA

Karen M. Emmons Department of Society, Human Development, and Health, Dana-Farber Cancer Institute, Harvard School of Public Health, Boston, MA

Stephanie M. Fullerton Department of Medical History and Ethics and Center for Genomics and Healthcare Equality, University of Washington, Seattle, WA

Alan Geller Division of Public Health Practice, Harvard School of Public Health, Boston, MA

Barbara Gottlieb Harvard Medical School and Harvard School of Public Health, Boston, MA

Amy Harley Harvard School of Public Health, Department of Society, Human Development and Health; Dana-Farber Cancer Institute, Center for Community-Based Research, Boston, MA

Lokie Harmond Behavioral Research Center, American Cancer Society, National Home Office, Atlanta, GA

Michelle Holmes Harvard Medical School, Boston, MA

Ahmedin Jemal Behavioral Research Center, American Cancer Society, National Home Office, Atlanta, GA

Christine M. Judge Division of Public Health Practice, Harvard School of Public Health, Boston, MA

Howard K. Koh Harvey V. Fineberg Professor of the Practice of Public Health, Associate Dean for Public Health Practice, Director, Division of Public Health Practice, Harvard School of Public Health, Boston, MA

Nancy Krieger Department of Society, Human Development, and Health, Harvard School of Public Health, Boston, MA

Kenneth Olden Laboratory of Molecular Carcinogenesis, National Institute of Environmental Health Sciences, National Institutes of Health, Research Triangle Park, NC

Barbara D. Powe Behavioral Research Center, American Cancer Society, National Home Office, Atlanta, GA

Lisa Quintiliani Harvard School of Public Health, Department of Society, Human Development and Health; Dana-Farber Cancer Institute, Center for Community-Based Research, Boston, MA

Eric C. Schneider Harvard School of Public Health, Boston, MA

Grace Sembajwe Harvard School of Public Health, Department of Society, Human Development and Health; Dana-Farber Cancer Institute, Center for Community-Based Research, Boston, MA

Alexandra E. Shields Harvard/MGH Center on Genomics, Vulnerable Populations, and Health Disparities, and Institute for Health Policy, Massachusetts General Hospital/Partners HealthCare; Department of Medicine, Harvard Medical School, Boston, MA

Sarah Massin Short Division of Public Health Practice, Harvard School of Public Health, Boston, MA

Glorian Sorensen Harvard School of Public Health, Department of Society, Human Development and Health; Dana-Farber Cancer Institute, Center for Community-Based Research, Boston, MA

K. Viswanath Dana-Farber Cancer Institute, Harvard School of Public Health, Boston, MA

Deborah Klein Walker Health Division, Abt Associates, Inc., Cambridge, MA

David Williams Department of Society, Human Development, and Health, Harvard School of Public Health, Boston, MA

Sherrie Flynt Wallington Harvard School of Public Health, Boston, MA

Part I
Dimensions of Cancer Disparities

Chapter 1
Defining, Investigating, and Addressing Cancer Inequities: Critical Issues

Nancy Krieger, Karen M. Emmons, and David Williams

Abstract Research and action to address social disparities in cancer require clarity about what constitutes and causes these persistent and onerous inequities in health. Currently, both scientific literature and government documents exhibit important disagreements, confused terminology, and considerable, if not deliberate, vagueness about the meaning of the phrase "cancer disparities." To help clarify what is meant by social disparities in cancer and what this means for efforts to investigate their causes and act to rectify them, this chapter offers a definition of cancer inequities that is premised on the causal contention that health inequities, by definition, arise from social inequity and considers its implications for developing a multidisciplinary research agenda for investigating and addressing social inequalities in cancer. Tackling this issue will require rigorous and critical frameworks, questions, and methods derived from multiple disciplines and will necessarily involve epidemiologic, clinical, and intervention research, both quantitative and qualitative. At issue is making conscious research choices about which types of disparities we study, in relation to which aspect of cancer, so as to improve the likelihood our research will help inform a society-wide discourse about the extent of, origins of, and remedies for social injustices in cancer, thereby aiding efforts to eliminate health inequities.

Research and action to address social disparities in cancer require clarity about what constitutes and causes these persistent and onerous inequities in health (Krieger 2005a). Marked socioeconomic and racial/ethnic inequalities in cancer incidence, survival, and mortality have been documented since the early twentieth century in the UK, the US, and other countries (Kogevinas et al. 1997;

This chapter is in part based on an article by Nancy Krieger previously published in Cancer Causes and Control (vol 16, pp, 5–14, 2005), © 2005 Springer; the publisher (Springer) has given permission for text to be included from this prior article.

N. Krieger (✉)
Department of Society, Human Development, and Health, Harvard School of Public Health, Kresge 717, 677 Huntington Avenue, Boston, MA 02115, USA
e-mail: nkrieger@hsph.harvard.edu

H.K. Koh (ed.), *Toward the Elimination of Cancer Disparities*,
DOI 10.1007/978-0-387-89443-0_1, © Springer Science+Business Media, LLC 2009

Singh et al. 2003; Trans-HHS Cancer Disparities Progress Review Group [THCDPRG] 2004). This "unequal burden of suffering and death due to cancer" (THCDPRG 2004, p. vi) remains with us still, as documented in the March 2004 report of the US Department of Health and Human Services' (HHS) Trans-HHS Cancer Health Disparities Progress Review Group (2004), which found that "minority and underserved populations ... are significantly more likely to be diagnosed with and die from preventable cancers, be diagnosed with late-stage disease for cancers detectable through screening in the early stage, receive either no treatment or treatment that does not meet currently accepted standards of care, die of cancers that are generally curable, and suffer from cancer without the benefit of pain control and other palliative care" (THCDPRG 2004, p. 2).

Agreement on these sorry facts of social inequities in cancer, however, does not necessarily entail accord as to their causes (Krieger 2001, 2005a). Indeed, since the rise of the modern public health movement in the mid-nineteenth century, important debates have focused on the ever-present question of who and what is responsible for these health disparities: Bad genes? Bad behaviors? Bad (or non-existent) health care, plus a failure to act on relevant knowledge? Or bad living and working conditions born of social inequity that become embodied as social inequities in health, including cancer (Patterson 1987; Porter 1999; Krieger 2001)? This article accordingly reviews critical issues relevant to cohering understanding of what is meant by "cancer disparities," offers a definition, and considers its implications for developing a multidisciplinary research agenda on social inequalities in cancer.

Definitions and Debates

The meaning of the phrase "social disparities in cancer" and the related term "social disparities in health," while perhaps seemingly self-evident, is in fact contentious. Review of the relevant scientific literature and government documents reveals a complex mix of important disagreements, confused terminology, and considerable, if not deliberate, vagueness (Whitehead 1990; Carter-Pokras and Bacquet 2002; Braveman and Gruskin 2003; Graham 2007, pp. 3–18). Words commonly employed, in reference to cancer and other health outcomes, include "health disparities," "social disparities in health," "health inequalities," "social inequalities in health," "health inequities," "health variations," and "health differences." Yet, while at first glance these myriad terms may appear to be synonymous, they are not – and the distinctions in meaning are important, not simply semantic. At issue are profound questions of who and what is accountable for social inequalities in health and thus what sorts of remedies should be developed, by whom, to address and ultimately eliminate them.

In brief, the argument boils down to the distinctions between inequity and difference. As clarified in the considerable literature generated by and in response to the World Health Organization on this issue, the concept of inequity involves notions of fairness and injustice, while difference simply means difference – with no normative judgment (Whitehead 1990; Carter-Pokras and Bacquet 2002; Braveman and Gruskin 2003; Graham 2007, pp. 3–18). As translated to health (Whitehead 1990),

(1) *Inequities in health* "… are unnecessary and avoidable, but in addition, are also considered unfair and unjust" while *Equity in health* means "everyone has the fair opportunity to attain their full health potential"; by contrast
(2) *Inequalities in health* as a term, is not explicit about injustice or fairness and instead could refer to differences that do not necessarily arise from inequity.

For example, social injustice is *not* a determinant of only men being at risk of getting prostate cancer and only women being at risk of getting cervical cancer. This difference in risk, by biological sex, however, is strictly that – a difference. Even so, social injustice – for example, involving class, racism, and gender – can nevertheless play an important role in determining the risk and outcome of each of these types of cancers, respectively, *among* men and *among* women.

Despite the clear-cut distinction between inequity and difference, however, confusion arises because the literature employs a welter of different and over-lapping terms. For example, while the phrase "social inequalities in health" clearly is intended to refer to health inequities, it sometimes – especially in the UK – is shortened to simply "health inequalities" (Davey Smith 2003; Graham 2007). Moreover, several prominent official documents have sought to use the term "health inequalities" and kindred phrases to *avoid* referring to issues of inequity. Thus, the WHO's *World Health Report 2000* (WHO 2000) explicitly defined "health inequalities" as solely differences in health among individuals and asserted these individual differences should be the object of study, rather than differences in health across social groups. Their argument was that examining data categorized in relation to a priori groups, say, by income level, was to "prejudge" the evidence in relation to notions of inequity. Similarly, the 1995 UK report *Variations in Health* (Variations Sub-Group 1995) deliberately spoke solely of "variations," likewise to avoid implications involving injustice. Continuing in this vein, the December 2003 version of the US *National Healthcare Disparities Report* (Agency for Healthcare Research and Quality [AHRQ] 2003), bearing a legally mandated title, asserted "Where we find variation among populations, this variation will simply be described as a difference. By allowing the data to speak for themselves, there is no implication that these differences results in adverse health outcomes or imply prejudice in any way."

Of note, all three reports stirred up major controversies (Braveman et al. 2000; Gakidou et al. 2000; Almeida et al. 2001; Braveman et al. 2001; Murray 2001; Bloche 2004; Steinbrook 2004). The upshot, reflected in the WHO's *World Health Report 2003* (WHO 2003), the 1998 UK *Independent Inquiry into Inequalities in Health Report*, also known as the *Acheson Report* (Acheson et al. 1988), and the re-issued February 2004 version (AHRQ 2004) of the US *National Healthcare Disparities Report* (AHRQ 2003), which includes text on health disparities that was deliberately deleted from the December 2003 edition, is renewed affirmation that equity is fundamental to the mission of improving population health. Consequently, health inequities must be addressed explicitly.

Within the US, however, explicit reference to equity and inequity is uncommon in our health research and reports. Instead, virtually uniquely among nations, our official and scientific discourse chiefly uses the phrase "health disparities," with an implicit understanding that these disparities are in some way unjust (Carter-Pokras and Bacquet 2002). Most typically, as with the official definitions used at the National Institutes of Health (NIH) (see Table 1.1), the term "health disparities" is used, often euphemistically, as a shorthand for "racial/ethnic disparities in health," albeit without ever referring to racism or

Table 1.1 US official definitions of "health disparities"

Source	Definition
National Institutes of Health (NIH, 1999)	"Health disparities are differences in the incidence, prevalence, mortality and burden of diseases and other adverse health conditions that exist among specific population groups in the United States. The NIH Program of Action initially will focus on racial and ethnic minority populations: African Americans, Asians, Pacific Islanders, Hispanics and Latinos, Native Americans and Native Alaskans. Research on health disparities related to socioeconomic status will also be addressed."
NIH National Center on Minority Health and Health Disparities (2007)	Mission concerned with: "reducing the profound disparity in health status of America's racial and ethnic minorities, Appalachian residents, and other health disparity populations, compared to the population as a whole."
US Department of Health and Human Services, *Healthy People 2010* (2000)	Second overarching goal: "to eliminate health disparities among segments of the population, including differences that occur by gender, race or ethnicity, education or income, disability, geographic location, or sexual orientation."
National Cancer Institute (NCI) Division of Cancer Control and Population Sciences (2007)	"Health disparities are differences in the incidence, prevalence, mortality, and burden of cancer and related adverse health conditions that exist among specific population groups in the United States. These population groups may be characterized by gender, age, ethnicity, education, income, social class, disability, geographic location, or sexual orientation."

injustice explicitly. Sometimes, however, it also refers to socioeconomic disparities in health and, less often, to additional health disparities involving gender,
sexuality, and other aspects of social position related to social inequality, as with
the definitions (see Table 1.1) offered by *Healthy People 2010* (US Department of
Health and Human Services 2000) and the National Cancer Institute (NCI)
Cancer Control and Population Sciences website (2007). Despite a welcome
greater specificity as to which groups are included, these more comprehensive
definitions nevertheless offer little insight into why these particular groups are at
issue; the definitions remain descriptive, not analytic. Also noteworthy in the
US discourse is that notions of "population groups" and "special populations"
figure prominently (Table 1.1), without any explicit explanation of why certain
"population sub-groups" are singled out and considered "special" (Krieger
1994). One hint, however, is that these "special populations" – women, children,
people of color, the disabled, the elderly, lesbian and gays, the poor, and people
in rural areas – include just about everyone other than white, relatively affluent,
urban, able-bodied, heterosexual, middle-aged white men (Krieger 2005a).

An alternative approach is to clarify terminology premised on the causal
contention that social disparities in health, by definition, arise from social
inequity. From this standpoint, Table 1.2 provides a conceptual and analytic
definition (Krieger 2005a) that clarifies causes and consequences, in relation to
social inequality and its expression in social inequalities in health. By doing so,
it offers a sharper focus for a research agenda, as we will next delineate.

Table 1.2 Analytic definition of "cancer disparities" (Krieger 2005a)

"Social disparities in cancer refer to health inequities spanning the full cancer continuum,
across the lifecourse. These cancer disparities involve social inequalities in the prevention,
incidence, prevalence, detection and treatment, survival, mortality, and burden of
cancer and other cancer-related health conditions and behaviors. They arise from
inequities involving, singly and in combination, adverse working and living conditions
and inadequate health care, as linked to experiences and policies involving socioeconomic
position (e.g., occupation, income, wealth, poverty, debt, and education) and
discrimination. This discrimination, both institutional and interpersonal, can be based
on race/ethnicity, socioeconomic position, gender, sexuality, age, language, literacy,
disability, immigrant status, insurance status, geographic location, housing status,
and other relevant social categories."

Critical Components of a Research Agenda on Cancer Inequities

Premised on the proposed definition of cancer inequities, a corresponding
research agenda would encompass research on *theory, monitoring, etiology,
treatment*, and *prevention* – as they pertain to investigating *cancer disparities*,
not just cancer per se. At issue is the "why" and not just the "how" of disease

occurrence and prevention, even as both types of knowledge are essential for understanding and addressing cancer inequities.

To clarify this distinction, consider the example of tobacco-related cancers. A focus on disease causation would be concerned with mechanisms to answer the "how" questions – that is, "how," via what mechanisms, does exposure to tobacco increase risk of cancer, at several anatomic sites? By contrast, research on disease distribution and health inequities would be concerned with the "why" questions – that is, "why" are there social inequities in tobacco-related cancers? – and hence, presumptively, to exposure to tobacco, and possibly to factors that increase susceptibility to tobacco-related carcinogenesis. A logical follow-up question would be as follows: are patterns of social inequities in tobacco-related cancers invariant or do they change over time or differ across diverse sectors of the population? The importance of asking this question is illustrated by the changing class gradient in smoking, which in both the US and the UK was more common in the early twentieth century among the affluent but then shifted and subsequently become more concentrated among working class and impoverished populations (Graham 2007, pp. 86–93). Presumably, the mechanisms by which tobacco causes cancer have not changed, even as social disparities in exposure to tobacco and its consequences have.

Theory. As suggested by the distinction between the "why" and "how" questions, clarification and development of theoretical frameworks and constructs is needed to improve how cancer researchers define and frame the problem of cancer inequities, identify relevant determinants, conceptualize germane interventions, and ensure the validity of our methods, measures, analyses, and interpretations. Controversies abound, for example, over how best to conceptualize and measure race/ethnicity, racism, socioeconomic position (SEP), gender, sexuality, disability, and the other domains of inequity included in our definition – not to mention when they should be measured, at what points in the lifecourse, and at which levels of social organization (Krieger 1994, 1999, 2003; Williams 1996; Krieger et al. 1997; Lynch and Kaplan 2000; Meyer 2001; Mays et al. 2003; Lollar and Crews 2003). Debates also concern choice of reference group and whether the focus should be on absolute versus relative differences, measures of effect that contrast only the extremes versus measures that take into account the full distribution, and measures that focus on changes in the average level of health versus changes in the gaps between specified groups (Wagstaff et al. 1993; Harper and Lynch 2005; Graham 2007, pp. 19–35). Resolving these issues will require both theoretical and substantive research.

Also needed is theoretical development pertaining to theories of disease distribution and theories to design public health interventions. In the case of disease distribution, theory can help clarify principles for asking the "why" questions concerning population distributions of disease. For example, the analytic definition offered above of "social disparities in cancer" is premised on ecosocial theory (see Fig. 1.1) and its focus on **"who and what drives social inequalities in health"** (Krieger 1994, 2001, 2008). Building on the axiom that health inequities arise from social inequities, key aspects of ecosocial theory

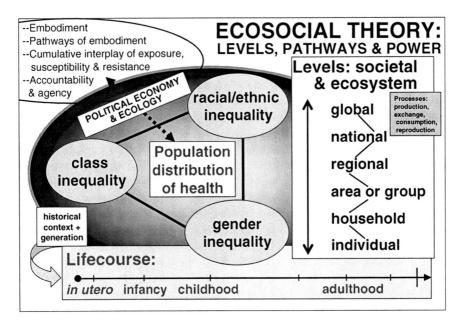

Fig. 1.1 Embodying inequality: an ecosocial approach to analyzing disease distribution, population health, and health inequities (Source: Krieger 1994, 2001, 2008; reprinted with permission from the American Journal of Public Health)

include its core construct of "embodiment," its emphasis on the cumulative interplay of social and biological exposure, susceptibility, and resistance at multiple levels across the lifecourse, and the question of accountability and agency: both for social inequalities in health and the ways they are – or are not – addressed.

More specifically, "embodiment" is a concept referring to how we literally incorporate, biologically, the material and social world in which we live, from in utero to death; a corollary is that no aspect of our biology can be understood without the knowledge of history and individual and societal ways of living (Krieger 2005b, 2008). Epidemiologically, "embodiment" is thus best understood: (a) as a construct, process, and reality, contingent upon bodily existence; (b) as a multilevel phenomenon, integrating soma, psyche, and society, within historical and ecological context, and hence an antonym to disembodied genes, minds, and behaviors; (c) as clue to life histories, hidden and revealed; and (d) as reminder of entangled consequences of diverse forms of social inequality. At issue are historically contingent trajectories of biologic and social development, structured by societal arrangements of power, property, and contingent patterns of production, consumption, and reproduction, and that involve gene expression, not just gene frequency.

The accountability and agency specified by ecosocial theory consequently refer to (1) who and what is responsible for health inequities and for rectifying them and (2) epidemiologists and other scientists' responsibility for the theories and evidence used and ignored to explain social inequalities in health. A corollary is that, given likely complementary causal explanations at different levels and spatiotemporal scales, scientific investigations should explicitly name and consider the benefits and limitations of their particular scale and level of analysis. For example, research on temporal changes in the rates of health outcomes and the magnitude of health inequities over, say, the past century would require considering changing societal factors, rather than genetics, as key drivers of changing patterns of population health and social inequalities in health, since it is unlikely gene frequencies would shift rapidly over a few generations. Key contingent hypotheses are as follows: (1) population patterns of health and disease constitute the embodied biological expression of historically contingent ways of living and working differentially afforded by each society's political economy and political ecology; and (2) policies and practices that benefit and preserve the economic and social privileges of dominant groups simultaneously structure and constrain the living and working conditions they impose on everyone else, thereby shaping particular pathways of embodiment. Suggesting these types of questions are increasingly being asked by researchers world-wide, Table 1.3 provides a related list of theoretically informed questions relevant to promoting equity in health, developed by Equinet (1998), a network of health researchers in South Africa focused on issues of health equity.

Table 1.3 Questions for research on promoting health equity, developed in 1998 by Equinet, the Network for Equity in Health in Southern Africa (1998)

Topic	Research questions
i	"the definition, extent and dimensions of difference in health status that are unnecessary, avoidable, and unfair";
ii	"the determinants of these inequalities in health, whether they arise at a social, economic or health sector level and how they are affected by policies within and beyond the health sector";
iii	"the specific differences in the distribution of health inputs (in and beyond the health sector) to people whose health needs are different, addressing those differences in need (vertical equity)";
iv	"the manner in which policies aimed at redistributing societal and health resources address the areas of vertical equity...";
v	"the extent to which different groups of people in the region are able to make choices over health inputs, have the capacity to use these choices towards health and the manner in which policies and measures affects such capacities";
vi	"the extent to which different groups of people have the opportunity for participation and the power to direct resources towards their health needs, and the policies that influence this."

In addition to theories that focus on determinants, it is important to consider theoretical models that can inform health-focused interventions designed to reduce health inequities. Sorensen et al. (2004) proposed a conceptual framework

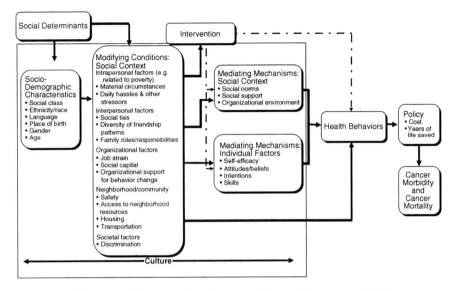

Fig. 1.2 Social contextual framework – a heuristic (Source: Sorensen et al. 2004; reprinted with permission from the American Journal of Public Health)

(see Fig. 1.2) that draws on a range of social and behavioral theories to explicate the social contextual pathways leading to health inequities by influencing health behaviors. As a first step, this framework defines a set of *modifying conditions*, that is, factors that independently impact on outcomes, but which are not influenced by the intervention, and *mediating mechanisms*, defined as variables along the pathway between the intervention and the outcomes. The mediating mechanisms have been identified from social and behavioral theory and prior research as factors that are important to behavior change and that are potentially modifiable (e.g., social norms, self-efficacy). Social context, including life experiences, social relationships, organizational structures, and societal influences, may function as either modifying conditions or mediating mechanisms, depending on the location within or outside the causal pathway between the intervention and the outcomes. The specific mediating and moderating variables included in applications of this framework will change based on the specific intervention being planned and populations/settings included.

An important component of this framework is its emphasis on multiple levels of influence (Sallis and Owen 2002; McLeroy et al. 1988; McKinlay 1993; Stokols 1996). Examples of socially determined *individual factors* might include material circumstances that are associated with income, such as debt load, owning one's own car, or having adequate resources for child care, and the daily hassles and worries that arise from living in disadvantaged situations. *Interpersonal factors* may include variables such as social ties, the diversity of friendship patterns, and family roles and responsibilities. *Organizational factors* may include the work organization such as job strain, which has been linked to health behaviors, such as tobacco use and physical inactivity (Johansson et al. 1991; Landsbergis et al. 1998; Eakin 1997), and the occupational culture and norms associated with health behaviors or factors in the health care setting that facilitate access to care and effective communication with one's physician (Eakin 1997; Freeborn and Pope 1994; Greenlick 1971). *Neighborhood and community factors* may include having – or not having – a safe place to exercise, access to neighborhood resources such as ready access to fresh produce at reasonable prices, housing, and transportation. For example, studies have shown that middle-class neighborhoods have proportionally more pharmacies, restaurants, banks, specialty stores, and greater access to high-quality fruits and vegetables, while low-income neighborhoods have more fast food restaurants, check cashing stores, liquor stores, laundromats, and little or no access to affordable and good produce (Troutt 1993; Zenk et al. 2006). Larger *societal forces*, e.g., public policy or racial discrimination, may also shape interventions by defining a range of social contextual factors and influencing results of efforts to change health behaviors (Patrick and Wickizer 1995). Finally, *culture*, which is the learned and shared knowledge, beliefs, and rules that people use to interpret experience and to generate social behavior, e.g., as pertaining to social norms, social networks, and specific health behaviors (such as eating), permeates multiple domains across this conceptual framework (Helman 2000; Keesing and Strathern 1997). It is important to emphasize that culture is dynamic and changes as individuals are exposed to new experiences and influences – and also not to confuse "culture" with constraints imposed by economic deprivation (as discussed in critiques of the literature on the alleged "culture of poverty" (Crawford 1977)).

Consequently, ideas about what constitute determinants of population health and health inequities and the ways in which they might be intervened upon, by whom, are not simply self-evident. They require theoretical elaboration both at a general level and in relation to specific cancer inequities.

Monitoring. Research is needed to improve monitoring of social disparities in cancer. Data on population trends not only reveal whether health inequities are increasing or decreasing over time, but also stand as critical tests of our etiologic hypotheses. More specifically, if we cannot explain the observed patterns, our knowledge is likely incomplete and our interventions potentially misguided (Krieger 1994, 2001).

In the case of research on monitoring, one set of complex questions, noted previously, pertains to the theoretically thorny issues of categories and contrasts, that is, who is to be compared, categorized how, and in relation to what parameters. Another set concerns measurement error and selection bias, e.g., in relation to race/ethnicity, which can affect both the cancer data and the population data from which we often derive our denominators (Williams 1996; US Cancer Statistics Working Group 2002; Mays et al. 2003). Also needed is research on how to incorporate key data typically not included in cancer registries due to their omission from medical records, such as data on SEP and social context (see Krieger et al. 1997, 2002a; Singh et al. 2003). Suggesting such research could be useful are results of the recent US *Public Health Disparities Geocoding Project* (Krieger et al. 2002a, 2005a). This project sought to ascertain which census-derived area-based socioeconomic measures, at which level of geographic (block group, census tract, or ZIP code), would be most apt for monitoring socioeconomic disparities in health, using geocoded public health surveillance data. Key findings based on analysis of not only cancer incidence and mortality data but also birth data, childhood lead poisoning, sexually transmitted infections, tuberculosis, non-fatal weapons-related injury, and overall mortality were that, among the 18 different area-based socioeconomic measures investigated, the census tract poverty measures (a) consistently detected expected socioeconomic gradients in health across a wide range of health outcomes, among both the total population and diverse racial/ethnic-gender groups, (b) yielded maximal geocoding and linkage to area-based socioeconomic data (compared to the block group and ZIP code data), and (c) was readily interpretable to and could feasibly be used by state health department staff.

Methodologically, in addition to demonstrating the importance of ensuring accuracy (and not just completeness) of geocoding, the project also revealed how serious bias could arise due to spatiotemporal mismatches between ZIP codes and census data. For example, we showed that if one used tract or block group data, results indicated the expected socioeconomic gradient for colon cancer, but the gradient was reversed using ZIP code data (Krieger et al. 2002b). Reflecting a type of selection bias, the discrepancy arose because of non-inclusion of cases who resided in ZIP codes created after and thus not included in the decennial census – a finding highly relevant to etiologic, not just monitoring, research.

Monitoring plays a particularly important role in understanding the complexity of factors influencing cancer inequities and is critical if we are to track progress related to efforts designed to reduce these disparities. The example of breast cancer illustrates these complexities extremely well, whereby economic advantage is associated with higher breast cancer incidence but is associated also with better survival and lower mortality (Krieger 2002; Singh et al. 2003; Krieger et al. 2006). Similar patterns play out by race/ethnicity, whereby in the US breast cancer incidence is highest among white non-Hispanic women, followed by black, Hispanic, Asian and Pacific Islander, and American Indian women – yet survival is highest among white women and, despite lower incidence, mortality is highest among black women (Krieger 2002; Singh et al. 2003; Krieger et al. 2006; Espey et al. 2007). Of note, this inequity in mortality persists despite efforts successfully closing the gap in mammography screening between African-American and white women (Adams et al. 2007). The implication is that, at least in the case of breast cancer, decreasing gaps in detection is not sufficient to decrease inequities in survival and mortality. Monitoring of incidence, survival, and mortality, as well as access to and uptake of early detection activities, is consequently critical in order to understand the complexity of patterns of population-level cancer inequities.

Etiology. Etiologic research, in turn, is necessary for testing hypotheses about the causes of social inequalities in the population distribution of cancer incidence, survival, and mortality, and also access to and provision of appropriate health care. This research necessarily must grapple with disease mechanisms as well as disease distribution (Krieger 1994, 2001). Etiologic research concerned with societal determinants of health is accordingly increasingly paying heed to issues of (a) cumulative economic deprivation, (b) exposure, susceptibility, and resistance across the lifecourse, and (c) gene expression, not simply gene frequency (Krieger 2001, 2005b; Davey Smith 2003; Kuh and Ben-Shlomo 2004).

To highlight the complexity of research gaps requiring attention, we next explore in some detail the needed research on one of the most important but also most neglected aspects of racism and cancer – institutional racism. Racism is viewed here as an organized system that categorizes and ranks human population groups and differentially allocates desirable resources to socially defined "races" (Bonilla-Silva 1996). It is based on an ideology of inferiority which regards some population groups as superior to others. As conceptualized in both the social science and population health literature, racism encompasses negative attitudes and beliefs toward racial outgroups (prejudice and stereotypes), as manifested in differential and unfair treatment of members of these groups by both individuals (interpersonal discrimination) and social institutions (institutional discrimination) (Krieger 1999; Williams and Collins 2001; National Research Council 2004). Racial prejudice and discrimination, measured at the individual level, are often used as indicators of racism in a society, but racism can exist in institutional structures and policies in the absence of racial prejudice at the level of individuals. At issue are both disparate treatment (including not only intentional and explicit but also what has been termed "subtle" discrimination) and disparate impact, with or without conscious intent (National Research Council 2004, pp. 56–65). The latter results from embedded institutional or structural processes, e.g., bank lending rules for mortgages that may at the surface appear "neutral" but in fact perpetuate differential racial treatment as typically linked to past histories of racism (National Research Council 2004, pp. 63–65). There consequently are multiple pathways by which racism can adversely affect the health of non-dominant racial/ethnic groups over the life course (Krieger 1999; Williams and Collins 2001). Most importantly, institutional discrimination can affect health by creating racial/ethnic differences in residential environments, SEP, and access to goods and services.

In the US institutional racism, as reflected in adverse residential segregation, is one of the fundamental determinants of racial inequities in social inequality and thus health, including cancer (Williams and Collins 2001). Although the discrimination in housing that created segregation was ruled illegal in the 1960s, the 2000 Census documented the persistence of extremely high levels of segregation in the US (Glaeser and Vigdor 2001; National Research Council 2004). As noted by the National Research Council report on *Measuring Racial Discrimination*, the institutional processes involved in perpetuating this type of segregation can include "the process by which housing is advertised," "subtle forms of racial steering" by real estate agents, and "apparently neutral rules regarding mortgage approvals that too often result in a higher level of loan refusals for persons in lower-income black neighborhoods than for equivalent white applicants" (National Research Council 2004, p. 64). Also at issue is explicit discrimination, as revealed by the numerous "audit" studies carried out by the US Department of Housing and Urban Development (HUD), in which two testers who differ on race/ethnicity (e.g., one black, one white) but matched on other characteristics (e.g., educational level, economic level, even type of clothing) and provided with identical documentation (e.g., on rental history) provide real-life "experimental" evidence of continued discrimination in the housing market (National Research Council, pp. 104–108). These types of adverse discrimination, and their links to economic and social deprivation, are important to differentiate from potentially positive – and possibly health promoting – aspects of social cohesion that can arise from the residential clustering of racial/ethnic (and other) groups subjected to discrimination (Abada et al. 2007; Bell et al. 2006; Sanders 2002; Mills et al. 2001).

Reflecting the entrenched realities of adverse residential segregation, small declines in segregation in recent decades have not reduced the residential isolation of most African Americans or the concentration of urban poverty (Glaeser and Vigdor 2001). Other data reveal increasing residential segregation of Latinos in the US (Orfield 1996). Segregation matters for cancer risk because it shapes socioeconomic conditions at the levels of the individual, the household, and the community. It restricts socioeconomic attainment for African Americans and other geographically isolated groups by determining access to education and employment opportunities (Massey and Denton 1993). One study found that the elimination of residential segregation would completely erase black–white differences in income, education, and unemployment and reduce racial differences in single motherhood by two thirds (Cutler et al. 1997). It is consequently the concentration of social disadvantage and not racial composition that is at the crux of the problems created by segregation.

Thus, racial inequities in cancer among adults must be understood within a lifecourse framework in which current racial inequalities in SEP and cancer reflect the unequal educational and consequent employment opportunities that have characterized and continue to characterize the American society. These inequities are reflected in the current non-equivalence of individual SEP indicators across race (Williams 1996; Krieger et al. 1997; Kaufman et al. 1997; Lynch and Kaplan 2000). For example, compared to whites, black high-school graduates have fewer job skills; employed blacks and Hispanics have lower median income at every level of education; college-educated blacks are more likely to be unemployed; middle-class African Americans and Puerto Ricans reside in poorer quality neighborhoods; and blacks and Hispanics have lower levels of wealth at comparable levels of household income (Williams 2004). Of particular relevance to cancer risks, employed blacks are more likely than their white peers to be exposed to occupational hazards and carcinogens, even after adjusting for job experience and education (Robinson 1984; Frumkin and Pransky 1999), with the patterning of occupational hazards even among low-income workers varying by race/ethnicity (Quinn et al. 2007).

Segregation also creates pathogenic residential conditions. Segregated areas have been characterized by a disinvestment of economic resources and poorer quality services provided by municipal authorities. The consequent decline in the urban infrastructure and physical environment can lead to increased exposure to environmental toxins and poor-quality housing (Bullard 1994). These conditions make it more challenging for residents of these areas to practice desirable health behaviors (Williams and Collins 2001). The higher cost and poorer quality of grocery items in economically disadvantaged neighborhoods can lead to poorer nutrition (Galvez et al. 2007). The saturation of tobacco and alcohol advertising in poor communities can facilitate substance use and the absence of recreation facilities, and concerns about personal safety can discourage physical exercise. The concentration of poverty also leads to elevated exposure to multiple stressors including economic hardship, loss of loved ones, criminal victimization, neighborhood violence, and chronic relationship stressors. The weakened community and neighborhood infrastructure in segregated areas can also adversely affect interpersonal relationships and trust among neighbors – social resources that can potentially reduce at least some of the negative effects of stress on health (Schulz et al. 2002).

This cursory overview of institutional racism has several implications for future efforts on understanding the contribution of social factors to cancer risk. First, given the multidimensional nature of SEP and the non-equivalence of specific SEP indicators across race/ethnicity, researchers must be wary of claiming to have successfully "adjusted" for SEP in racial/ethnic comparisons, especially when using only a single measure of SEP, even as investigating the impact of racial/ethnic socioeconomic inequities on racial/ethnic health inequities is critical (Krieger 1994, 1999; Williams 1996). Second, given the dynamic nature of racism, research on racism and health must continue to monitor the changing nature of racism and multiple pathways by which racism, especially in its institutional manifestations, can adversely affect health. In particular, research needs to conceptualize and assess all of the race-related factors embedded in residential segregation that can potentially have consequences for the onset and/or the progression of specific types of cancer. Third, research seeking to characterize the effects of institutional racism on health should optimally use longitudinal designs, a life-course perspective, and models that seek to capture the accumulation of the multiple adversities over time. Fourth, individuals and populations exposed to multiple pathogenic risk factors often have other co-occurring illnesses. Research reveals, for example, that most of the deaths among breast cancer patients are due to causes other than breast cancer (Tammemagi et al. 2005). Research on social contextual factors and cancer risk should consider co-morbidity and also devote greater attention not only to the determinants of disease progression and mortality but also to the impact that these factors have on disparities in the quality of life (Garofalo et al.

2006). Fifth, studies of the pathogenic consequences of factors linked to residential segregation must understand them within the context of other risk factors, including other aspects of racism that can affect health. For example, there is interest in the ways in which stress can differentially affect risk of cancer onset and progression (Nielsen and Gronbaek 2006). But this literature has failed to comprehensively assess cumulative exposure to multiple life stressors, especially the adverse impact of experiences of discrimination (Krieger 1999; Williams et al. 2003). The contribution of discrimination to the risk of cancer incidence, survival, and mortality has received little research attention (Krieger 2005a; Krieger et al. 2005b).

Treatment. Racial/ethnic disparities in treatment illustrate the multiple ways in which institutional and individual discrimination can affect both access to care and the quality and intensity of medical treatment. By reducing access to employment opportunities and to jobs with health insurance benefits, institutional discrimination can determine access to medical care. Compared to whites, African Americans, Latinos, and some Asian populations have lower levels of direct private employer-based insurance coverage, insurance coverage indirectly through a spouse's employment, and higher levels of uninsurance and public health insurance coverage (Smedley et al. 2003; Hogue et al. 2000; NIH 1998). They are also more likely than whites to receive care in non-optimal organizational settings (such as the emergency room) and to lack continuity in the health care received. Between 1977 and 1996, the black–white gap in access and the use of health services did not narrow and the gap between Hispanics and whites widened (Weinick and Zuvekas 2000). In addition, there are large racial/ethnic differences in having a usual source of care and in receiving ambulatory care in the prior year that are not accounted for by income and health insurance coverage (Weinick and Zuvekas 2000).

Research reveals that there are systematic racial differences in the quality and intensity of medical care across a broad spectrum of therapeutic interventions (Smedley et al. 2003). This research indicates that even after adjusting for differences in health insurance, SEP, stage and severity of disease, comorbidity, and the type of medical facility, blacks and other minorities are less likely to receive medical procedures and to experience poorer quality medical care than whites. These disparities exist for multiple types of cancer (Smedley et al. 2003). Moreover some evidence suggests that racial disparities in treatment account for at least part of the racial disparities in mortality for breast (Bickell et al. 2006), rectal (Morris et al. 2004), esophageal (Steyerberg et al. 2005), and prostate cancer (Underwood et al. 2004).

Research is needed to identify the sources of these disparities in care and the optimal intervention strategies to eliminate them. It is likely that geographic variations in the rates of medical procedures and the quality of medical care in the US, linked to residential segregation, are a contributor to these patterns (Baicker et al. 2004). Some evidence suggests that health-care facilities are more likely to close in poor and minority communities than in other areas (Whiteis 1992) and that pharmacies in minority neighborhoods may be less likely to be

adequately stocked with medication (Morrison et al. 2000). Moreover, blacks
and Latinos are more likely than whites to be treated in contexts such as large
inner-city urban hospitals that are often the place of final resort for the poor
(Smedley et al. 2003). In these contexts, physicians are less likely to be board-
certified and less able to provide high-quality care and referrals to specialty care
(Mukamel et al. 2000; Bach et al. 2004). Research also suggests that provider
bias linked to negative stereotypes of socially stigmatized racial and ethnic
groups is also likely to contribute to the observed disparities in care (Smedley
et al. 2003; Green et al. 2007). Health care providers are a part of the larger
society that views racial/ethnic minorities negatively on multiple social dimensions and the typical health-care encounter contains at least some of the factors
that enhance the likelihood of the use of stereotypes. Research indicates that
stereotypes are more likely to be activated when there is time pressure, the need
to make quick judgments, cognitive overload, task complexity, and when the
emotions of anger or anxiety are present (van Ryn 2002). At the present time,
we do not have a clear sense of the relative contribution of geographic and
provider level race-related factors to social disparities in care for specific types
of cancer. Future research needs to identify the determinants of inequities in
care and examine how they combine with other risks factors and resources to
account for differential progression of cancer across population groups.

Prevention. One motivation for etiologic research is to generate knowledge
useful for designing efforts to prevent disease. Research for prevention consequently is needed to develop, evaluate, and improve methods to assess two
kinds of programs, projects, and policies that affect cancer disparities. The
first involves efforts explicitly intended to address social inequalities in
cancer, typically initiated by public health practitioners. The second pertains
to the beneficial and adverse health consequences of "non-health" policies
and programs, including those arising in the economic, trade, labor, housing,
education, transportation, agriculture, and military sectors. Both types of
activities are relevant – and are at the core of the principal recommendations
of the March 2004 Trans-HHS Cancer Disparities Progress Review report
(THCDPRG 2004).

Thus, the report's first priority recommendation calls for supporting "culturally competent evidence-based programs that are effective in addressing cancer
health disparities" (THCDPRG 2004, p. 4), with much of the document discussing the kinds of research needed to build this evidence base, including
community-based participatory research. Suggesting this type of research is
necessary as racial/ethnic and socioeconomic inequities are growing in two
important risk factors for several types of cancer: obesity and smoking. For
example, between 1976 and 2000, obesity among non-Hispanic black women
increased more than 60%, from 31% to 50% (Jemal et al. 2004), and they are
more than twice as likely to be obese, compared to non-Hispanic white women
(Ogden et al. 2006). New research highlights the societal determinants that
contribute to inequities in obesity, including economic and geographic barriers
to obtaining and preparing affordable nutritious meals (Devine et al. 2006;

Moore and Diez Roux 2006; Galvez et al. 2007). Similarly, in the case of cigarette smoking, since the mid-twentieth century prevalence has been higher among the US working class compared to professional populations (33% versus 18%) (Barbeau et al. 2004), and non-Hispanic black men have higher smoking prevalence than non-Hispanic white men (26.7% versus 24%) (CDC 2005). Moreover, despite similar if not higher numbers of attempts to quit, the working class smokers are less likely to successfully quit smoking (15% versus 21% former smokers) when compared to professional populations (Barbeau et al. 2004), as is also the case for black compared to white populations (35.4% versus 50.5%) (van de Mheen et al. 1998). The implication is that more refined interventions are required, designed with the specific context of each population in mind.

The report's second priority recommendation in turn calls for creation of a "Federal Leadership Council on Cancer Health Disparities led by the HHS Secretary in partnership with the Secretaries of other appropriate Federal departments to mobilize available resources in a comprehensive national effort to eliminate cancer health disparities" (THCDPRG 2004, p. 5). Ascertaining connections between non-health policies, population health, and health disparities is a huge research question of its own (Graham 2007, pp. 160–181) and there is a rapidly growing body of work, termed "health impact assessment," which seeks to do just this (Krieger et al. 2003; Morgan 2003; Kemm et al. 2004), with clear relevance to cancer inequities.

A Systematic Approach to Identifying Research Questions: "The Cancer Disparities Research Grid"

The research agenda linked to the proposed definition of cancer inequities is, not surprisingly, enormous. As shown in Table 1.4, however, it can be reformulated into a "grid" (Krieger 2005a) that can be used to identify, systematically, where research has or has not been done in relation to diverse domains of social inequality (the rows) across the cancer continuum, from prevention to death (the columns).

An initial version of this grid (Krieger 2005a) was used at a workshop held in January 2004 that was organized by the Cancer Disparities program-in-development of the Dana Farber/Harvard Cancer Center, located in Boston, MA (Krieger et al. 2005b). This workshop was geared toward developing a multidisciplinary research agenda on cancer disparities. One component included formal presentations, during which one speaker analyzed social inequities in breast cancer in relation to the "grid"; another consisted of break-out sessions for which team leaders had prepared preliminary versions of the "grid" for cervix, colon, and prostate cancers. These preliminary grids served as the basis for several articles on these four cancer sites (Bigby and Holmes 2005; Gilligan 2005; Newman and Garner 2005; Palmer and Schneider 2005).

Table 1.4 "Cancer disparities" analytic grid (Krieger 2005a)

DOMAINS OF SOCIAL INEQUALITY:	CANCER CONTINUUM									
singly & combined, involving adverse conditions & discrimination at multiple levels (person, place, institutional, societal), across the lifecourse	Prevention (primary, secondary, tertiary)	Incidence	Etiology	Screening	Diagnosis	Access to clinical trials	Treatment	Survival	Morbidity	Mortality
Race/ethnicity & racism										
Socioeconomic position										
Gender										
Sexuality										
Age										
Language										
Literacy										
Disability										
Immigrant status										
Insurance status										
Geography (urban/rural)										
Housing status										

Note: research on cancer disparities encompasses epidemiologic, clinical, and intervention research; filling out the grid can highlight areas requiring emphasis (either because of the identified burden or because of gaps in knowledge), plus point to research requiring interdisciplinary expertise, premised on a population health perspective.

Several useful lessons emerged from the exercise of working with the "grid." Among these are the following:

(1) The "grid" proved helpful in systematically highlighting, for each site, where work has been done, where major controversies exist, where findings suggest the largest burdens of cancer inequities fall *and persist* (raising the question of why knowledge is not being translated into effective action to address these disparities) – as well as where we have no idea if inequities exist because the research has not been done;

(2) The "grid" underscored the importance of disease specificity by demonstrating how the patterning of knowledge, ignorance, and population burden of cancer inequities varied considerably by type of cancer; and

(3) The process of filling out the "grid" emphasized connections between diverse domains of inequality and the accumulation of cancer inequities across the continuum, since often a single study rated inclusion in more than one "cell."

Thus, as emphasized by ecosocial theory, embodiment matters and our bodies do not separately parse our lived experiences (Krieger 1994, 2001, 2005b). It is not as if, say, one day someone is poor, another day a woman, another day Latina, another day heterosexual, another day an immigrant, another day uninsured, and still another day exposed to HPV, and ultimately is diagnosed with and dies from invasive cervical cancer. Or, related, recognition that black men are disproportionately burdened by prostate cancer necessarily suggests that increased resources should be directed to this group – but still leaves open the question as to whether risk of prostate cancer *among black men* varies by SEP, immigrant status, sexuality, access to health care, etc. The scientific challenge is thus to investigate which, if any, of these social determinants – individually and in combination – result in health inequities, so as to improve understanding of etiology and grounds for action.

Conclusion: Research for Health and Cancer Equity

In conclusion, defining and investigating cancer inequities is essential, both because of the inequities they embody and because of their persistence, suggesting that much work needs to be done. Tackling this issue will require rigorous and critical frameworks, questions, and methods derived from multiple disciplines and will necessarily involve epidemiologic, clinical, and intervention research, both quantitative and qualitative. Careful attention to core constructs can help cohere such a research agenda, thereby assisting us in making conscious research choices – about which types of inequities we study, in relation to which aspect of cancer. That initiatives to address social inequities in cancer will require collaboration between individuals and groups both in and outside of the health sector only serves to underscore the unique and critical contribution that cancer researchers can make. Our task is to generate the scientific evidence relevant to informing a society-wide discourse about the extent, origins of, and remedies for social injustices in cancer, thereby aiding efforts to eliminate social inequalities in health.

Acknowledgments The first author wrote the original article upon which this chapter is based (see Krieger 2005a). Preparation of the original article was in part supported by the Dana Farber/Harvard Cancer Center (DF/HCC) Cancer Disparities "program-in-development." Preliminary versions were presented at the DF/HCC workshop on "Social Disparities in Cancer: Developing a Multidisciplinary Research Agenda" (DF/HCC, Boston, MA, January 23, 2004) and as part of an invited symposium on "In the Era of Genomics and Persistent Social Inequities in Cancer," held at the American Society of Preventive Oncology, 28th annual meeting, Washington, DC, March 16, 2004. Helpful comments on both the content of the grid and the wording of the definition of cancer inequities, initially conceived and developed by the first author, were provided by members of the Executive Committee of the DF/HCC Cancer Disparities program-in-development. Additional support was provided by NIH grants: 1K05CA124415-01A1 and 5P01CA7308.

References

Abada, T., Hou, F., and Ram, B. 2007. Racially mixed neighborhoods, perceived neighborhood social cohesion, and adolescent health in Canada. Soc Sci Med 65:2004–2017.

Acheson, D., Barker, D., Chambers, J., Graham, H., Marmot, M., and Whitehead, M. 1998. Independent Inquiry into Inequalities in Health. London: The Stationary Office.

Adams, E.K., Breen, N., and Joski, P. 2007. Impact of the National Breast and Cervical Cancer Early Detection Program on mammography and Pap test utilization among white, Hispanic, and African American women: 1996–2000. Cancer 109(2 Suppl):348–358.

Agency for Healthcare Research and Quality (AHRQ). 2003. National Healthcare Disparities Report. Prepublication Copy. Rockville, MD: US Department of Health and Human Services, Agency for Healthcare Research and Quality, December. Accessed on January 6, 2004 at: http://www.qualitytools.ahrq.gov/disparitiesreport/download_report.aspx (as of November 26, 2007, no longer available on-line).

Agency for Healthcare Research and Quality (AHRQ). 2004. National Healthcare Disparities Report. July 2003 (original report, released in February 2004 to replace the edited version released in December 2003). Rockville, MD: US Department of Health and Human Services, Agency for Healthcare Research and Quality, December. Accessed on November 26, 2007 at: http://www.ahrq.gov/qual/nhdr03/nhdr03.htm

Almeida, C., Braveman, P., Gold, M., Szwarcwald, C.L., Ribeiro, J.M., Miglionico, A., Millar, J.S., Porto, S., Costa, N.R., Rubio, V.O., Segall, M., Starfield, B., Travessos, C., Uga, A., Valente, J., and Viacava, F. 2001. Methodological concerns and recommendations on policy consequences of the World Health Report 2000. Lancet 357:1692–1697.

Bach, P.B., Pham, H.H., Schrag, D., Tate, R.C., and Hargraves, J.L. 2004. Primary care physicians who treat blacks and whites. New Engl J Med 351:575–584.

Baicker, K. Chandra,A., Skinner, J.S., and Wennberg, J.E. 2004. Who are you and where you live: how race and geography affect the treatment of medicare beneficiaries. Health Affairs Suppl Web Exclusives:VAR33–34.

Barbeau, E., Krieger, N., and Soobader, M-J. 2004. Working class matters: Socioeconomic deprivation, race/ethnicity, gender and smoking in NHIS 2000. Am J Public Health 94:269–278.

Bell, J.F., Zimmerman, F.J., Mayer, J.D., Almgren, G.R., and Huebner, C.E. 2006. Birth outcomes among urban African-American women: a multilevel analysis of the role of racial residential segregation. Soc Sci Med 63:3030–3045.

Bickell, N.A., Wang, J.J., Oluwole, S., Schrag, D., Godfrey, H., Hiotis, K., Mendez, J., and Guth, A.A. 2006. Missed Opportunities: racial disparities in adjuvant breast cancer treatment. J Clin Oncol 24:1357–1362.

Bigby, J., Holmes, M. 2005. Disparities across the breast cancer continuum. Cancer Causes Control 16:35–44.

Bloche, M.G. 2004. Health care disparities – science, politics, and race. New Engl J Med 350:1568–1570.

Bonilla-Silva E. 1996. Rethinking racism: toward a structural interpretation. Am Sociol Rev 62:465–480.

Braveman, P., and Gruskin, S. 2003. Poverty, equity, human rights and health. Bull World Health Organ 81:539–545.

Braveman, P., Krieger, N., and Lynch, J. 2000. Health inequalities and social inequalities in health. Bull World Health Organ 78:232–234.

Braveman, P., Starfield, B., and Geiger, H.J. 2001. World Health Report 2000: how it removes equity from the agenda for public health monitoring and policy. BMJ 323:678–681.

Bullard, R.D. 1994. Urban infrastructure: social environmental, and health risks to African Americans. In Handbook of Black American Health: The Mosaic Conditions, Issues, Policies, and Prospects, ed. I. Livingston, pp. 315–330. Westport, Connecticut: Greenwood Publishing.

Carter-Pokras, O., and Bacquet, C. 2002. What is a "Health Disparity"? Public Health Reports 117:426–434.

Centers for Disease Control and Prevention (CDC). 2005. Morbidity and Mortality Weekly Report. Tobacco Use Among Adults—US, 2005. 42:1145.

Crawford, R. 1977. You are dangerous to your health: the ideology and politics of victim blaming. Int J Health Serv 7:663–680.

Cutler, D.M., Glaeser, E.L., and Vigdor, J.L. 1997. Are ghettos good or bad? Q J Econ 112: 827–872.

Davey Smith, G., ed. 2003. Health Inequalities: Lifecourse Approaches. Bristol, UK: Policy Press.

Devine, C.M., Jastran, M., Jabs, J., Wethington, E., Farell, T.J., and Bisogni, C.A. 2006. "A lot of sacrifices": work-family spillover and the food choice coping strategies of low-wage employed parents. Soc Sci Med 63:2591–2603.

Eakin, J. M. 1997. Work-related determinants of health behavior, in Handbook of Health Behavior Research I: Personal and Social Determinants, ed. D. S. Gochman, pp. 337–357. New York, NY: Plenum Press.

Equinet: Regional Network for Equity in Health in Southern Africa. 1998. Equinet Policy Series 2. Equity in Health in Southern Africa: Overview and Issues from annotated bibliography. Accessed on November 26, 2007 at: http://www.equinetafrica.org/workequity.php

Espey, D.K., Wu, X.C., Swan, J., Wiggins, C., Jim, M.A., Ward, E., Wingo, P.A., Howe, H.L., Ries, L.A., Miller, B.A., Jemal, A., Ahmed, F., Cobb, N., Kaur, J.S., and Edwards, B.K. 2007. Annual report to the nation on the status of cancer, 1975–2004, featuring cancer in American Indians and Alaska Natives. Cancer 110:2119–2152.

Freeborn, D. K., and Pope, C. R. 1994. Promise and Performance in Managed Care. Baltimore, MD: John Hopkins University Press.

Frumkin, H., and Pransky, G. 1999. Special Populations in Occupational Health. Volume 14, No 3 of. Occupational Medicine State of the Art Reviews. Philadelphia: Hanley & Belfus, Inc.

Gakidou, E.E., Murray, C.J.L., and Frenk, J. 2000. Defining and measuring health inequality. Bull World Health Organ 78:42–54.

Galvez, M.P., Morland, K., Raines, C., Kobil, J., Siskind, J., Gobold, J., and Brenner, B. 2007. Race and food store availability in an inner-city neighbourhood. Public Health Nutr Oct 15;1–8 [Epub ahead of print]

Garofalo, J.P., Hamann, H.A., Ashworth, K., and Baum, A. 2006. Stress and the quality of life in African American cancer survivors. Ethn Dis 16:732–738.

Gilligan, T. 2005. Social disparities and prostate cancer: mapping the gaps in our knowledge. Cancer Causes Control 16:45–53.

Glaeser, E.L., and Vigdor, J.L. 2001. Racial segregation in the 2000 Census: Promising news. Washington, DC: The Brookings Institution, Survey Series.

Graham, H. 2007. Unequal Lives: Health and Socioeconomic Inequalities. Berkshire, England: Open University Press.

Green, A.R., Carney, D.R., Pallin, D.J., Ngo, L.H., Raymond, K.L., Iezzoni, L.I., and Banaji, M.R. 2007. Implicit bias among physicians and its prediction of thrombolysis decisions for black and white patients. J Gen Intern Med 22:1231–1238.

Greenlick, M. R. 1971. Medical services to poverty groups. In The Kaiser Permanent Medical Care Program: A Symposium. ed. A. B. Somers, pp. 38–51. New York, NY: The Commonwealth Fund, New York.

Harper, S., and Lynch, J. 2005. Methods for Measuring Cancer Disparities: Using Data Relevant to Healthy People 2010 Cancer-Related Objectives. NCI Cancer Surveillance Monograph Series, Number 6. Bethesda, MD: National Cancer Institute, 2005. NIH Publication No. 05-5777. Accessed on November 26, 2007 at: http://seer.cancer.gov/publications/disparities/

Helman, C. 2000. Culture, Health and Illness. Oxford, UK: Butterworth-Heinemann.

Hogue, C.J., Hargraves, M.A., and Collins, K.S. 2000. Minority Health in America: Findings and Policy Implications from the Commonwealth Fund Minority Health Survey. Baltimore: Johns Hopkins University Press.

Jemal, A., Clegg, L.X., Ward, E., Ries, L.A., Wu, X., Jamison, P.M., Wingo, P.A., Howe, H.L., Anderson, R.N., and Edwards, B.K. 2004. Annual report to the nation on the status of cancer, 1975–2001, with a special feature regarding survival. Cancer 101:3–27.

Johansson, G., Johnson, J. V., and Hall, E. M. 1991. Smoking and sedentary behavior as related to work organization. Soc Sci Med 32:837–846.

Kaufman, J.S., Cooper, R.S., and McGee, D.L. 1997. Socioeconomic status and health in blacks and whites: The problem of residual confounding and the resiliency of race. Epidemiology 8:621–628.

Keesing, R., and Strathern, A. 1997. Cultural Anthropology: A Contemporary Perspective. Forth Worth, TX: Harcourt Brace.

Kemm, J., Parry, J., and Palmer, S., eds. 2004. Health impact assessment: concepts, theory, techniques, and applications. Oxford: Oxford University Press.

Kogevinas, M., Pearce, N., Susser, M., and Boffetta, P. 1997. Social inequalities and cancer: a summary by the editors. In Social Inequalities and Cancer, eds. M. Kogevinas, N. Pearce, M. Susser, and P. Boffetta, pp. 1–15. Lyon: International Agency for Research on Cancer (IARC Scientific Publications No. 138).

Krieger, N. 1994. Epidemiology and the web of causation: has anyone see the spider? Soc Sci Med 39:887–903.

Krieger, N. 1999. Embodying inequality: a review of concepts, measures, and methods for studying health consequences of discrimination. Int J Health Services 29:295–352; slightly revised and updated as: Krieger, N. 2000. Discrimination and health. In Social Epidemiology, ed., L. Berkman and I. Kawachi, pp. 36–75. Oxford: Oxford University Press.

Krieger, N. 2001. Theories for social epidemiology in the 21st century: an ecosocial perspective. Int J Epidemiol 30:668–677.

Krieger, N. 2002. Breast cancer: a disease of affluence, poverty, or both?—the case of African American women. Am J Public Health 92:611–613.

Krieger, N. 2003. Genders, sexes, and health: what are the connections—and why does it matter? Int J Epidemiol 32:652–657.

Krieger, N. 2005a. Defining and investigating social disparities in cancer: critical issues. Cancer Causes Control 16:5–14.

Krieger, N. 2005b. Embodiment: a conceptual glossary for epidemiology. J Epidemiol Community Health 59:350–355.

Krieger, N. 2008. Proximal, distal and the politics of causation: What's level got to do with it? Am J Public Health 98:221–230.

Krieger, N., Chen, J.T., Waterman, P.D., Rehkopf, D.H., and Subramanian, S.V. 2005a. Painting a truer picture of US socioeconomic and racial/ethnic health inequalities: the Public Health Disparities Geocoding Project. Am J Public Health 95:312–323.

Krieger, N., Chen, J.T., Waterman, P.D., Rehkopf, D.H., Yin, R., and Coull, B.A. 2006. Race/ethnicity and changing US socioeconomic gradients in breast cancer incidence: California and Massachusetts, 1978–2002. Cancer Causes Control 17:217–226.

Krieger, N., Chen, J.T., Waterman, P.D., Soobader, M.J., Subramanian, S.V., and Carson, R. 2002a. Geocoding and monitoring of US socioeconomic inequalities in mortality and cancer incidence: does the choice of area-based measure and geographic level matter? The Public Health Disparities Geocoding Project. Am J Epidemiol 156:471–482.

Krieger, N., Emmons, K.M., and Burns White, K. 2005b. Cancer disparities: developing a multidisciplinary research agenda – preface. Cancer Causes Control 16:1–3.

Krieger, N., Northridge, M., Gruskin, S., Quinn, M., Kriebel, D., Davey Smith, G., Bassett, M.T., Rehkopf, D.H., Miller, C., and the HIA "promise and pitfalls" conference group. 2003. Assessing health impact assessment: multidisciplinary & international perspectives. J Epidemiol Community Health 57:659–662.

Krieger, N., Waterman, P., Chen, J.T., Soobader, M-J, Subramanian, S.V., and Carson, R. 2002b. ZIP Code caveat: bias due to spatiotemporal mismatches between ZIP Codes and US census-defined areas—the Public Health Disparities Geocoding Project. Am J Public Health 92:1100–1102.

Krieger, N., Williams, D., and Moss, N. 1997. Measuring social class in US public health research: concepts, methodologies and guidelines. Annu Rev Public Health 18:341–378.

Kuh, D., and Ben-Shlomo, Y., eds. 2004. A Lifecourse Approach to Chronic Disease Epidemiology: Tracing the Origins of Ill-Health from Early to Adult Life. 2nd ed. Oxford: Oxford University Press.

Landsbergis, P.A., Schnall, P.L., Deitz, D.K., Warren, K., Pickering, T.G., and Schwartz, J.E. 1998. Job strain and health behaviors: Results of a prospective study. Am J Health Promotion 12:237–245.

Lollar, D.J., and Crews, J.E. 2003. Redefining the role of public health in disability. Annu Rev Public Health 24:195–208.

Lynch, J., and Kaplan, G. 2000. Socioeconomic position. In Social Epidemiology, ed. L. Berkman and I. Kawachi, pp. 13–35. Oxford: Oxford University Press.

Massey, D.S., and Denton, N.A. 1993. American Apartheid: Segregation and the Making of the Underclass. Cambridge, Massachusetts: Harvard University Press.

Mays, V.M., Ponce, N.A., Washington, D.L., and Cochran, S.D. 2003. Classification of race and ethnicity: implications for public health. Annu Rev Public Health 24:83–110.

McKinlay, J. B. 1993, The promotion of health through planned sociopolitical change: Challenges for research and policy. Soc Sci Med 36:109–117.

McLeroy, K., Bibeau, D., Steckler, A., and Glanz, K. 1988. An ecological perspective on health promotion programs. Health Educ Q 15:351–377.

Meyer, I.H. 2001. Why lesbian, gay, bisexual, and transgender public health? Am J Public Health 91:856–859.

Mills, T.C., Stall, R., Pollack, L., Paul, J.P., Binson, D., Canchola, J., and Catania, J.A. 2001. Health-related characteristics of men who have sex with men: a comparison of those living in "gay ghettos" with those living elsewhere. Am J Public Health 91:980–983.

Moore, L.V., and Diez Roux, A.V. 2006. Associations of neighborhood characteristics with the location and types of food stores. Am J Public Health 96:325–331.

Morgan, R.K. 2003. Health impact assessment: the wider context. Bull World Health Organ 81:390.

Morris, A.M., Billingsley, K.G., Baxter, N.N., and Baldwin, L. 2004. Racial disparities in rectal cancer treatment: a population-based analysis. Arch Surg 139:151–155.

Morrison, R.S., Wallenstein, S., Natale, D.K., Senzel, R.S., and Huang, L.L. 2000. "We don't carry that": failure of pharmacies in predominantly nonwhite neighborhoods to stock opioid analgesics. New Engl J Med 342:1023–1026.

Mukamel, D.B., Murthy, A.S., and Weimer, D.L. 2000 Racial differences in access to high-quality cardiac surgeons. Am J Public Health 90:1774–1777.

Murray, C.J.L. 2001. Commentary: comprehensive approaches are needed for full understanding. BMJ 323:680–681.

National Cancer Institute (NCI) Cancer Control and Population Sciences, National Institutes of Health. 2007. Overview of Health Disparities Research: Health Disparities Definition. Accessed on November 26, 2007 at: http://cancercontrol.cancer.gov/od/hd-overview.html

National Center on Minority Health and Health Disparities (NCMDH), National Institutes of Health. 2007. About NCMHD: Mission, Vision. Accessed on November 26, 2007 at: http://www.ncmhd.nih.gov/about_ncmhd/mission.asp

National Institute of Health (NIH). 1998. Women of Color Health Data Book: Adolescents to Seniors. Bethesda, MD: Office of Research on Women's Health.

National Research Council. 2004. Measuring Racial Discrimination. Panel on Methods for Assessing Discrimination. Rebecca M. Blank, Marilyn Dabady, and Constance F. Citro, Editors. Committee on National Statistics, Division of Behavioral and Social Sciences and Education. Washington, D.C.: The National Academies Press.

Newman, S., and Garner, E. 2005. Social inequities along the cervical cancer continuum: a structured review. Cancer Causes Control 16:55–61.

Nielsen, N.R., and Gronbaek, M. 2006. Stress and breast cancer: a systematic update on the current knowledge. Nat Clin Pract Oncol 3:612–620.

Ogden, C.L., Carroll, M.D., Curtin, L.R., McDowell, M.A., Tabak, C.J., and Flegal, K.M. 2006. Prevalence of overweight and obesity in the United States, 1999–2004. JAMA 295:1549–1555.

Orfield, G. 1996. Turning back to segregation. In Dismantling Desegregation: The Quiet Reversal of Brown v. Board of Education, eds. G. Orfield and S.E. Eaton, pp. 1–22. New York: The New Press.

Palmer, R.C., and Schneider, E.S. 2005. Social disparities across the continuum of colorectal cancer: a systematic review. Cancer Causes Control 16:55–61.

Patrick, D. L., and Wickizer, T. M. 1995. Community and Health. In Society and Health, ed. B. C. Amick, S. Levine, A. R. Tarlov, and D. C. Walsh, pp. 46–92. Oxford, UK: Oxford University Press.

Patterson, J.T. 1987. The Dread Disease: Cancer and Modern American Culture. Cambridge, MA: Harvard University Press.

Porter, D. 1999. Health, Civilization and the State: A History of Public Health from Ancient to Modern Times. London: Routledge.

Quinn, M.M., Sembajwe, G., Stoddard, A.M., Kriebel, D., Krieger, N., Sorensen, G., Hartman, C., Naishadham, D., and Barbeau, E.M. 2007. Social disparities in the burden of occupational exposures: results of a cross-sectional study. Am J Ind Med 50:861–875.

Robinson, J. 1984. Racial Inequality and the Probability of Occupation-Related Injury or Illness. Milbank Mem Fund Q 62:567–593.

Sallis, J. F., and Owen, N. 2002. Ecological models of health behavior. In Health Behavior and Health Education: Theory, Research and Practice, 3rd edition, ed. K. Glanz, B. K. Rimer, and F. M. Lewis, pp. 462–484. San Francisco, CA: Jossey-Bass.

Sanders, J.M. 2002. Ethnic boundaries and identity in plural societies. Annu Rev Sociol 28:327–357.

Schulz, A.J., Williams, D.R., Israel, B.A., and Lempert, L.B. 2002. Racial and spatial relations as fundamental determinants of health in Detroit. Milbank Q 80:677–707.

Singh, G.K., Miller, B.A., Hankey, B.F., and Edwards, B.K. 2003. Area Socioeconomic Variations in US Cancer Incidence, Mortality, Stage, Treatment, and Survival, 1975–1999. Bethesda, MD: National Cancer Institute, 2003, NCI Cancer Surveillance Monograph Series, Number 4, NIH Pub. No. 03-5417.

Smedley, B.D., Stith, A.Y., and Nelson, A.R. 2003. Unequal Treatment: Confronting Racial and Ethnic Disparities in Health Care. Washington, DC: National Academies Press.

Sorensen, G., Barbeau, E., Hunt, M.K., and Emmons, K.M. 2004. Reducing social disparities in tobacco use: A social contextual model for reducing tobacco use among blue-collar workers. Am J Public Health 94:230–239.

Steinbrook, R. 2004. Disparities in health care – from politics to policy. New Engl J Med 350:1486–1488.

Steyerberg, E.W., Earle, C.C., Neville, B.A., and Weeks, J.C. 2005. Racial differences in surgical evaluation, treatment, and outcome of locoregional esophageal cancer: a population-based analysis of elderly patients. J Clin Oncol 23:510–517.

Stokols, D. 1996. Translating social ecological theory into guidelines for community health promotion. Am J Health Promot 10:282–298.

Tammemagi, C.M., Nerenz, D., Neslund-Dudas, C., Feldkamp, C., and Nathanson, D. 2005. Comorbidity and survival disparities among black and white patients with breast cancer. JAMA 294:1765–1772.

Trans-HHS Cancer Health Disparities Progress Review Group (THCDPRG). 2004. Making Cancer Health Disparities History. Submitted to the Secretary, US Department of Health and Human Services, March 2004. Washington, DC: US Department of Health and Human Services.

Troutt, D. D. 1993. The thin red line: How the poor still pay more. San Francisco, CA: Consumers Union of the United States.

US Department of Health and Human Services. 2000. Healthy People 2010: Understanding and Improving Health. 2nd ed. Washington, DC: US Government Printing Office, November. Accessed November 26, 2007 at: http://www.healthypeople.gov/Document/html/uih/uih_2.htm#goals

US National Institutes of Health. 1999. What are Health Disparities. Accessed on January 5, 2004 at: http://healthdisparities.nih.gov/whatare.html (as of November 26, 2007, no longer available on line).

Underwood, W., DeMonner, S., Ubel, P., Fagerlin, A., Sanda, M.G., and Wei, J.T. 2004. Racial/ethnic disparities in the treatment of localized/regional prostrate cancer. J Urol 171:1504–1507.

van de Mheen, H., Stronks, K., Looman, C.W., and Mackenbach, J.P. 1998. Does childhood socioeconomic status influence adult health through behavioural factors? Int J Epidemiol 27:431–437.

van Ryn, M. 2002. Research on the provider contribution to race/ethnicity disparities in medical care. Med Care 40:I140–I151.

Variations Sub-Group of the Chief Medical Officer's Health of the Nation Working Group. 1995. Variations in Health: What Can the Department of Health and the NHS Do? London: The Department of Health.

Wagstaff, A., Paci, P., and van Doorslaer, E. 1993. On the measurement of inequalities in health. Soc Sci Med 33:545–557.

Weinick, R.M., and Zuvekas, S.H. 2000. Racial and ethnic differences in access to and use of health care services 1977 to 1996. Med Care Res Rev 57:36–54.

Whitehead, M. 1990. The Concepts and Principles of Equity and Health. Copenhagen, WHO Regional Office for Europe (document EUR/ICP/RDP/414). Accessed on November 26, 2007 at: http://www.euro.who.int/Document/PAE/conceptsrpd414.pdf

Whiteis, D.G. 1992. Hospital and community characteristics in closures of urban hospitals, 1980–87. Public Health Rep 107:409–416.

Williams, D.R. 1996. Race/ethnicity and socioeconomic status: measurement and methodological issues. Int J Health Serv 26:s483–505.

Williams, D.R. 2004. Closing the Gap: Improving the Health of Minority Elders in the New Millennium. Washington, DC: Gerontological Society of America.

Williams, D.R., and Collins, C.A. 2001. Racial residential segregation: a fundamental cause of racial disparities in health. Public Health Rep 116:404–415.

Williams, D.R., Neighbors, H.W., and Jackson, J.S. 2003. Racial/ethnic discrimination and health: findings from community studies. Am J Public Health 93:200–208.

World Health Organization (WHO). 2000. The World Health Report 2000: The World Health Report 2000 Health Systems: Improving Performance. Geneva: World Health Organization. Accessed on November 26, 2007 at: http://www.who.int/whr/2000/en/index.html

World Health Organization (WHO). 2003. The World Health Report 2003: Shaping the Future. Geneva: World Health Organization. Accessed November 26, 2007 at: http://www.who.int/whr/2003/en/index.html

Zenk, S.N., Schulz, A.J., Israel, B.A., James, S.A., Bao, S., and Wilson, ML. 2006. Fruit and vegetable access differs by community racial composition and socioeconomic position in Detroit, Michigan. Ethn Dis 16:275–280.

Chapter 2
Cancer Disparities: Data Systems, Sources, and Interpretation

Barbara D. Powe, Ahmedin Jemal, Dexter Cooper, and Lokie Harmond

Overall cancer death rates in the United States have continued to decrease since the early 1990s largely because of reduction in smoking and improved treatment for many cancers. However, this overall decrease masks the continued and often increasing gaps in cancer incidence, mortality, and survivorship between and within racial/ethnic minority groups as well as other specific population groups in this country. These differences extend across the cancer continuum of prevention, detection, diagnosis, treatment, survivorship, and end of life.

Evidence for these disparities has been mounting since 1973, when Hensechke et al. documented increasing cancer mortality among African Americans over the previous 25 years (Hensechke et al., 1973). Then, in 1985, the Heckler report formally called the nation's attention to the fact that there were significant differences in health care outcomes for African Americans, Native Americans, Hispanics, and Asian/Pacific Islanders compared to Caucasians and that these poorer outcomes resulted in higher death rates (US Department of Health and Human Services, 1985). Freeman, in a special report on cancer in the socioeconomically disadvantaged (Freeman, 1989), concluded that the poorer outcome in African Americans compared to Caucasians is primarily linked to lower socioeconomic status. Further, the report concluded that poor Americans, irrespective of race, have a 10–15% lower 5-year cancer survival rate than more affluent Americans. Based on this type of mounting evidence, US Surgeon General David Satcher refocused the nation's attention by setting a national goal of eliminating disparities (US Department of Health and Human Services, 2001).

Reaching this goal, however, continues to be a challenge. The issue of disparities is complex, and effectively examining the magnitude of and progress toward decreasing disparities depends on the ability to collect, analyze, and interpret relevant data appropriately. To that end, this chapter outlines current data tracking systems (domestic and international) and provides an overview of existing disparities in cancer burden by race/ethnicity, socioeconomic status, and country. It will also discuss the implications of these findings for future research.

B.D. Powe (✉)
Behavioral Research Center, American Cancer Society, National Home Office, Atlanta, GA
e-mail: Barbara.Powe@cancer.org

H.K. Koh (ed.), *Toward the Elimination of Cancer Disparities*,
DOI 10.1007/978-0-387-89443-0_2, © Springer Science+Business Media, LLC 2009

Definitions of Disparities and Implications for Data Interpretation

There are many definitions and terms used in the global discussion of disparities. In Chapter 1 of this book, Krieger and colleagues review such definitions in a detailed way. Consistent and universally accepted definitions are crucial because the way in which "disparities" and related terms are defined can significantly influence what questions are asked, how data are collected, how data are interpreted, and how the results of this interpretation are applied to efforts to reduce disparities. Other factors that have to be considered when defining, monitoring, and interpreting disparities are whether the interest lies in total disparities, whether the measurement emphasis should be on absolute or relative disparities, and who is considered to be the referent group. Because of the complexity of these types of data, this chapter uses (1) the NIH definition of disparities that focuses on group disparities; (2) Caucasians as the reference group in describing racial/ethnic disparities; (3) educational attainment as a marker for socioeconomic status; and (4) relative and absolute disparities when presenting data. Below is a brief overview of the generally accepted meanings of these key terms.

Disparities and Group Disparities. Several federal and public health agencies in the United States define health disparities as differences in the incidence, prevalence, survival, mortality, and burden of diseases and other adverse health conditions that exist in specific population groups. According to the 106th Congress of the United States, health disparities exist ". . .if there is a significant disparity in the overall rate of disease incidence, prevalence, morbidity, mortality, or survival rates in the population as compared to the health status of the general population. In addition, such a term includes populations for which there is a considerable disparity in the quality, outcomes, cost, or use of health care services or access to or satisfaction with such services as compared to the general population" (106th Congress of the United States, 2000). One form of disparity, for example, might be "excess deaths" in a minority population, i.e., the difference between the number of deaths observed in the minority population and the number of deaths that would have been expected in that population if they had the same age- and sex-specific death rate as the nonminority population (US Department of Health and Human Services, 1985).

Disparities can involve biological, environmental, and behavioral factors, as well as income and education, and may be characterized by gender, age, ethnicity, education, income, social class, disability status, geographic location, or sexual orientation (National Cancer Institute, 2007; Centers for Disease Control and Prevention, Division of Cancer Prevention and Control, 2007; US Department of Health and Human Services, 2001). See Chapter 1 of this book for a more detailed discussion of these dimensions.

Social Disparities/Group Disparities Versus Total Disparity. When these differences in health conditions or outcomes are linked to specific groups (e.g., race/ethnicity, poverty, education, social status), they are referred to as "social disparities" or "group disparities." For example, in the United States, group disparities have been cited between the racial and ethnic minority populations of African Americans, Asians, Pacific Islanders, Hispanics and Latinos, Native Americans, and Native Alaskans—specific groups that have been identified as disparate populations with regard to cancer incidence, mortality, and survival (National Cancer Institute, 2007b). In contrast, the measure "total disparity" reflects the univariate distribution of health among all individuals in a population without regard to their group membership (Harper & Lynch, 2005).

Absolute Versus Relative Disparity. Disparities can be estimated in different ways, depending on the purpose of the measurement. The term "absolute disparity" is the raw numeric difference between the rates or other values of two groups. For example, the absolute disparity in cancer mortality rates between males and females would be the numerical difference between their respective rates (Harper & Lynch, 2005). "Relative disparity," on the other hand, is the percentage difference or ratio between two groups. This measure allows two groups to be compared without regard to the magnitude of the rates. Thus, even if rates of stomach cancer decreased for both males and females, the relative disparity, or ratio of male-to-female mortality, could simultaneously increase (Harper & Lynch, 2005). An absolute disparity measure can be used to indicate the number of people affected and to evaluate the public health impact of this number by comparing it to a standard or target rate; a relative disparity measure, in contrast, can be used to indicate how much one group differs from another and thus compare various health indicators or evaluate changes in disparities over time.

Inequality and Inequity. Terms such as inequality and inequity are also used when referring to disparities (See Chapter 1). While these terms and definitions have similarities, they are often interpreted quite differently, which can lead to differences in data collection and analysis. Although sometimes used synonymously with "inequity," "inequality" is more accurately a generic term used to designate differences, variations, and disparities in the health of individuals and groups (Kawachi et al., 2002) without judgment about the fairness or controllability of the differences. For example, the World Health Organization (WHO) defines inequality as differences in health status or in the distribution of health determinants between different population groups, some of these health inequalities "attributable to biological variations or free choice... [and] others ... to the external environment and conditions mainly outside the control of the individuals concerned" (World Health Organization, 2007). In contrast, the term "health inequity" relies not only on an observed difference in outcomes but also on a moral/judgment about justice, usually related to social, political, or ethical beliefs (Harper & Lynch, 2005; Peter & Evans, 2001). These inequitable differences are deemed unnecessary and avoidable, and also considered unfair and/or to stem from injustice (Kawachi et al., 2002), a term that is taken to mean a "denial or violation of economic, sociocultural, political, or civil rights by certain population groups within a society (Levy & Sidel, 2006). The crux of the distinction between inequality and inequity is that the identification of health inequities entails normative judgment premised upon (a) one's theory of justice, (b) one's theories of society, and (c) one's reasoning underlying the genesis of health inequalities (Public Health Agency of Canada, 2007). The chapter by Krieger et al. in this volume closely examines these critical terms (see Chapter 1).

Excess Deaths. This term is defined as the difference between the number of deaths observed in a minority population and the number of deaths which would have been expected in a minority population if they had the same age- and sex-specific death rate as the non-minority population (US Department of Health and Human Services, 1985).

Overview of Current Data Tracking Systems

Inconsistencies and gaps in how and what data health care systems collect undermine efforts to obtain data that allow effective and full evaluation of the extent of disparities (Ver Ploeg & Perrin, 2004). For example, in the United States there are insufficient linkages to facilitate data sharing confidentially across systems (i.e., national, state, local government agencies). Furthermore, medical records submitted from hospitals, clinics, and other health facilities to cancer registries are often missing data points, including information on socioeconomic status. There is also a substantial time lag in getting this data from the patient to the hospital record system and finally, to a state's cancer registry. Further, national surveys often omit data about certain racial/ethnic minority groups. In fact, prior to 1970 cancer mortality data were generally classified based on only three racial/ ethnic groups: "black," "white," and "other" (Ver Ploeg & Perrin, 2004).

Current data that describe disparities in cancer incidence, survival, and mortality in the United States are available from the Surveillance, Epidemiology, and End Results (SEER) Program of the National Cancer Institute (NCI), the National Program of Cancer Registries (NPCR) of the Centers for Disease Control and Prevention (CDC), and the National Center for Health Statistics (NCHS). Data on trends in international cancer disparities, as well as several other published reports, are available from the International Agency for Research on Cancer (IARC). A brief description of these data sources follows.

SEER. Between 1973 and 1975, the SEER Program collected population-based cancer incidence and survival data in nine geographic areas, covering 10% of the United States population. Since then, this NCI-sponsored program has continued to collect data on patient demographics, primary tumor site, tumor morphology and stage at diagnosis, first course of treatment, and follow-up for vital status (National Cancer Institute, 2007a). In 1992, SEER began collecting this data by expanded racial/ethnic categories and has since expanded its coverage to 18 registries covering 25% of the nation's population.

NPCR. Administered by the CDC, the NPCR was established in 1992 through the Cancer Registries Amendment Act. The NPCR collects and codes data on the incidence, type, extent, and location, as well as the initial treatment of the cancer (Centers for Disease Control and Prevention Division of Cancer Prevention and Control, 2007). Currently, this program supports cancer registries in 45 states, the District of Columbia, Puerto Rico, the Republic of Palau, and the Virgin Islands. These state-based cancer registries collect, manage, and analyze data from medical facilities (hospitals, physicians' offices, therapeutic radiation facilities, freestanding surgical centers, and pathology laboratories) and report these data to a central cancer registry. The NPCR and SEER programs collectively monitor cancer occurrence for approximately 96% of the population (Centers for Disease Control and Prevention Division of Cancer Prevention and Control, 2007).

NCHS. The NCHS, housed in the CDC, is another leading source for statistical health data. National mortality data have been abstracted from death certificates annually since 1930. These data are classified according to the current International Classification of Diseases (ICD) codes and selection rules of underlying cause of death at the year of death (National Center for Health Statistics, 2007).

IARC. Lastly, international data on cancer incidence and mortality can be accessed from the IARC, which is a part of the WHO. Its mission is to "coordinate and conduct research on the causes of human cancer, the mechanisms of carcinogenesis, and to develop scientific strategies for cancer control" (International Agency for Research on Cancer, 2007). The IARC monitors cancer incidence data for approximately 20% and mortality data for approximately 30% of the world's population.

Cancer Disparities by Race/Ethnicity and Socioeconomic Status

This section provides data on the disparities in cancer rates and trends in incidence, mortality, and survival among the major racial/ethnic groups in the United States. Data are provided for all cancers combined and for selected cancer sites. Trend data are provided for Caucasians and African Americans from 1975 to 2004. The trend data for the other racial/ethnic groups are only provided for all cancers combined because the year-to-year rates for specific cancer types were unstable over time. This section also provides limited information on cancer disparity by socioeconomic status (SES) using educational attainment and health insurance status as indicators of SES, although data showing the SES cancer disparity over time are lacking.

African Americans. African Americans are more likely to develop and die from all cancers combined than any other racial or ethnic population (Tables 2.2 and 2.3). The death rate from cancer among African American males is about 37% higher than among white males; for African American females, it is about 17% higher than among white females. Importantly, the disparities in mortality rates between African Americans and whites have widened over the years for all cancers combined as well as for most of the major cancers (Figs. 2.1–2.6).

Hispanics. Hispanics have lower incidence rates for all cancers combined and for most common types of cancer than whites, but they generally have higher

Table 2.1 Definitions of terms[*]

Disparities

Differences in the incidence, prevalence, mortality, and burden of cancer and related adverse health conditions that exist among specific population groups in the United States. These population groups may be characterized by gender, age, ethnicity, education, income, social class, disability, geographic location, or sexual orientation (National Cancer Institute, 2007).

Differences that occur by gender, race or ethnicity, education, or income, disability, living in rural localities or sexual orientation (US Department of Health and Human Services, 2001).

Health disparities occur when one group of people has a higher incidence or mortality rate than another, or when survival rates are less for one group than another. Disparities are most often identified along racial and ethnic lines that show that African Americans, Hispanics, Native Americans, Asian Americans, Alaska Natives, and whites have different disease rates and survival rates. Disparities are determined and measured by three health statistics—incidence rates (the number of newly diagnosed cancers in a specified population over a defined time period), mortality rates (the number of cancer deaths in a specified population over a defined time period), and survival rates (the length of survival following diagnosis of cancer). Disparities can involve biological, environmental, and behavioral factors, as well as differences based on income and education (Centers for Disease Control and Prevention Division of Cancer Prevention and Control, 2007)

A population is a health disparity population if there is a significant disparity in the overall rate of disease incidence, prevalence, morbidity, mortality, or survival rates in the population as compared to the health status of the general population. In addition, such term includes populations for which there is a considerable disparity in the quality, outcomes, cost, or use of health care services or access to, or satisfaction with such services as compared to the general population (106th Congress of the United States, 2000).

Excess Deaths

Difference between the number of deaths observed in a minority population and the number of deaths which would have been expected in a minority population if they had the same age- and sex-specific death rate as the non-minority population (US Department of Health and Human Services, 1985).

Inequities

Relies on a moral, ethical judgment about justice and thus is not unambiguously measurable or observable. Judgments concerning inequity rely on social, political, and ethical discourse about what a society believes is unfair (Harper & Lynch, 2005; Harper & Lynch, 2005; Peter & Evans, 2001).

Inequities in health that are deemed to be unfair or stemming from some form of injustice. The crux of the distinction between equality and equity is that (a) the identification of health inequities entails normative judgment premised upon one's theory of justice, (b) one's theories of society, and (c) one's reasoning underlying the genesis of health inequalities (Public Health Agency of Canada, 2007).

Those inequalities in health deemed to be unfair or to stem from injustice. The dimensions of being avoidable or unnecessary have often been added to this concept (Kawachi et al., 2002).

Inequality

Differences in health status or in the distribution of health determinants between different population groups. Differences are unnecessary, avoidable, and considered unfair and unjust. Some health inequalities are attributable to biological variations or free choice and others are attributable to the external environment and conditions mainly outside the control of the individuals concerned (World Health Organization, 2007).

A generic term used to designate differences, variations, and disparities in the health of individuals and groups (Kawachi et al., 2002).

Injustice

Denial or violation of economic, sociocultural, political, or civil rights by certain population groups within a society (Levy & Sidel, 2006).

Table 2.1 (continued)

Absolute Disparities

Reflects the difference in values. For example, the actual difference between male and female stomach cancer mortality rates is the absolute disparity (Harper & Lynch, 2005).

Relative Disparities

Reflects differences in outcome ratios. For example, as rates of stomach cancer decreased for males and females, the ratio of male-to-female mortality increased (Harper & Lynch, 2005).

Total Disparity

Reflects the univariate distribution of health among all individuals in a population without regard to their group membership (Harper & Lynch, 2005).

Social-Group Disparities

Reflects differences between groups based on an identified parameter such as race/ethnicity or education, to name a few (Harper & Lynch, 2005).

[*]See also Chapter 1

Table 2.2 Cancer incidence rates by site, race, and ethnicity, US, 2000–2004

Incidence	White	African American	Asian American/ Pacific Islander	American Indian/Alaska Native[†]	Hispanic/ Latino[†§]
All sites					
Males	556.7	663.7	359.9	321.2	421.3
Females	423.9	396.9	285.8	282.4	314.2
Breast (female)	132.5	118.3	89.0	69.8	89.3
Colon & rectum					
Males	60.4	72.6	49.7	42.1	47.5
Females	44.0	55.0	35.3	39.6	32.9
Kidney & renal pelvis					
Males	18.3	20.4	8.9	18.5	16.5
Females	9.1	9.7	4.3	11.5	9.1
Liver & bile duct					
Males	7.9	12.7	21.3	14.8	14.4
Females	2.9	3.8	7.9	5.5	5.7
Lung & bronchus					
Males	81.0	110.6	55.1	53.7	44.7
Females	54.6	53.7	27.7	36.7	25.2
Prostate	161.4	255.5	96.5	68.2	140.8
Stomach					
Males	10.2	17.5	18.9	16.3	16.0
Females	4.7	9.1	10.8	7.9	9.6
Uterine cervix	8.5	11.4	8.0	6.6	13.8

Per 100,000 population, age adjusted to the 2000 US standard population. [†] Data based on Contract Health Service Delivery Areas (CHSDA), 624 counties comprising 54% of the US American Indian/Alaska Native population; [‡] Persons of Hispanic/Latino origin may be of any race. [§] Data unavailable from the Alaska Native Registry and Kentucky. Data unavailable from Minnesota, New Hampshire, and North Dakota (Ries et al., 2007).

Table 2.3 Cancer death rates by site, race, and ethnicity, US, 2000–2004

Mortality	White	African American	Asian American Pacific Islander	American Indian/Alaska Native[†]	Hispanic/ Latino[‡¶]
All sites					
Males	234.7	321.8	141.7	187.9	162.2
Females	161.4	189.3	96.7	141.2	106.7
Breast (female)	25.0	33.8	12.6	16.1	16.1
Colon & rectum					
Males	22.9	32.7	15.0	20.6	17.0
Females	15.9	22.9	10.3	14.3	11.1
Kidney & renal pelvis					
Males	6.2	6.1	2.4	9.3	5.4
Females	2.8	2.8	1.1	4.3	2.3
Liver & bile duct					
Males	6.5	10.0	15.5	10.7	10.8
Females	2.8	3.9	6.7	6.4	5.0
Lung & bronchus					
Males	72.6	95.8	38.3	49.6	36.0
Females	42.1	39.8	18.5	32.7	14.6
Prostate	25.6	62.3	11.3	21.5	21.2
Stomach					
Males	5.2	11.9	10.5	9.6	9.1
Females	2.6	5.8	6.2	5.5	5.1
Uterine cervix	2.3	4.9	2.4	4.0	3.3

Per 100,000 population, age adjusted to the 2000 US standard population. [†]Data based on Contract Health Service Delivery Areas (CHSDA), 624 counties comprising 54% of the US American Indian/Alaska Native population; [‡]Persons of Hispanic/Latino origin may be of any race. Data unavailable from the Alaska Native Registry and Kentucky. [¶] Data unavailable from Minnesota, New Hampshire, and North Dakota (Ries et al., 2007).

rates of cancers associated with infection, such as uterine, cervix, liver, and stomach cancers. For example, incidence rates of liver cancer are twice as high in Hispanic men and women as in non-Hispanic Caucasians.

Asian Americans and Pacific Islanders. Similar to Hispanics, Asian Americans and Pacific Islanders have lower incidence rates than whites for the most common cancer sites but have a higher incidence of many of the cancers related to infection. On the other hand, this population has the highest incidence and death rates from liver and stomach cancers of all racial/ethnic groups in both men and women, with the exception of deaths from stomach cancer in men.

American Indians and Alaska Natives. Incidence and death rates from kidney cancer in American Indian and Alaska Native men and women are higher than in any other racial/ethnic population. Cancer rates for American Indians and Alaska Natives should be interpreted with caution, however, because available

Table 2.4 Trends in 5-year relative survival rates (%) by race and year of diagnosis, US, 1975–2003

	White			African American			All Races		
	1975–1977	1984–1986	1996–2003	1975–1977	1984–1986	1996–2003	1975–1977	1984–1986	1996–2003
All sites	51	55	67†	40	41	57†	50	54	66†
Brain	23	28	34†	27	33	37†	24	29	35†
Breast (female)	76	80	90†	62	65	78†	75	79	89†
Colon	52	60	66†	46	50	55†	51	59	65†
Esophagus	6	11	18†	3	8	11†	5	10	16†
Hodgkin lymphoma	74	80	87†	71	75	81†	74	79	86†
Kidney	51	56	66†	50	54	66†	51	56	66†
Larynx	67	68	66	59	53	50	67	66	64
Leukemia	36	43	51†	34	34	40	35	42	50†
Liver#	4	6	10†	2	5	7†	4	6	11†
Lung & bronchus	13	14	16†	12	11	13†	13	13	16†
Melanoma of the skin	82	87	92†	60‡	70§	77	82	87	92†
Myeloma	25	27	34†	31	32	32	26	29	34†
Non-Hodgkin lymphoma	48	54	65†	49	48	56	48	53	64†
Oral cavity	55	57	62†	36	36	41	53	55	60†
Ovary¶	37	39	45†	43	41	38	37	40	45†
Pancreas	3	3	5†	2	5	5†	2	3	5†
Prostate	70	77	99†	61	66	95†	69	76	99†
Rectum	49	58	66†	45	46	58†	49	57	66†
Stomach	15	18	22†	16	20	24†	16	18	24†
Testis	83	93	96†	82‡	87‡	88	83	93	96†

Table 2.4 (continued)

	White			African American			All Races		
	1975–1977	1984–1986	1996–2003	1975–1977	1984–1986	1996–2003	1975–1977	1984–1986	1996–2003
Thyroid	93	94	97[†]	91	90	94	93	94	97[†]
Urinary bladder	75	79	81[†]	51	61	65[†]	74	78	81[†]
Uterine cervix	71	70	74[†]	65	58	66	70	68	73[†]
Uterine corpus	89	85	86[†]	61	58	61	88	84	84[†]

Survival rates are adjusted for normal life expectancy and are based on cases diagnosed in the SEER 9 areas from 1975–77, 1984–86, and 1996 to 2003 and followed through 2004. [†] The difference in rates between 1975–1977 and 1996–2003 is statistically significant ($p<0.05$). [‡] The standard error of the survival rate is between 5 and 10 percentage points. [§] The standard error of the survival rate is greater than 10 percentage points. [¶] Recent changes in classification of ovarian cancer, namely excluding borderline tumors, have affected 1996–2002 survival rates. [#] Includes intrahepatic bile duct (Ries et al., 2007).

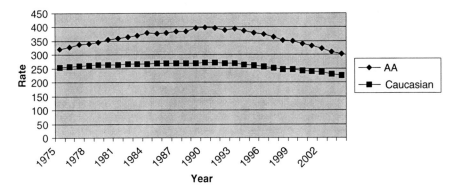

Fig. 2.1 Trends in age-standardized death rates for males (All Malignant Cancers) by race, 1975–2004
Underlying mortality data provided by the National Center for Health Statistics. Rates are per 100,000 and age adjusted to the 2000 US Std Population (19 age groups—Census P25-1130) standard; AA = African American.

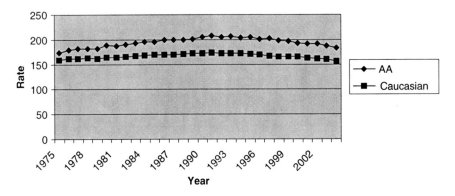

Fig. 2.2 Trends in age-standardized death rates for females (All Malignant Cancers) by race, 1975–2004
Underlying mortality data provided by the National Center for Health Statistics. Rates are per 100,000 and age adjusted to the 2000 US Std Population (19 age groups—Census P25-1130) standard; AA = African American.

data are not considered representative. To resolve this issue, a linkage of cancer registry data and the Indian Health Service patient database has been developed.

In addition to the variation in cancer burden between different racial/ethnic groups, significant disparities exist among sub-populations. For example, incidence rates for cervical cancer are almost three times higher in Vietnamese American women than in Chinese and Japanese Americans; this is partly because the Vietnamese, in general, immigrated more recently, are poorer, and have less access to cervical cancer screening. Trend data for

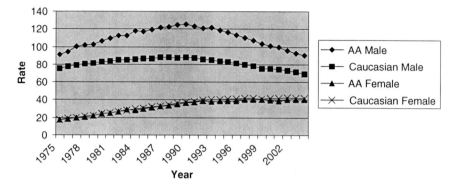

Fig. 2.3 Lung cancer: Trends in age-standardized death rates by race and sex, 1975–2004 Underlying mortality data provided by the National Center for Health Statistics. Rates are per 100,000 and age adjusted to the 2000 US Std Population (19 age groups—Census P25-1130) standard; AA = African American.

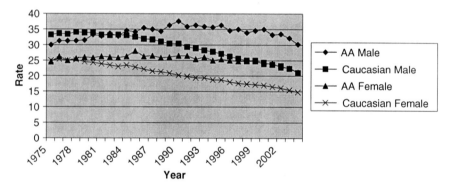

Fig. 2.4 Colorectal cancer: Trends in age-standardized death rates by race and sex, 1975–2004 Underlying mortality data provided by the National Center for Health Statistics. Rates are per 100,000 and age adjusted to the 2000 US Std Population (19 age groups—Census P25-1130) standard; AA = African American.

other racial/ethnic minority groups are unstable over time due to lack of data and therefore are not presented.

Factors contributing to these disparities are complex and will be explored in depth throughout the remainder of this book. Overall, however, it is clear that many disparities are related to the many obstacles faced by various racial and ethnic minorities in receiving health care services relating to cancer prevention, early detection, and high-quality treatment. These obstacles include low income; inadequate health insurance; geographic, cultural, and language barriers; racial bias; and stereotyping. For example, poverty influences both the prevalence of underlying risk factors for cancer (such as tobacco use and

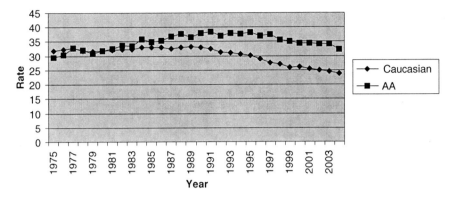

Fig. 2.5 Female breast cancer: Trends in age-standardized death rates by race and sex, 1975–2004
Underlying mortality data provided by the National Center for Health Statistics. Rates are per 100,000 and age adjusted to the 2000 US Std Population (19 age groups—Census P25-1130) standard; AA = African American.

obesity) and the access to health care services. Compared with just 11% of whites, 25% of African Americans and 22% of Hispanics/Latinos live below the poverty line. Moreover, 18% of African Americans and 33% of Hispanics/Latinos are uninsured, compared to only 12% of whites. These differences have considerable relevance to health disparities, given that low-income and uninsured people in particular are more likely to be diagnosed with cancer at later stages, receive substandard clinical care and services, and die from cancer. Not surprisingly, then, the 5-year relative survival rate for all cancers combined is lower for African Americans (57%) than it is for whites (67%).

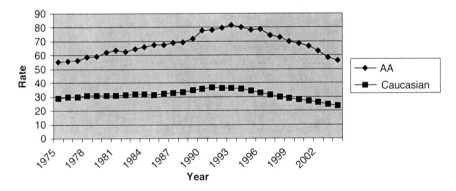

Fig. 2.6 Prostate Cancer: Trends in age-standardized death rates by race and sex, 1975–2004
Underlying mortality data provided by the National Center for Health Statistics. Rates are per 100,000 and age adjusted to the 2000 US Std Population (19 age groups—Census P25-1130) standard; AA = African American.

Table 2.5 Cancer death rates by educational attainment, race, and sex, US, 2001*

	Men			Women		
	Black	Non-Hispanic white	Absolute difference	Black	Non-Hispanic white	Absolute difference
All sites						
<= 12 years of education	214.43	163.78	50.65	148.10	128.79	19.31
> 12 years of education	90.14	73.00	17.14	103.30	73.02	30.28
RR (95% CI)	2.38 (2.33–2.43)	2.24 (2.23–2.26)	–	1.43 (1.41–1.46)	1.76 (1.75–1.78)	–
Absolute difference	124.29	90.78	–	44.80	55.77	–
Lung						
<= 12 years of education	73.23	60.99	12.24	30.82	37.06	-6.24
> 12 years of education	25.78	18.13	7.65	17.92	14.20	3.72
RR (95% CI)	2.84 (2.69–3.00)	3.36 (3.30–3.43)	–	1.72 (1.61–1.84)	2.6 (2.53–2.67)	–
Absolute difference	47.45	42.86	–	12.90	22.86	–
Colorectal						
<= 12 years of education	20.59	14.23	6.36	14.13	9.36	4.77
> 12 years of education	11.30	7.88	3.42	10.82	5.44	5.38
RR (95% CI)	1.81 (1.63–2.02)	1.81 (1.73–1.89)	–	1.31 (1.18–1.45)	1.72 (1.63–1.82)	–
Absolute difference	9.29	6.35	–	3.31	3.92	–
Prostate						
<= 12 years of education	10.52	3.26	7.26	NA		
> 12 years of education	4.80	2.22	2.58			
RR (95% CI)	2.17 (1.82–2.58)	1.47 (1.34–1.62)	–			
Absolute difference	5.72	1.04	–			
Breast						
<= 12 years of education	NA			36.06	25.20	10.86
> 12 years of education				31.13	18.50	12.63
RR (95% CI)				1.16 (1.10–1.22)	1.36 (1.32–1.40)	–
Absolute difference				4.93	6.70	–

*Rates are for individuals 25–64 years at death, per 100,000, and age-adjusted to the 2000 US standard population (Albano et al., 2007).
RR=relative risk; CI = confidence interval; NA=not applicable.

Socioeconomic Status

Factors associated with SES contribute to substantial differences in cancer incidence and mortality within and among racial/ethnic groups. SES is highly correlated with cancer risk and outcomes across the continuum from prevention to palliative care (Woods et al., 2006). Some of the explanations for these disparities may be that persons with lower SES are more likely to engage in behaviors such as tobacco use and physical inactivity, that increase cancer risk in part because of marketing strategies that target these populations and environmental or community influences, such as opportunities for physical activity and access to fresh fruits and vegetables. Lower SES is also associated with financial, structural, and personal barriers to health care, including lack of or inadequate health insurance, reduced access to recommended preventive care and treatment services, lower literacy rates, and lower levels of education.

Cancer mortality rates among both African American and Caucasian men with 12 or fewer years of education are more than twice those of men with higher levels of education (Table 2.5). In the United States, moreover, approximately 26% of African Americans and 45% of Hispanics do not graduate high school, compared to 15% of Caucasians and 17% of Asian Americans. In fact, potentially avoidable factors associated with lower educational status may account for almost half of all deaths, not only cancer deaths, among working-aged adults in the United States, regardless of race (Jemal et al., 2008). Death rates for each of the four major cancer sites are higher in less-educated black and white men and women than in those with more years of education. Furthermore, there is a clear link between educational attainment and rates of poverty. Specifically, African Americans who do not graduate high school have a 37% poverty rate compared to a rate of 31% for Hispanics, 16% for Asian Americans, and 22% for Caucasians with equivalent educational level (US Census Bureau, 2007a; US Census Bureau, 2007b). Moreover, findings suggest that African American patients between ages 18 and 56 years who resided in ZIP codes with low proportions of high-school graduates or low median household incomes were more likely to be diagnosed with advanced disease and/or larger tumors than their counterparts in other racial/ethnic groups (Chen et al., 2007b,a; Halpern et al., 2007).

The presence of health insurance—a factor interrelated with poverty and educational attainment—is another key contributor to the cancer disparities. More than 45 million Americans under the age of 65 lack health insurance or are underinsured (Ward et al., 2008). For several cancers, those who are uninsured are less likely to receive recommended cancer screening tests and more likely to be diagnosed with later stage disease and to have lower survival rates than those with private insurance (Ward et al., 2008). Several studies, for example, have found that patients with advanced-stage cancer (breast, laryngeal, oropharyngeal) at diagnosis were more likely to be uninsured or covered by Medicaid than those with private insurance. Similarly, patients were more likely to present with the largest tumors if they were uninsured or covered by Medicaid (Chen et al., 2007a,b; Halpern et al., 2007). Ward and colleagues (Ward et al., 2008) also found that among Caucasian women diagnosed with all stages of breast cancer, only 76% of those who were uninsured survived 5 years compared to 89% of those with private insurance. Yet among the African American women in this study, 65% of those who were uninsured survived 5 years compared to 81% of those who were privately insured. In Hispanic women, moreover, the 5-year survival rate was 83% for uninsured versus 86% for insured patients. Therefore, while insurance status clearly plays a role in survival rates, this factor alone cannot explain remaining disparities between racial/ethnic groups.

International Cancer Disparities

The burden of cancer strikingly varies across countries as well, largely due to differences in prevalence of major risk factors and the availability of screening and treatment services. In Eastern European Countries and China, for example, lung cancer is the most common cancer among men, in contrast to prostate cancer in North America, North and Western Europe, and Australia, and liver cancer and Kaposi Sarcoma (AIDS-related cancer) in many African countries (Fig. 2.7). Among women, the most common cancer is breast cancer in North America, Europe, Australia, and parts of South America, and North America; cervix cancer in South Asia, parts of Sub-Saharan Africa, and parts of South America; and stomach cancer in China. In general, cancers related to smoking (lung), reproductive factors (breast), screening (breast and prostate), and dietary factors (colon) predominate in economically developed countries; whereas cancers related to infections (e.g., cervix, liver, Kaposi sarcoma, and stomach) predominate in economically developing countries. For example, the incidence rate of cervical cancer in some African countries is five times as high as in the United States and North and West European countries where routine pap testing has been in place for many decades (Kogevinas et al., 1997).

Furthermore, the burden of cancers related to smoking, dietary habits, and reproductive factors—such as lung, breast, and colorectal cancers—is also increasing in economically developing countries as people in these countries live longer and adopt Western life styles (Mackay et al., 2006). In fact, tobacco-attributable deaths are projected to double from 3.4 million in 2007 to 6.8 million in 2050 in low- and middle-income countries (American Cancer Society, 2007).

Lack of screening services for early detectable cancers (e.g., cervix, breast, colon, and rectum) as well as lack of treatment for treatable cancers (e.g., leukemia, lymphoma, testis, breast, colon and rectum) also contribute to relatively lower survival rate of cancer after diagnosis in developing countries. The 5-year survival rate for breast cancer, for example, is less than 40% in many African and Asian countries, compared to over 80% in the United States

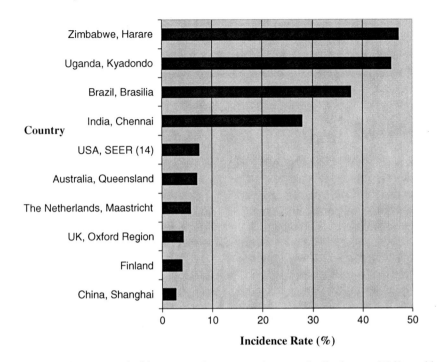

Fig. 2.7 Cervical cancer incidence rates by country (age-standardized rates (1960 world standard population); Mackay et al., 2006)

and Northern and Western European countries. Moreover, the 5-year survival rate for childhood cancers rose to over 70% in Northern and Western Europe and the United States over the past four decades because of improved treatment (e.g., chemotherapy), while survival remains low in many developing countries. The worldwide disparity in the availability of cancer treatment is best described by the considerable global variation in distribution of radiotherapy centers, appropriate for treating approximately 50% of all cancer patients (Mackay et al., 2006). Economically developing countries comprise more than 80% of the world population but possess only 20% of all electron accelerator machines and 70% of all cobalt machines (Kogevinas et al., 1997). Several countries in African and Asia lack even one such machine.

In addition to disparities between countries, there are disparities in the burden of cancer based on race/ethnicity or socioeconomic position among population groups within various countries (Woods et al., 2006; Kogevinas et al., 1997). For example, in Australia cancers of the liver and cervix are more than three times as high in indigenous (i.e., Aborigines and Torres Strait Islanders) than in non-indigenous populations (Condon, 2003). One review of socioeconomic differential in incidence and mortality for all cancers combined and for 24 types of cancer in 20 countries found that men with lower SES consistently show excess risk for smoking-related cancers (i.e., lung, larynx, oral cavity and pharynx, and esophagus) as well as stomach and liver cancers (Kogevinas et al., 1997). Excess risk was also noted among women of lower SES for cancers of the stomach, esophagus, and cervix. These disparities have widened over time in many countries including the United Kingdom and the United States.

Implications

Despite growing knowledge about disparities between Caucasians and African Americans, numerous gaps in data monitoring and tracking still need to be addressed to better understand the source of these disparities so that effective and targeted interventions can be implemented. Furthermore, data tracking systems still have not systematically collected data over time on racial/ethnic minority groups other than African Americans and have not tracked disparities within subgroups of these minorities. For example, Hispanics are currently categorized into one group, despite the fact that persons classified as Hispanic may be from any of a variety of cultures (e.g., Puerto Rico, Cuba, Mexico, or the Dominican Republic), with the burden of cancer varying significantly within these subpopulations. The same case can be made for persons of Asian descent or for rural versus urban dwellers. Collecting detailed data will provide greater insight into differences in cancer mortality as well as screening and treatment issues that could translate into more effectively tailored interventions.

While not discussed in detail in the current chapter, other sociocultural factors (e.g., language barriers, geographic region, behaviors, lifestyles, discrimination, segregation, and culture, to name a few) play a role in disparities. Unfortunately, however, data on these factors are not currently tracked for a variety of reasons. Among them, many of the national data systems rely on telephone interviews, a method that may not be the optimally effective method for some underserved racial/ethnic minority groups who may mistrust interviewers, speak little or no English, and/or lack a telephone altogether—resulting in missing and unreliable data. Moreover, despite the high proportion of uninsured and underinsured persons within certain racial/ethnic minority groups, no clear method of collecting and monitoring insurance trends and their influence on disparities has yet been developed. While quality of care is clearly another key indicator in monitoring disparities—given that the ability to receive state-of-the-art care has a direct impact on mortality and survivorship rates—there is still no method for systematically collecting data on quality of care and its relationship to disparities among various racial/ethnic minority groups.

Lastly, international data systems have to be better utilized. Hardly limited to the United States, cancer is a global concern and utilizing as many domestic and international resources as possible to assess disparities between countries would be in everyone's best interest. Initiatives such as the Joint Canada/United States Survey of Health (JCUSH) may provide the opportunity to explore similarities and differences with regard to cancer disparities.

Conclusion

Eliminating disparities in the cancer burden between different segments of the United States population is one of the overarching themes of Healthy People 2010. Effectively tracking and monitoring data trends is crucial to evaluating efforts to reduce disparities on a national (as well as international) level. Yet the complex, interrelated causes of these health disparities are unlikely to be determined by race/ethnicity alone. Instead, these disparities are most likely fueled by socioeconomic disparities in work, wealth, income, education, housing and overall standard of living, and other economic and social barriers to high-quality cancer prevention, early detection, and treatment services, as well as the impact of racial and ethnic discrimination on all of these factors. Elucidating and eventually counteracting these factors will first require the researchers, educators, public health providers, and policy makers who rely on these data trends to speak the same language and develop consistent methodologies with regard to defining disparities, tracking disparities, and monitoring progress toward eliminating the disparities.

References

106th Congress of the United States (2000). Minority Health and Health Disparities Research and Education Act of 2000. *Public Law*, 2495–2511.

Albano, J. D., Ward, E., Jemal, A., Anderson, R., Cokkinides, V. E., Murray, T., et al. (2007). Cancer mortality in the United States by education level and race. *Journal of National Cancer Institute*, 99(18), 1384.

American Cancer Society (2007). Global cancer facts & figures 2007. American Cancer Society. Available: http://www.cancer.org/docroot/stt/stt_0.asp

Centers for Disease Control and Prevention Division of Cancer Prevention and Control (2007a). Health disparities in cancer. Available: http://www.cdc.gov/cancer/healthdisparities/basic_info/

Centers for Disease Control and Prevention Division of Cancer Prevention and Control (2007b). National program of cancer registries. Available: http://www.cdc.gov/cancer/npcr/about.htm

Chen, A. Y., Schrag, N. M., Halpern, M., & Ward, E. M. (2007a). The impact of health insurance status on stage at diagnosis of oropharyngeal cancer. *Cancer*, 110, 395–402.

Chen, A. Y., Schrag, N. M., Halpern, M., Stewart, A., & Ward, E. M. (2007b). Health insurance and stage at diagnosis of laryngeal cancer: Does insurance type predict stage at diagnosis? *Archives of Otolaryngology-Head & Neck Surgery*, 133, 784–790.

Condon, J. R. (2003). Cancer in indigenous Australians: A review. *Cancer Causes Control*, 14, 109–121.

Freeman, H. (1989). *Cancer and the socioeconomic disadvantaged*. Atlanta: American Cancer Society.

Halpern, M., Bian, J., Ward, E. M., Schrag, N. M., & Chen, A. Y. (2007). Insurance status and stage of cancer at diagnosis among women with breast cancer. *Cancer*, 110, 403–411.

Harper, S., & Lynch, J. (2005). *Methods for measuring cancer disparities: Using data relevant to Healthy People 2010 cancer-related objectives*. NCI Cancer Surveillance Monograph Series, Number 6. Bethesda, MD: National Cancer Institute. NIH Publication No. 05-5777.

Hensechke, U. K., Leffall, L. D., Mason, C. H., Reinhold, A. W., Schneider, R. L., & White, J. E. (1973). Alarming increase of the cancer mortality in the US Black populations (1950–1967). *Cancer*, 31, 753–768.

International Agency for Research on Cancer (2007). About IARC. International Agency for Research on Cancer. Available: http://www.iarc.fr/

Jemal, A., Thun, M., Ward, E., Henley, S. J., Cokkinides, V. J., & Murray, T. E. (2008). Mortality from leading causes by education and race in the United States, 2001. *American Journal of Preventive Medicine*, 34, 1–8.

Kawachi, I., Almeida-Filho, N., & Subramanian, S. V. (2002). A glossary for health inequalities. *Journal of Epidemiology and Community Health*, 56, 647–652.

Kogevinas, M., Pearce, N., Susser, M., & Boffetta, P. (1997). *Social inequalities and cancer*. Lyon: IARC Scientific Publications.

Levy, B. S. & Sidel, V. W. (2006). *Social injustice and public health*. New York City: Oxford.

Mackay, J., Jemal, A., Lee, N. C., & Parkin, D. M. (2006). *The cancer atlas*. Atlanta: Ga.

National Cancer Institute (2007a). About SEER. Available: http//www.seer.cancer.gov/about

National Cancer Institute (2007b). How are cancer health disparities defined? Available: http://crchd.cancer.gov/definitions/defined.html

National Center for Health Statistics (2007). Surveys and Data Collection Systems. National Center for Health Statistics. Available: http://www.cdc.gov/nchs/express.htm

Peter, F. & Evans, T. (2001). Ethical dimensions of health equity. In *Challenging Inequities in Health: From Ethics to Action*. New York: Oxford.

Public Health Agency of Canada (2007). Crossing sectors – experiences in intersectoral action, public policy and health. Available: http://www.phac-aspc.gc.ca/publicat/2007/cro-sec/9app_e.html

Ries, L. A. G., Miller, B. A., Melbert, D., Krapcho, M., Mariotto, A., Feuer, E. J., et al. (2007). SEER cancer statistics review, 1975–2004. Available: http://seer.cancer.gov/csr/1975_2004/

US Census Bureau (2007a). Current population survey, 2006: Annual social and economic supplement. Available: http://www.census.gov/population/socdemo/education/cps2006/tab01-01.xls

US Census Bureau (2007b). Income, poverty, and health insurance coverage in the United States, 2004. [On-line] Available: http://www.census.gov/compendia/statab/tables/07s0697.xls

US Census Bureau (2007c). People without health insurance coverage by race and Hispanic origin using 3-Year average: 2004 to 2006. Available: http://www.census.gov/hhes/www/hlthins/hlthin06/p60no233_table7.pdf

US Department of Health and Human Services (1985). *Report of the secretary's task force on Black and minority health*. Washington, DC: U.S. Government Printing Office.

US Department of Health and Human Services (2001). *Healthy People 2010: Understanding and improving health*. Washington, DC: U.S. Government Printing Office.

Ver Ploeg, M. & Perrin, E. (2004). *Eliminating health disparities: Measurement and data needs*. Washington, DC: The National Academies Press.

Ward, E., Halpern, M., Schrag, N. M., Cokkinides, V., DeSantis, C., Brandi, P., et al. (2008). Association on insurance with cancer care utilization and outcomes. *CA: A Cancer Journal for Clinicians*, 58, 9–31.

Woods, L. M., Rachet, B., & Coleman, M. P. (2006). Origins of socio-economic inequalities in cancer survival: A review. *European Society for Medical Oncology*, 17, 5–19.

World Health Organization (2007). Health impact assessment (HIA). Available: http://www.who.int/hia/about/glos/en/index1.html

Chapter 3
Genes, Environment, and Cancer Disparities

Alexandra E. Shields, Stephanie M. Fullerton, and Kenneth Olden

Eliminating health disparities is a national priority, as reflected in numerous federal initiatives (Institute of Medicine 2002; Kaiser Commission on Medicaid and the Uninsured 2003; Mayberry et al. 2000). The IOM "Crossing the Quality Chasm" (Institute of Medicine 2001) report cited the elimination of health disparities as one of its six priority goals for improving the quality of health care in the US, while the subsequent IOM report, "Unequal Treatment," provided exhaustive documentation of racial/ethnic health disparities across a wide range of health care settings, diseases (including cancer), and clinical settings (Institute of Medicine 2002). Healthy People 2010 named the elimination of health disparities as one of two primary national goals for improving the health of Americans and explicitly called for reducing the number of new cancer cases as well as the illness, disability, and death caused by cancer (US Department of Health and Human Services 2000). Despite national efforts, however, important disparities persist in cancer incidence, stage at diagnosis, severity, and survival (Bradley 2006; Freeman and Chu 2005; Phillips and Williams-Brown 2005; Raghavan 2007).

Part of the problem is that we do not fully understand the causal factors underpinning cancer disparities, or health disparities more broadly. While access to and quality of health care continue to account for many cancer disparities, much of what affects cancer risk and cancer outcomes lies *beyond the medical model*. Most prominent among these are social and environmental factors that shape an individual's propensity toward health and risk of disease, and reflect the complex ways in which systematic disadvantage (Powers and Faden 2006) translates into the places individuals live, the kinds of environmental toxins they are exposed to, the level of stress they experience, and the degree of access they have to social and material resources that affect health.

A robust literature has documented the role of socioeconomic position (SEP) (Chu et al. 2007; Krieger et al. 1999; Schwartz et al. 2003) and environmental assaults on cancer risk (Clapp 2000), cancer severity, and outcomes (Bach et al.

A.E. Shields (✉)
Harvard/MGH Center on Genomics, Vulnerable Populations, and Health Disparities, and Institute for Health Policy, Massachusetts General Hospital/Partners HealthCare; Department of Medicine, Harvard Medical School, Boston, MA 02115, USA

H.K. Koh (ed.), *Toward the Elimination of Cancer Disparities*,
DOI 10.1007/978-0-387-89443-0_3, © Springer Science+Business Media, LLC 2009

2002; Curtis et al. 2008). Much recent research has also focused on the role of genetics in cancer risk and outcomes to provide additional insight into the complex interactions of social, environmental, and genetic factors in determining cancer risk (Dong et al. 2008; Clavel 2007). There are two dominant lines of genomics research pertinent to understanding cancer disparities. One line of research seeks to identify genetic variants that increase cancer risk or affect response to treatment, investigating the extent to which risk allele frequencies vary among populations of different geographical ancestry. The other line of research focuses on complex gene–gene and gene–environment interactions (GEIs) that may explain differential cancer risk or outcomes, and the extent to which key environmental exposures that interact with genes to modify cancer risk are differentially distributed across populations.

Although previous research has identified numerous environmental exposures that have a direct impact on cancer, GEI research may identify new exposures or change our understanding of the importance of known environmental factors for cancer risk. In some cases, a particular genetic variant may be highly prevalent across all populations and have little impact on cancer risk, but become deleterious only in the presence of a particular environmental exposure that is differentially distributed across the population due to residential segregation, racism, cultural differences, or class. In other cases, a known genetic risk factor for cancer may be amplified or even become protective in the presence of a certain environmental exposure. To the extent that environmental exposures that modify genetic risk are socially or racially patterned, GEI research may provide new levers with which to tackle cancer disparities by redirecting attention to high priority environmental exposures and the need to develop effective regulatory and public health policies to protect all communities from them.

This new focus on genomics research as a focal point for understanding racial disparities in health has been met with skepticism by some investigators (Cooper et al. 2003; Sankar et al. 2004; Krieger 2005). We have, after all, identified many environmental factors that directly confer significant and demonstrable risk for developing cancer, yet have failed to implement public health policies and interventions to translate this knowledge into reduced risks. For some, the turn to factors "inside the body" to explain racial disparities in health obviates a focus on the importance of SEP and racism in explaining cancer disparities. However, we believe that, while social and environmental factors will often swamp the effect of genetic susceptibility in determining risk for cancer, there is no "one size fits all" approach. In some cases genetic factors alone, or in combination with particular environmental conditions, will account for a large portion of inter-individual variation in cancer risk, as in the case of 8q24 risk variants explaining a significant portion of prostate cancer risk in black men (Haiman et al. 2007). All new information should thus be mined for its potential to help us understand and address cancer disparities. Despite noted disciplinary tensions in understanding the etiology of cancer disparities, most can agree that new tools are needed to disentangle the complex and inter-related roles of biological, environmental, social, and behavioral factors in producing cancer disparities.

In this chapter, we assess the potential for genomics research, and GEI research in particular, to inform efforts to reduce cancer disparities, and call for actions we believe likely to increase the potential of GEI research to meaningfully inform efforts to reduce disparities. We first examine population differences in the prevalence of genetic variants believed to increase (or decrease) risk for several types of cancer. We then examine recent work identifying GEIs that have significant implications for cancer risk. We offer a schema for assessing the potential contribution of genomics research to understanding the etiology of racial/ethnic differences in health disparities, and provide illustrative examples of the varying constellations of genetic, social, and environmental factors that together define cancer risk. We argue that the greatest contribution is likely to come from GEI research that incorporates measures of social and environmental exposures believed to play a role in disease risk and known to be socially patterned by race/ethnicity and SEP. It is here that we see the greatest opportunities for new knowledge to inform the development of more nuanced and sophisticated prevention efforts. We conclude with a set of recommendations aimed at increasing the potential of GEI research to produce new insights into the etiology of cancer disparities and thus new leverage points for addressing them.

Role of Genetics in Explaining Cancer Risk and Cancer Disparities

Cancer has long been recognized as a heterogenous disease category, with varying incidence primarily attributable to the influence of environmental determinants, particularly naturally occurring and synthetically derived carcinogens (Adami et al. 2008). The early recognition that members of the same family could be subject to a higher-than-average risk of developing certain cancers like breast or colorectal cancer, however, combined with elucidation of the role of oncogenes in tumor initiation and progression, contributed to sustained efforts to identify germline genetic mutations that might contribute to cancer susceptibility (Fearon 1997; Peto 2001). Such efforts, at both a familial- and population-level, have been extremely productive, so that today the role of genetic variation in mediating cancer risk is widely accepted and increasingly well understood.

Until recently, the most reliable data on cancer susceptibility were generated from the analysis of hereditary cancer syndromes within high-risk families. Mutations identified in such families are invariably rare (sometimes so rare as to be restricted to one or a few pedigrees), disrupt the function of a single protein, and typically are of very high penetrance (i.e., if the predisposing mutation is inherited, its bearer will very likely go on to develop the associated cancer). The best known high penetrance cancer mutations are those that occur in the *BRCA1* and *BRCA2* genes and contribute to breast and/or ovarian cancer (Narod and Foulkes 2004; Sarin 2006), or in the *MLH1*, *MSH2*, and *MSH6* genes involved in hereditary nonpolyposis colorectal cancer (HNPCC) (Lynch and de la Chapelle 1999). While the general population has a lifetime risk of breast cancer of 13% (Jemal et al. 2004), a germline mutation in *BRCA1* or *BRCA2* confers risks through age 75 of 35–84% for breast and 6–55% for ovarian cancers (Antoniou et al. 2003; Garber and Offit 2005; Nelson et al. 2005). Similarly, the general population risk of developing colorectal cancer is approximately 5%, compared to a lifetime risk of 80% or more among those carrying an HNPCC mutation (Strate and Syngal 2005). Several hundred disease-causing mutations are currently recognized for each class of inherited cancer (Couch 2004; Lucci-Cordisco et al. 2003).

Although much is known about genetic contributions to cancer etiology in high-risk families, high-penetrance susceptibility variants account for only a small proportion (typically less than 5%) of cancers (Hemminki et al. 2008), with little effect on the pervasive problem of cancer disparities. Investigation has thus shifted to the consideration of more common, less penetrant, susceptibility variants, which are shared more broadly among non-related individuals and may contribute to subtle differences in the likelihood of developing particular cancers. Two major classes of genetic epidemiological investigation can be used to identify such genetic effects: (1) candidate gene analysis, where variants within genes with a biologically plausible connection to cancer susceptibility are prioritized (Dong et al. 2008), and (2) genome-wide investigation, where a large number of random genetic markers (typically several hundred thousand) are simultaneously considered for their association with cancer risk (Ambrosone 2007; Manolio et al. 2008). Both types of investigation involve comparison of many thousands of individuals and have benefited from technological advances that have allowed cheaper, faster, and more accurate genotyping, hence the identification of human genetic variation at unprecedented levels of detail. Genome-wide association studies (GWAS), in particular, have become feasible only since the completion of the International Haplotype Map (HapMap) Project in 2005 (International HapMap Consortium 2005).

To what extent might current knowledge about population differences in low penetrance susceptibility variants explain cancer disparities? Using data from the National Cancer Institute, we identified five cancers marked by significant racial/ethnic disparities for which reliable information about genetic susceptibility were available: breast, colorectal, gastric, lung, and prostate cancer. We then identified data describing the risks of disease associated with known susceptibility variants for these cancers and used previously reported gene frequency information to measure the extent to which the susceptibility variants differ in prevalence among several different human populations.

Caution is warranted in applying these and related data to understanding the etiology of health disparities as currently measured in the United States. Most relevantly, there is a clear distinction to be drawn between populations of differing geographical ancestry, a genetically meaningful term used by population geneticists, and self-identified race or ethnicity, a complex term that correlates to population ancestry to varying degrees (Shriver et al. 2003) and is an amalgam of ancestry, culture, and community identity. As such, self-identified race is far from an ideal measure of human genetic heterogeneity (Lee et al. 2008; Shields et al. 2005). National data tracking health disparities, however, are almost always categorized according to self-identified race/ethnicity labels used in the US Census and pro-scribed by OMB Directive 15 (Office of Management and Budget 1997). This disconnect between how data on health disparities is collected and measured and what genomics research has to offer in efforts to understand differential risk of cancer across various human populations is no small matter and has been the subject of much commentary (Lee et al. 2008; Risch 2006; Shields et al. 2005).

In Table 3.1, we summarize what is currently known about the role of common genetic variants in contributing to risk for (or protection from) the five cancers marked by the most dramatic racial/ethnic disparities: breast (23 variants), color-ectal (10), gastric (6), lung (11), and prostate (15). In most cases, the gene involved in the observed association is indicated. Most of these genes encode proteins involved in DNA repair or carcinogen metabolism and detoxification. However, 19 of the 65 associations (29%), all of which were identified by recent GWAS, do not fall within any recognized gene region, including a large number of variants identified in the chromosomal region 8q24. Thus, robust statistical associations with cancer susceptibility have been demonstrated that are currently impossible to relate to specific biological pathways. The remaining polymorphisms were iden-tified in the context of replicated candidate gene investigations. Odds ratios (ORs), which measure the odds of disease for an individual with the risk genotype versus individuals without the risk genotype, range in the table from 0.7 to 2.36 (ORs less than 1 reflect a protective effect of the allele arbitrarily chosen for comparison). Estimates represent average effects identified by meta-analysis of independent samples (Dong et al. 2008) or by replicated GWAS (Manolio et al. 2008) and more recent reports, as cited in the table.

The frequency of each associated risk allele, as observed in normal individuals sampled as part of the HapMap Project (populations of Northern and Western European ancestry (CEU, $n = 120$), West African ancestry (YRI, $n = 120$), and Asian ancestry (CHB+JPT, $n = 178$, representing the combined Han Chinese and Japanese samples) and reported in the Single Nucleotide Polymorphism database dbSNP (http://www.ncbi.nlm.nih.gov/projects/SNP/), is summarized to provide an estimate of the population heterogeneity of the cancer susceptibility variants. A commonly used standardized measure of allele frequency difference, F_{ST} (Wright 1942), was calculated to measure the extent of population heterogeneity at any specific locus (i.e., the degree to which a specific genetic variant is found at different frequencies in different populations) and permit comparisons of hetero-geneity across genetic variants. As shown, F_{ST} values for the set of cancer suscept-ibility variants range from 0.010 to 0.667. While F_{ST} can theoretically vary between 0 and 1, with 0 indicating no frequency differences among samples, F_{ST} values typically average about 15% (Tishkoff and Verrelli 2003) and one recent analysis has reported a genome-wide average of 0.110 (Barreiro et al. 2008). Twenty-six of the 65 replicated associations (40%) examined here have F_{ST} values greater than 0.150, suggesting a greater-than-average degree of population differ-entiation. Note that this is a descriptive assessment only and not a claim that these risk-associated alleles are unusually differentially distributed (in a statistically significant sense) among the populations studied.

Table 3.1 Population Frequencies of Replicated Common Cancer Susceptibility Variants

Gene	Variant	OR	Risk Allele	Allele Frequency from dbSNP				Reference
				European (CEU)	West African (YRI)	Asian (CHB+JPT)	F_{ST}	
Breast Cancer								
ATP1B2	-8852T>C	0.88*	G	0.867	0.367	0.657	**0.271**	(Dong et al. 2008) unless otherwise noted
CASP8	Asp302His	0.89*	C	0.125	0.017	0.000	0.102	
COMT	Met158Val	1.14	G	0.483	0.708	0.752	0.091	(Manolio et al. 2008)
CYP17	rs4919682	1.16	T	0.308	0.092	0.124	0.094	(Manolio et al. 2008)
CYP17	rs4919687	1.17	A	0.331	0.083	0.184	0.098	
CYP1A1	A2455G (exon 7)	0.72	G	0.067	0.000	0.228	**0.155**	
CYP1B1	Leu432Val	1.50	G	0.442	0.850	0.112	**0.549**	
FGFR2	rs1219648	1.20*	G	0.417	0.467	0.331	0.020	(Manolio et al. 2008)
FGFR2	rs2981582	1.26*	C	0.583	0.483	0.749	0.076	(Manolio et al. 2008)
GATA3	rs570613	0.85*	G	0.350	0.425	0.320	0.013	
IGFBP3	-202C>A	0.92	A	0.409	0.667	0.667	0.091	
LSP1	rs3817198	1.07*	T	0.658	0.875	0.878	0.101	(Manolio et al. 2008)
MAP3K1	rs889312	1.13*	A	0.692	0.672	0.478	0.059	(Manolio et al. 2008)
POR	Gly5Gly	1.58	G	0.000	0.292	0.000	**0.323**	
PTGS2	rs5275	0.80	C	0.371	0.669	0.174	**0.257**	
TNRC9	rs3803662	1.20*	C	0.700	0.467	0.366	0.118	(Manolio et al. 2008)
WDR79	Arg68Gly	1.60	G	0.842	0.083	0.715	**0.667**	
WDR79	Phe150Phe	1.15*	A	0.100	0.308	0.278	0.072	
XRCC1	Arg399Gln	1.60	A	0.580	0.100	0.276	**0.271**	
2q35	rs13387042	1.20*	A	0.633	0.775	0.122	**0.472**	(Manolio et al. 2008)
5p12	rs10941679	1.19*	G	0.242	0.233	0.472	0.085	(Stacey et al. 2008)
8q24	rs13281615	1.08*	T	0.542	0.567	0.411	0.028	(Manolio et al. 2008)
16q12	rs3803662	1.28*	T	0.300	0.533	0.634	0.118	(Manolio et al. 2008)

Table 3.1 (continued)

Gene	Variant	OR	Risk Allele	Allele Frequency from dbSNP			F_ST	Reference
				European (CEU)	West African (YRI)	Asian (CHB + JPT)		
Colorectal Cancer								
CCND1	G870A	1.18*	A	0.517	0.158	0.467	**0.160**	
GSTT1**	null	1.37	null	0.335	0.485	0.735	**0.164**	
MTHFR	C677T	0.83	T	0.242	0.108	0.438	0.142	
MTHFR	A1298C	0.81	C	0.358	0.102	0.189	0.100	
NQO1	Pro187Ser	1.18	T	0.217	0.192	0.461	0.107	
SMAD7	rs4939827	1.16*	T	0.508	0.233	0.231	0.116	(Manolio et al. 2008)
XPC	Lys939Gln	1.32*	C	0.408	0.258	0.361	0.026	
8q24	rs6983267	1.27*	G	0.458	0.983	0.365	**0.463**	(Manolio et al. 2008)
8q24	rs10505477	1.17*	T	0.442	0.900	0.360	**0.345**	(Manolio et al. 2008)
11q23	rs3802842	1.11*	C	0.242	0.342	0.338	0.015	(Tenesa et al. 2008)
Gastric Cancer								
CDH1	−160C>A	0.81	A	0.258	0.175	0.215	0.010	
GSTT1**	null	1.27	null	0.335	0.485	0.735	**0.164**	
MTHFR	C677T	1.52	T	0.242	0.108	0.438	0.142	
P53	Arg72Pro	0.84	G	0.767	0.331	0.551	**0.192**	
PSCA	rs2976392	1.71	A	0.417	0.250	0.448	0.048	(Sakamoto et al. 2008)
TNF-A	−308G>A	1.49	A	0.217	0.061	0.028	0.111	
Lung Cancer								
CYP1A1	MspI (T3801C)	2.36	C	0.100	0.200	0.417	0.144	
CYP1A1	A2455G (exon 7)	1.61	G	0.067	0.000	0.228	**0.155**	
GSTT1**	null	1.28	null	0.335	0.485	0.735	**0.164**	

Table 3.1 (continued)

Gene	Variant	OR	Risk Allele	European (CEU)	West African (YRI)	Asian (CHB + JPT)	F_{ST}	Reference
mEH	His113Tyr	0.70	C	0.325	0.100	0.455	**0.156**	
MPO	G463A	0.71	T	0.237	0.167	0.167	0.011	
XPA	G23A	0.73*	G	0.586	0.763	0.533	0.062	
XPC	Lys939Gln	1.30	C	0.408	0.258	0.361	0.026	
XPD	Lys751Gln	1.30	G	0.333	0.183	0.070	0.110	
XRCC1	Arg399Gln	1.34	A	0.580	0.100	0.276	**0.271**	
15q24	rs1051730	1.31*	T	0.400	0.110	0.022	**0.268**	(Thorgeirsson et al. 2008)
15q25	rs8034191	1.21*	C	0.433	0.142	0.028	**0.272**	(Hung et al. 2008)
Prostate Cancer								
CDH1	−160C>A	1.31	A	0.258	0.175	0.215	0.010	
CYP17	rs2486758	1.07*	C	0.250	0.033	0.314	0.136	
CYP17	rs6892	1.08*	C	0.175	0.000	0.236	0.127	
RNASEL	Asp541Glu	1.27	G	0.625	0.217	0.741	**0.304**	
TCF2	rs4430796	1.22*	A	0.467	0.400	0.678	0.084	(Manolio et al. 2008)
2p15	rs721048	1.15*	A	0.117	0.000	0.033	0.076	(Gudmundsson et al. 2008)
8q24	rs1447295	1.86*	A	0.067	0.342	0.157	0.128	(Ghoussaini et al. 2008)
8q24	rs6983267	1.26*	G	0.458	0.983	0.365	**0.463**	(Manolio et al. 2008)
8q24	rs6983561	2.11*	C	0.025	0.583	0.219	**0.402**	(Ghoussaini et al. 2008)
8q24	rs7000448	1.23*	T	0.392	0.783	0.267	**0.290**	(Ghoussaini et al. 2008)
8q24	rs10090154	1.32*	T	0.059	0.179	0.118	0.034	(Haiman et al. 2007)
8q24	rs13254738	1.12*	C	0.350	0.725	0.672	**0.169**	(Ghoussaini et al. 2008)

Table 3.1 (continued)

Gene	Variant	OR	Risk Allele	Allele Frequency from dbSNP			Fst	Reference
				European (CEU)	West African (YRI)	Asian (CHB + JPT)		
8q24	rs16901979	1.79*	A	0.025	0.542	0.234	**0.346**	(Manolio et al. 2008)
17q24	rs1859962	1.20*	G	0.508	0.208	0.346	0.099	(Manolio et al. 2008)
Xp11.22	rs5945572	1.23*	A	0.400	0.358	0.079	**0.152**	(Gudmundsson et al. 2008)

OR = odds ratio, defined as the odds of disease for an individual with the risk genotype versus individuals without the risk genotype. Per allele ORs are indicated by *s. All other ORs (e.g., those which involve contrasts between homozygous risk genotypes versus homozygous wild type genotypes) are as reported in Dong et al. (2008). F_{ST} for each site was calculated as var(p)/[p-avg *(1-p-avg)], where p = frequency of the risk allele (Wright 1942). Values of F_{ST} greater than 0.150 are highlighted in bold. ** = allele frequencies taken from Moyer et al. (2007), for Caucasian Americans, African Americans, and Han Chinese Americans.

The degree to which such population differences in the frequency of susceptibility alleles contribute to recognized cancer disparities is uncertain. The attributable fraction of disease explained by a risk factor is dependent on the size of the risk effect and the prevalence of the risk factor in a given population (Hemminki et al. 2008). Thus, we might speculate that variants with larger average effect sizes and greater degrees of population differentiation could contribute disproportionately to cancer disparities. Figure 3.1 illustrates the relationship between variant effect size (as estimated by the ORs summarized in Table 3.1) and the degree of population differentiation (as reflected in the derived F_{ST} estimates). As shown, only a minority of the observed susceptibility variants (7 out of 65, or 11%) have both an OR greater than 1.5 and an F_{ST} value greater than 0.150. Four of the outliers are polymorphisms implicated in breast cancer susceptibility (CYP1B1 Leu432Val, POR Gly5Gly, WDR79 Arg68Gly, and XRCC1 Arg399Gln), one is associated with lung cancer risk (CYP1A1 A2455G), and two are involved in prostate cancer predisposition (8q24 rs6983561 and rs16901979).

The reported effect sizes are, however, averages based on meta-analysis and the effect size of any given variant could vary from population to population, so the exact contribution, if any, of these frequency differences to cancer disparities remains to be determined. Where population-specific effect sizes have been well estimated, differences in association across populations are typically more modest than differences in allele frequency (Ioannidis et al. 2004). The best recognized such example involves the association of 8q24 variants with prostate cancer risk.

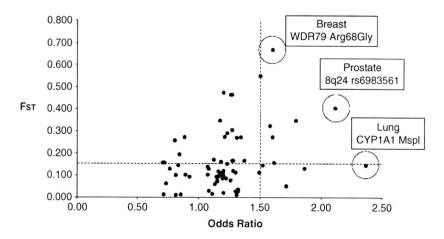

Fig. 3.1 Average effect size (odds ratio) versus population heterogeneity (F_{ST}) of the common cancer susceptibility variants presented in Table 3.1. The odds ratio (OR) measures the odds of disease for an individual with the risk genotype versus individuals without the risk genotype. F_{ST}, a standardized measure of allele frequency difference, describes the degree to which frequencies of the risk variant differ among samples of European, West African, and Asian ancestry (Table 3.1). A horizontal dashed line marks the average F_{ST} value of 0.150. The vertical dashed line distinguishes variants whose OR is less than or greater than 1.5. Three outlier variants are identified

When a combination of variants in the region (including rs6983561, rs13254738, rs10090154, rs6983267, and rs7000448, as per Table 3.1) is considered, most of which predispose to cancer to the same degree across populations but are found at higher frequency in individuals of African ancestry, as much as 68% of the cancer burden in a cohort of self-identified African Americans was potentially explained (Haiman et al. 2007). In contrast, the same variants explained only 32% of prostate cancer risk in a sample of European Americans.

Taken together, these data emphasize the complexity of our emerging understanding of genetic contributions to cancer susceptibility. A large and growing number of common genetic risk factors for the cancers subject to the most important disparities are now recognized, although many of these variants have yet to be linked to a defined biological pathway. A large proportion of these variants also display higher-than-average degrees of allele frequency differentiation among populations. While the individual increase in risk associated with any single variation might be quite low, the large number of individuals harboring such variations, and their potential to increase risk via interaction with specific environmental triggers (as discussed below), make them of special significance to the investigation of cancer disparities.

Gene–Environment Interaction Research and Its Application to the Investigation of Cancer Risk

While a sizeable number of genetic variants are now recognized as contributing to cancer susceptibility, individual genetic determinants are either rare (hence likely to contribute little to the overall population burden of disease) or more common but contribute to cancer risk to a much smaller degree and/or only in the presence of defined behavioral and environmental exposures (Fig. 3.2).

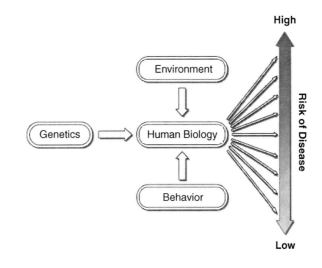

Fig. 3.2 Cancer risk is determined by the interaction of genes, environmental exposures, and behaviors

While many new polymorphisms have been identified as associated with increased cancer risk, the real challenge is to understand the mechanisms and pathways through which these genetic variants act to affect an individual's risk of developing cancer. Genetic variants are most often acting in concert with other genes or environmental factors inside and outside the body to increase risk of cancer and determine the trajectory of disease. Increasing attention has thus been directed to the investigation of GEIs and their role in understanding cancer.

Gene–environment interaction research represents a broad class of genetic research focused on understanding how human genetic variability is associated with differential responses to environmental exposures, and with differential effects depending on variations in other genes. The concept of gene–gene interactions and GEIs is not new. Garrod (1902) was one of the first to suggest that the effects of genes could be modified by the environment. He suggested that individual differences in genetics could play a role in variation in response to drugs and that the effect of genotype could be modified by the diet. While concerns about GEIs have had a long history (reviewed by Haldane 1946), the importance of understanding these interactions as a means to prevent complex diseases like cancer has only emerged over the past 15 years (Olden 1993, 1997; Olden et al. 2001; Schwartz and Collins 2007).

Gene–environment interaction studies rely on information about and measures of both genetic predisposition and environmental exposure. Genetic predisposition can be estimated from family history or phenotype, or determined directly by candidate gene or genome-wide analysis. Environmental and lifestyle factors can be measured using self-reported information collected from interviews or surveys, direct measures of participants' physical characteristics (e.g., anthropometry) or behaviors, or via biochemical detection of biomarkers of environmental exposures (Hunter 2005). Once such variables are collected, the main aim of research is to estimate the effects of both classes of risk factors at the same time in an effort to identify the underlying causal pathways contributing to disease risk. In the case of susceptibility to cancer, for example, it may be that a particular genetic mutation affects the ability of a metabolic enzyme to recognize and inactivate a chemical agent with known or suspected carcinogenic properties. Individuals with such a genotype would, as a consequence, be especially sensitive to the effects of the chemical and, if exposed to it, develop the associated cancer more often individuals whose genotypes rendered them resistant to the effects of the carcinogen. In the absence of the exposure, however, there would no discernable difference in cancer risk between the two classes of genotype (Fig. 3.3).

The identification of GEIs is of obvious value to understanding disease etiology and appropriately targeting public health interventions. As emphasized in the recent Institute of Medicine study on Genes, Environment and Behavior (2006), GEI research can (1) contribute to better estimates of the population-attributable risk for genetic and environmental risk factors by accounting for them jointly; (2) provide greater understanding of associations between environmental factors and diseases by examining these factors in genetically susceptible individuals; (3) improve the ability to explore disease mechanisms in humans by

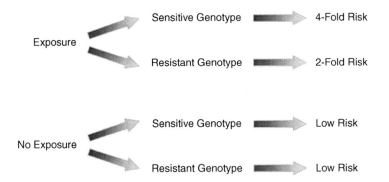

Fig. 3.3 Genetic modulation of environmental disease risk

using information on susceptibility and resistance genes to focus on the biological pathways most relevant to that disease, as well as the environmental factors most relevant to the biological pathways; (4) help identify specific compounds out of the complex mixtures of compounds that humans are exposed to, such as diet or air pollution, that cause disease; (5) use new knowledge about biological pathways to design preventive and therapeutic strategies; and (6) offer the opportunity for tailored preventive services based on the presence of susceptibility or resistance alleles (Institute of Medicine 2006).

The clear value of GEI investigation, however, is tempered by the considerable methodological challenges inherent in the identification of replicable (hence etiologically plausible) GEIs. Identifying interacting effects requires robust measurement of relevant exposures, thorough exploration of a range of statistical models of interaction, and consideration of very large numbers of individuals to achieve sufficient statistical power (Hunter 2005). For this reason, GEI studies have lagged behind the epidemiological investigation of genetic or environmental risk factors alone, and where GEI studies have been attempted, they have generally considered only a very limited range of genotypic and environmental exposure information.

Known or suspected instances of GEI reported for the same five cancers deemed high priority in terms of cancer disparities (Table 3.2) illustrate the relatively small number of environmental determinants that have been considered to date. Exposures encompassed in these studies fall in only three areas and are entirely limited to physical exposures within the body: smoking, diet (including fruit and vegetables, red meat, folate, and alcohol), and endogenous and exogenous hormones (i.e., estrogen). Missing from current cancer GEI investigations are community-level measures shown in the social epidemiology literature to have significant associations with cancer risk (e.g., community level inequality, community level violence, and crowding) or with exposures disproportionately visited upon low-income and minority communities due to racial and socioeconomic segregation in the US (e.g., differential exposure to diesel particles, stress hormones, poor quality diet, and/or poor housing stock).

Table 3.2 Gene-Environment Interactions Reported in the Context of Cancer Susceptibility

Gene	Variant	Environmental Exposure	Outcome and Nature of Interaction	Reference
Breast Cancer				
GSTM1	null	Alcohol	Alcohol-consuming premenopausal women lacking GSTT1 gene at increased risk.	(Park et al. 2000)
COMT	Met158Val	Estrogen	Carriers of variant genotypes show increased risk with greater duration from menarche to first full-term pregnancy.	(Lin et al. 2005)
CYP17	−34T->C	Estrogen	Postmenopausal women with WT genotype at increased risk if they had ever used hormone replacement therapy.	(Chang et al. 2005)
MTHFR	677TT	Folate	Lower intake of dietary folate increased risk associated with 677TT genotype.	(Suzuki et al. 2008)
MPO	G463A	Fruit and vegetable intake	Women who consumed higher amounts of total fruits and vegetables experienced greater protective effect of polymorphism. No effect among the low-consumption group.	(He et al. 2009)
XRCC1	Arg194Trp	Plasma carotenoids (vegetable intake)	Increased plasma carotenoid levels modify the effect of the Arg194Trp variant.	(Han et al. 2003)
CYP1A1	m1	Polypolychlorinated biphenyls	Risks associated with the variant genotype were highest for women with higher serum PCB levels.	(Zhang et al. 2004)
CYP1A1	MspI, exon 7	Smoking	Women smokers with variant genotypes (either) are at higher risk than wild type (WT) non-smokers.	(Ishibe et al. 1998)
GSTT1	null	Smoking	Postmenopausal smokers with GSTT1-null genotype at increased risk, especially if commenced smoking before age 18.	(Zheng et al. 2002)
XRCC1	Arg399Gln	Smoking	Risk of cancer was greater for non-smokers than smokers; for smokers, risk with genotype increases with pack-years.	(Pachkowski et al. 2006; Zhou et al. 2003)

Table 3.2 (continued)

Gene	Variant	Environmental Exposure	Outcome and Nature of Interaction	Reference
Colorectal Cancer				
MTHFR	677CC	Alcohol	Alcohol consumption associated with significantly reduced risk for carriers of 677CC genotype.	(Matsuo et al. 2005)
MTHFR	Ala222Val	Folic acid intake	Homozygotes for the low activity Ala222Val variant are at different risk of colorectal cancer and adenomas if nutritional folate status is low.	(Chen et al. 1999)
NAT2	Rapid versus slow acetylator	Heterocyclic amines in cooked meat	Red meat intake is more strongly associated with colorectal cancer among rapid acetylators.	(Chen et al. 1998)
P53	Arg72Pro	NSAIDs	A protective effect of non-steroidal anti-inflammatory drug use was observed for homozygous carriers of the 72Arg allele.	(Tan et al. 2007)
CYP1B1	1294G	Smoking	Smokers with CYP1B1 1294G polymorphism at increased risk.	(Fan et al. 2007)
GSTT1	null	Smoking	Smokers with the GSTT1-null genotype at increased risk.	(Laso et al. 2002)
Gastric Cancer				
GSTT1, SULT1A1, NAT2	various	Smoking	GSTT1, SULT1A1 and NAT2 polymorphisms modulate susceptibility to gastric cancer with smoking.	(Boccia et al. 2007)

Table 3.2 (continued)

Gene	Variant	Environmental Exposure	Outcome and Nature of Interaction	Reference
Lung Cancer				
XRCC1	Arg194Trp	Antioxidant intake	Arg194Trp variant modifies the association between serum antioxidants and lung cancer risk.	(Ratnasinghe et al. 2003)
GSTM1	null	Environmental Tobacco Smoke	Individuals with GSTM1 null genotype and high-dose ETS exposure ($>/= 40$ pack-years by husbands) at significantly higher risk than GSTM1 non-null genotype and low-dose ETS exposure.	(Kiyohara et al. 2003)
XPA	G23A	Fruit intake	Fruit intake was associated with lower risk only among carriers of the variant genotype.	(Raaschou-Nielsen et al. 2008)
GSTM1	null	Fruit and vegetable intake	Fruit and vegetable intake reduced the risk of lung cancer only among carriers of at least one functional GSTM1 allele.	(Sorensen et al. 2007)
XPD	Arg156Arg	Never smoking	Variant A-allele associated with increased risk for lung cancer among never-smokers only.	(Yin et al. 2005)
CYP1A1	MspI	Non-smoking, light smoking	The association of the risk allele with lung cancer is only observed among non-smokers, not smokers.	(Clavel 2007; Ishibe et al. 1997)
APE1	148Glu	Light smoking	Risk associated with Glu/Glu genotype greater with light smoking.	(Ito et al. 2004)
MPO	G-463A	Smoking	Protective effect for the G/A and A/A genotypes in "ever smokers" only.	(Kiyohara et al. 2005)

Table 3.2 (continued)

Gene	Variant	Environmental Exposure	Outcome and Nature of Interaction	Reference
NAT2	rapid acetylator	Smoking	Risk with rapid acetylator genotype increased significantly as pack-years increased.	(Zhou et al. 2002)
NQO1	Pro187Ser	Smoking	The Pro187Ser variant genotypes were associated with slightly increased lung cancer risk in white "ever smokers" but not in white "never smokers."	(Chao et al. 2006)
mEH	His113Tyr	Smoking	Low activity mEH variant associated with increased risk in non-smokers and decreased risk in heavy smokers.	(Zhou et al. 2001)
Prostate Cancer				
GSTP1	Val(105)	Polycyclic aromatic hydrocarbons	Men who carry the GSTP1 Val(105) variant and are exposed at high levels to occupational PAH are at increased risk.	(Rybicki et al. 2006)
CYP1A1, mEH		Smoking	Smokers carrying susceptible genotypes are subject to higher risk than those carrying non-susceptible genotypes.	(Mittal and Srivastava 2007)

The current range of environmental exposures investigated in cancer GEI research is, of course, the by-product of a prior emphasis on candidate genes prioritized precisely because they were believed to be relevant to biochemical pathways involved in the metabolism or detoxification of recognized carcinogens. With the recent successful association by GWAS of new chromosomal regions with cancer risk, involving either unsuspected biological pathways or yet to be identified genes, there will be good methodological, as well as social justice, reasons to broaden consideration to a wider range of exposures. This will require concerted attention to the development of cheaper and more reliable methods of measuring environmental effects, and explicit commitment to considering such data alongside increasingly comprehensive sets of genetic information. The new Genes, Environment, and Health Initiative, jointly sponsored by the NIH National Institute of Environmental Health Sciences and National Human Genome Research Institute, has invested significant resources in the development of new monitoring technologies, aimed at better measuring diet, physical activity, psychosocial stress, biomarkers of environmental stress, and other environmental risk factors. This initiative and related efforts promise to enhance GEI research capacity and contribute to a wider appreciation of the interacting effects of genes and environments in cancer etiology. Within this initiative, however, there are no explicit efforts to prioritize developing sound methodological approaches for measuring known social and environmental factors that differentially affect poor and minority communities, and thus have greater potential to inform GEI research aimed at elucidating the etiology of cancer disparities.

Contribution of GEI Research to Reducing Cancer Disparities

Gene–environment interaction research not only promises to elucidate cancer etiology in important new ways, but may be especially valuable in identifying underlying contributions to persistent cancer disparities. GEI research can help us understand and disentangle causal pathways that explain ethnic and racial differences in cancer prevalence by identifying how genetic susceptibility and environmental exposures interact to promote disease. It can also provide a more complex and nuanced framework within which to consider the role of differential population exposures to either class of interacting risk factor (Fig. 3.4). Racial disparities in a highly prevalent cancer, for example, may be traceable to differential exposure to environmental factors that increase risk of developing the disease, but only in the presence of a specific genetic variant susceptibility. If the relevant susceptibility variant is common to most populations (i.e., population heterogeneity in genetic susceptibility is low), and interactions with differentially distributed environmental risk factors ignored, the underlying cause of differential disease burden could be overlooked and opportunities for effective

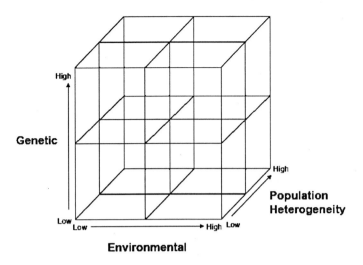

Fig. 3.4 Multidimensional matrix of cancer susceptibility. Cancer risk is determined by the joint impact of genetic susceptibility, environmental exposure, and the extent to which each risk factor is differentially distributed with regard to population background

intervention missed. On the other hand, there may be certain susceptibility variants that are disproportionately prevalent among persons of African or European descent that independently or in relationship to common environmental exposures affect disease etiology. In these cases, ensuring that individuals with a high risk genetic profile are able to take full advantage of all known prevention strategies would be particularly important.

Gene–environment interaction research may also help advance efforts to reduce cancer disparities by helping to identify how genes, social environment, and physical environment combine in complex ways to affect cancer severity and/or response to treatment. It may be, for example, that certain environmental exposures (e.g., air pollutants above a certain threshold) or social exposures (e.g., psychosocial stress) interact with genetic susceptibility to undermine the efficacy of chemotherapeutic regimens or other medications used prophylactically to prevent cancer recurrence. Poor and minority patients may be disproportionately exposed to these particular environmental exposures, and thus at greater risk for non-response to standard pharmacotherapy regimens and subsequent adverse health outcomes. Understanding these mechanisms of disease severity and treatment response will be critical to developing new, more effective treatment strategies for those affected.

To realize the potential for GEI research to address cancer disparities in these ways, information on the differential distribution of key environmental risk factors will need to be considered alongside evidence of population heterogeneity in genetic susceptibility and known or suspected forms of GEI. There is already good evidence to suggest that many well-recognized environmental cancer risk factors disproportionately affect racial/ethnic minority populations, including smoking (Barbeau et al. 2004; Moolchan et al. 2007), low consumption of fruits and vegetables (Blanck et al. 2008; Subar et al. 1995), and alcohol use (Russo et al. 2004). Relatively little attention has been directed to considering the ways in which such differences in environmental exposure might intersect with heterogeneity in genetic risk susceptibility to promote disparate cancer outcomes. Here we consider a continuum of examples (Fig. 3.5) that illustrate how attention to GEIs in the context of population differences in the distribution of genetic and/ or environmental factors may provide new avenues for research and new opportunities for intervention.

Prostate Cancer. At the far end of the continuum are cancer disparities for which there are currently inconsistent data about the role of environmental risk factors and, accordingly, little overt evidence of heterogeneity of risk exposure, yet good evidence for differentially distributed genetic susceptibility. Such cancers would be expected to fall in the rear upper-left corner of the matrix of GEI cancer susceptibility (Fig. 3.5), reflecting a high role for genetic susceptibility, the low impact of environmental exposure, and evidence that genetic susceptibility is differentially distributed with regard to population background. The best-recognized example in this category is prostate cancer, which is nearly two times as common among African American men than any other US ethnic group (Reddy et al. 2003). Chapter 8 of this book offers a detailed review of prostate cancer and disparities. Despite very high incidence and mortality rates, and sustained epidemiological attention, the only established risk factors for this cancer are age, area of residence, ethnic background, and family history (Mucci et al. 2008). As discussed above, however, recent investigation has identified a clear association between variations in the 8q24 region and prostate cancer risk, and several of the most important susceptibility variants occur at unusually high frequency in populations of African ancestry (Table 3.1, Fig. 3.1), providing a partial explanation for observed differences in cancer incidence. No studies have thus far attempted to investigate the interaction of 8q24 prostate cancer susceptibility variation with known or suspected environmental determinants. Using risk information from that gene region to stratify study cohorts could help identify environmental risk factors that have thus far eluded detection by other methods.

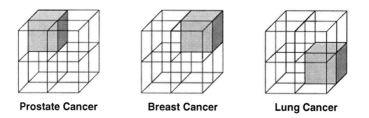

Prostate Cancer   **Breast Cancer**   **Lung Cancer**

Fig. 3.5 Example cancer disparities in relation to the cancer susceptibility matrix. Axes are as identified in Fig. 3.4

Breast Cancer. In an intermediate position in the continuum are cancer disparities where there is good evidence for both genetic and environmental contributions to disease risk that are each, in turn, differentially distributed with respect to population background. Such cancers would be expected to fall in the rear upper-right corner of the matrix of GEI cancer susceptibility (Fig. 3.5), reflecting a high role for genetic susceptibility, the high impact of environmental exposures, and high population heterogeneity associated with each class of risk factor. One well-studied example in this category is breast cancer, a cancer whose incidence and mortality varies considerably among racial/ethnic groups. Chapter 6 of this book reviews breast cancer disparities, particularly as they relate to socioeconomic status. Specifically, African American, Hispanic, Asian, and Native American women have lower incidence but higher mortality compared to non-Hispanic white women (Newman and Martin 2007). Unlike prostate cancer, a large number of reproductive and environmental risk factors have been shown to play a role in breast cancer risk, including postmenopausal hormone use, moderate alcohol intake, adult weight gain, and insufficient intake of fruits and vegetables (Hankinson et al. 2008). There is strong evidence that several of these risk factors are differentially distributed with respect to ethnic background (Blanck et al. 2008; Russo et al. 2004; Subar et al. 1995). There is also a long and growing list of common susceptibility variants that have been robustly linked to disease risk, a proportion of which show marked allele frequency differences among groups (Table 3.1). Indeed one of the breast cancer susceptibility variants identified in Table 3.1, the WDR79 Arg68Gly variant, is subject to the most pronounced allele frequency differences observed in that collection of variants.

No investigation has reported the interaction of the WDR79 variant with an environmental risk factor, but a number of studies have examined GEIs in the context of breast cancer risk (Table 3.2). One study with relevance to breast cancer disparities reported a positive interaction between the CYP1A1 m2 susceptibility variant (A2455G in Table 3.1) and exposure to polychlorinated biphenyls (PCBs), a known endocrine disruptor (Zhang et al. 2004). Specifically, for women with the m2 variant, the risk for breast cancer doubled (OR = 2.1), while with exposure to PCBs this risk tripled (OR = 3.6) in premenopausal and quadrupled (OR = 4.1) in postmenopausal women with the variant. These findings are consistent with the key role that cytochrome P-450 phase I metabolizing enzymes play in converting inactive chemicals into more active (i.e., carcinogenic) forms (Mucci et al. 2001). Furthermore, most CYP variant alleles, including the CYP1A1 and CYP1B1 variants associated with breast cancer risk in Table 3.1, show marked allele frequency differences among groups, suggesting that complex interactions between risk alleles and environmental exposures could contribute to breast cancer disparities. These findings point to another dimension affecting the complex matrix of cancer risk that is not reflected in our schematic—that of time. Environmental exposures are typically measured at a specific point in time, when what we would want ideally is an individual's lifetime exposure to a particular environmental assault. The life course of the human body thus provides a further dimension important to consider in GEI studies.

Lung Cancer. At the other end of the continuum are cancer disparities for which there are currently good data about the role of differentially distributed environmental risk factors, but relatively less information about the role of genetic contributions to disease risk. Such cancers would be expected to fall in the rear lower-right corner of the matrix of GEI cancer susceptibility (Fig. 3.5), reflecting a small role for genetic susceptibility, the high impact of environmental exposure, and evidence that environmental exposure is differentially distributed with regard to population background. An example in this category is lung cancer, which is common across all ethnic groups but disproportionately affects African Americans (Berger et al. 2007). The main environmental risk factor for lung cancer is cigarette smoking and other forms of tobacco exposure, including second hand smoke. Chapter 5 of this book closely examines disparities in tobacco use and lung cancer. A wide array of occupational agents, including asbestos, beryllium, and silica, have also been consistently associated with lung cancer risk (Boffetta and Trichopoulos 2008). These and related exposures are clearly differentially distributed with regard to racial/ethnic identity and socioeconomic background and these differences are likely a major contributory factor to lung cancer disparities (Barbeau et al. 2004; Moolchan et al. 2007).

Furthermore, while genes appear to play only a relatively minor role as independent risk factors, there is evidence for GEIs mediating the relationship between smoking and lung cancer risk (Table 3.2). One relevant example is the case of variation in the MPO (myeloperoxidase) gene, which codes for a phase I metabolizing enzyme similar to the cytochrome P-450s. A common G to A transition at position 463 reduces MPO expression with a consequent decreased risk of lung cancer associated, in a dose dependent manner, with the presence of the A allele (Kiyohara et al. 2005). Several studies have reported evidence of an interaction between MPO genotype, smoking, and lung cancer risk, with a protective effect for the G/A and A/A genotypes observed in "ever smokers" (OR = 0.63), but no effect among persons who have never smoked (OR = 1.14). Interestingly, the protective effect for the A/A genotype was also found only in groups with lower tobacco consumption (OR = 0.43), whereas heavy smoking abolished the MPO-related effect (OR = 1.03) (Kiyohara et al. 2005). Unlike other phase I metabolizing enzyme variation, however, allele frequencies at the MPO locus vary comparatively little among populations of European, West African, or Asian ancestry (Table 3.1), making the exact role of the interaction with respect to cancer disparities currently uncertain.

As these three brief examples illustrate, there is much scope for the active application of GEI research to the problem of cancer disparities. By directly measuring causal environmental variables that often track with self-identified race or SEP in our society, GEI research could help to disentangle the complex array of factors that interact to produce disease. Ultimately, the relative contribution of genetic factors to health disparities will only be answered by research designs that explicitly address the multiple factors that produce human illness and focus in particular on measuring environmental exposures that track with racial identity and SEP.

Leveraging GEI Research to Address Health Disparities

Emerging GEI research focused on a high-impact condition like cancer and motivated by a commitment to reduce cancer disparities creates a powerful nexus of opportunity for advancing efforts to reduce health disparities. Leveraging this potential, however, will require (1) identifying and addressing barriers to transdisciplinary GEI research on the role of genetic, social, environmental, and behavioral factors in producing cancer and (2) including measures most relevant to the lived experience of disadvantaged communities in such studies. The recent IOM study on Genes, Behavior, and the Social Environment (2006) made several recommendations to improve GEI research, as summarized in Table 3.3. Although implementation of these guidelines would surely advance the field of GEI research, the guidelines lack explicit focus on the development of measures, as well as methodological approaches to facilitate the inclusion of measures, that most significantly affect the lives of poor and minority communities. Below, we highlight several actions that we believe can increase the potential for future GEI studies to produce new insight into the etiology of racial/ethnic and socioeconomic disparities in cancer risk and outcomes and provide new traction in national efforts to reduce cancer disparities.

(1) **Expand capacity to incorporate a broader range of social and environmental measures in GEI studies, giving priority to measures of the social and physical environment known to affect racial/ethnic minority communities and persons of low SEP disproportionately.** Few diseases or conditions are caused purely or primarily by genetic factors. A large body of evidence indicates that nearly half of all causes of mortality in the US are linked to social and behavioral factors such as smoking, diet, alcohol use, sedentary lifestyle, and accidents (Haga et al. 2003), yet genetics research has only begun to address the multifactorial and common diseases that account for the majority of public health burden (Institute of Medicine 2003a). The limited number and scope of social and environmental measures included in GEI studies thus far points to the great difficulty in measuring these complex phenomena. As new capacity for measurement is developed, those measures of environmental exposures that are disproportionately visited upon racial/ethnic minority communities and those of lower SEP should be given priority.

(2) **Support the development of research infrastructure to support robust GEI research aimed at generating new insight into the etiology of cancer disparities.** Related to the inclusion of social and environmental measures in GEI studies that are especially pertinent to understanding cancer disparities is the need to develop national research infrastructure to support the

Table 3.3 Recommendations from "Genes, Behavior, and the Social Environment: Moving Beyond the Nature/Nurture Debate"

1: Conduct Transdisciplinary, Collaborative Research

The NIH should develop Requests for Applications (RFAs) to study the impact on health of interactions among social, behavioral, and genetic factors and their interactive pathways (i.e., physiological). Such transdisciplinary research should involve the genuine collaboration of social, behavioral, and genetic scientists. Genuine collaboration is essential for the identification, incorporation, analysis, and interpretation of the multiple variables used. (Chapter 6)

2: Measure Key Variables Over the Life Course and Within the Context of Culture

The NIH should develop RFAs for studies of interactions that incorporate measurement, over the life course and within the context of culture, of key variables in the important domains of social, behavioral, and genetic factors. (Chapter 6)

3: Develop and Implement New Modeling Strategies to Build More Comprehensive, Predictive Models of Etiologically Heterogeneous Disease

The NIH should emphasize research aimed at developing and implementing such models (e.g., pattern recognition, multivariate statistics, and systems-oriented approaches) for incorporating social, behavioral, and genetic factors and their interactive pathways (i.e., physiological) in testable models within populations, clinical settings, or animal studies. (Chapter 6)

4: Investigate Biological Signatures

Researchers should use genomic, transcriptomic, proteomic, metabonomic, and other high-dimensional molecular approaches to discover new constellations of genetic factors, biomarkers, and mediating systems through which interactions with social environment and behavior influence health. (Chapter 6)

5: Conduct Research in Diverse Groups and Settings

The NIH should encourage research on the impact of interactions among social, behavioral, and genetic factors and their interactive pathways (i.e., physiological) on health that emphasizes diversity in groups and settings. Furthermore, NIH should support efforts to ensure that the findings of such research are validated by replication in independent studies, translated to patient-oriented research, conducted and applied in the context of public health, and used to design preventive and therapeutic approaches. (Chapter 6)

6: Use Animal Models to Study Gene–Social Environment Interaction

The NIH should develop RFAs that use carefully selected animal models for research on the impact on health of interactions among social, behavioral, and genetic factors and their interactive pathways (i.e., physiological). (Chapter 7)

7: Advance the Science of the Study of Interactions

Researchers should base testing for interaction on a conceptual framework rather than simply the testing of a statistical model, and they must specify the scale (e.g., additive or multiplicative) used to evaluate whether or not interactions are present. If a multiplicative scale is used, consistency with an additive relation between the effects of different factors also should be evaluated. The NIH should develop RFAs for research on developing study designs that are efficient at testing interactions, including variations in interactions over time and development. (Chapter 8)

8: Expand and Enhance Training for Transdisciplinary Researchers

The NIH should use existing and modified training tools both to reach the next generation of researchers and to enhance the training of current researchers. Approaches include individual fellowships (F31, F32) and senior fellowships (F33), transdisciplinary institutional grants (T32, T90), and short courses. (Chapter 9)

Table 3.3 (continued)

9: Enhance Existing and Develop New Datasets
The NIH should support datasets that can be used by investigators to address complex levels of social, behavioral, and genetic variables and their interactive pathways (i.e., physiological). This should include the enhancement of existing datasets that already provide many, but not all, of the needed measures (e.g., the National Longitudinal Survey of Youth, ADDHealth) and the encouragement of their use. Furthermore, NIH should develop new datasets that address specific topics that have high potential for showing genetic contribution, social variability, and behavioral contributions—topics such as obesity, diabetes, and smoking. (Chapter 9)

10: Create Incentives to Foster Transdisciplinary Research
The NIH and universities should explore ways to create incentives for the kinds of team science needed to support transdisciplinary research. Areas to address include (1) hiring, promotion, and tenure policies that acknowledge the contributions of collaborators on transdisciplinary teams; (2) peer review that includes reviewers who have experience with inter- or transdisciplinary research and are educated about the complexity and challenges involved in such research; (3) mechanisms for peer review of research grants that ensure the appropriate evaluation of transdisciplinary research projects; and (4) credit for collaborators in teams, such as NIH acknowledgement of co-investigators and university sharing of incentive funds. (Chapter 9)

11: Communicate with Policymakers and the Public
Researchers should (1) be mindful of public and policy-makers' concerns, (2) develop mechanisms to involve and inform these constituencies, (3) avoid overstating their scientific findings, and (4) give careful consideration to the appropriate level of community involvement and the level of community oversight needed for such studies. (Chapter 10)

12: Expand the Research Focus
The NIH should develop RFAs for research that elucidate how best to encourage people to engage in health-promoting behaviors that are informed by a greater understanding of these interactions, how best to effectively communicate research results to the public and other stakeholders, and how best to inform research participants about the nature of the investigation (gene–environment interactions) and the uses of data following the study. (Chapter 10)

13: Establish Data-Sharing Policies That Ensure Privacy
IRBs and investigators should establish policies regarding the collection, sharing, and use of data that include information about (1) whether and to what extent data will be shared; (2) the level of security to be provided by all members of the research team as well as the research and administrative process; (3) the use of state-of-the-art security for collected data, including, but not limited to, NIH's Certificates of Confidentiality; (4) the use of formal criteria for identifying the circumstances under which individual research results will be revealed; and (5) how, before sharing data with others, recipients must agree to use data only in ways that are consistent with those agreed to by the research participants. Furthermore, if a mechanism to identify individual research participants is retained in the database, IRBs and investigators should consider whether to contact participants prior to initiating research on new hypotheses or other new research. (Chapter 10)

14: Improve the Informed Consent Process
Researchers should ensure that informed consent includes the following: (1) descriptions of the individual and social risks and benefits of the research; (2) the identification of which individual results participants will and will not receive; (3) the definition of the procedural protections that will be provided, including access policies and scientific and lay oversight; and (4) specific security, privacy, and confidentiality protections for the data and samples of research participants. (Chapter 10)

National Academy of Sciences. 2006. This executive summary, plus thousands more, available at http://www.nap.edu. Genes, Behavior, and the Social Environment, http://books.nap.edu/catalog/11693.html

development, dissemination, and use of such measures. The national dbGaP database currently makes data from NIH-funded GWAS studies and other large cohort studies publicly available to accelerate scientific discovery. A complementary national resource could be developed and supported to facilitate the inclusion of measures especially important to investigating health disparities, including data used to validate individual measures, technical specifications of measures, and links to national databases that currently exist but are not maximally utilized in research. The EPA and NIEHS, for example, both maintain national data bases on environmental exposures that are not well utilized by researchers, largely due a lack of familiarity with these data assets. These data may be useful for assessing differential concentrations of ambient air pollutants, for example, over large geographical areas. Because collecting more localized measures of ambient air pollution is expensive, financial support for such labor intensive data collection is essential when such measurement is critical to the science. If we expect genomics researchers to include additional measures important to understanding health disparities in their studies, then we also need to make available to them the data assets, analytic resources, and financial resources required to integrate such measures into their studies.

(3) **Discourage the use of self-identified race/ethnicity as a proxy for human genetic heterogeneity in GEI studies.** Although self-identified race can often serve as a fairly accurate proxy for human genetic variation, such use of self-identified variables should be discouraged in GEI studies and genetic studies more generally. Rather, incentives should be provided for researchers to include state-of-the-art measures of human genetic diversity and to measure other dimensions of human experience that often track with race/ethnicity directly, including social class, cultural practices, experiences of racism, quality of housing stock, quality of diet, and stress (Lee et al., 2008; Shields et al. 2005).

(4) **Build capacity for transdisciplinary research within the cancer research community.** Identifying the most robust measures of social, environmental, and behavioral factors affecting cancer risk will require the talents, methodological expertise, and insights of multiple disciplines. Leading researchers in epidemiology, environmental health sciences, public health, psychology, anthropology, demography, sociology, health disparities research, and other disciplines will need to partner with leading genomics and clinical researchers to design studies able to capture as much complexity as possible in examining the complex role of genetic, social, environmental, and behavioral factors in shaping cancer disparities. The National Cancer Institute has been one of the leaders in spurring transdisciplinary scientific research efforts, with highly visible successes, such as the Transdisciplinary Tobacco Research Centers. Transdisciplinary research involves broadly constituted teams of researchers that work across disciplines in the development of "the research questions to be addressed" (Institute of Medicine 2003b). While "interdisciplinary" research focuses on answering a question of mutual concern to those from various disciplines and "multidisciplinary" research

involves research on questions of both mutual and separate interest to participating investigators, "transdisciplinary" research implies the conception of research questions that transcend individual departments or specialized knowledge bases because solutions to these problems are, by definition, beyond the purview of individual disciplines (Institute of Medicine 2003b).

It has become clear that fulfillment of the potential for genomics research to improve public health will require integrating knowledge across multiple disciplines and levels of analysis in just this way (Khoury et al. 2004). Research emerging from the NIH-funded Transdisciplinary Tobacco Use Research Centers (TTURCs) highlights the new ideas, integrative models, institutional changes, and innovative policies that can emerge out of transdisciplinary research (Stokols et al. 2003; Stokols et al. 2005). With respect to developing a transdisciplinary model to guide GEI research aimed at generating new levers to address health disparities, the important contributions of genetic, social, environmental, and behavioral factors in producing disease will need to be integrated. Transdisciplinary research teams are needed to design studies that are both feasible and robust with respect to social and environmental factors that disproportionately affect the health of poor and minority communities. This will involve resolving disciplinary tensions regarding thresholds of evidence and standards for determining significance in the conduct of scientific studies.

These efforts could be greatly enhanced if NIH and other funding entities could support the development of a broad array of transdisciplinary research centers focused explicitly on cancer disparities. As with the TTURC experiment, only research teams representing the broad array of disciplines needed to design and execute sophisticated GEI studies aimed at understanding cancer risk, severity, and outcomes among low SEP and minority populations would be eligible for funding.

Summary

Disparities-focused GEI research holds unique potential to help us move beyond measuring cancer disparities to identifying new leverage points with which we can reduce such disparities. Exciting developments in genomics research promise new insight into the complex interplay of genetic and environmental factors in producing human disease and the differential patterning of disease across racial and/or ethnic groups, pointing to new and more effective interventions. Developing the tools, methods, data, and research infrastructure to study GEIs is at the cutting edge of genome science. The scientific challenges associated with understanding these complex relationships have captured the imaginations of scientists across diverse fields and spurred new public initiatives. GEI research seeks to disentangle the complex relationships between genes, social environment, and physical environment in order to understand not only which genes are associated with disease, but also the function of specific genes in the context of gene–gene interactions and GEIs that work together to produce human disease. GEI research is thus critical to understanding the role of genetics in all complex diseases, which by their nature are always determined by this complex interplay of genetic, social, and environmental factors. Because GEI is focused on this disentangling of the complex array of factors that interact to produce disease, it also holds great potential to help us dig below poorly specified racial descriptors to better understand the complex interplay of human genetic variation, environmental exposures, social environment, and behavior that leads to cancer disparities, and health disparities more broadly— providing new insight into health disparities and new leverage points to tackle disparities. GEI research thus holds the key both to translating the promise of genome research into improved public health and to applying genome research to national efforts to reduce health disparities. Given that nearly all diseases that affect large segments of the population, cancer included, are complex diseases, GEI research is also key to delivering on the promise of genome research to improve public health, including the goal of reducing the population burden of cancer.

We have a unique opportunity at this point in time to engage the GEI research community in the enormous and daunting task of reducing health disparities. By partnering with GEI researchers working in the area of cancer genetics, those committed to reducing cancer disparities could increase the potential for GEI research to provide new insight into the etiology of health disparities by generating and disseminating new transdisciplinary conceptual models, measures, and analytic support to accelerate disparities-focused transdisciplinary GEI research. Disparities-focused transdisciplinary research teams could greatly serve the public by accelerating the translation of cutting edge genome science into greater understanding of the complex factors that contribute to unacceptable disparities in disease prevalence, severity, and outcomes among minority and low-income persons.

Acknowledgments The authors would like to thank Sharon Kardia, Nick Patterson, and David Christiani for critical comments on earlier drafts of this manuscript. Richard Kwong, Rosemarie Ramos, and Sara Weiner provided excellent research assistance. This chapter was supported by NIH grant NHGRI P20 HG003400 (AS) and the Disparities Program of the Dana-Farber/ Harvard Cancer Center. SMF is supported, in part, by a grant to the Center for Genomics and Healthcare Equality (P50HG003374, National Human Genome Research Institute, Wylie Burke, PI).

References

Adami HO, Hunter D, Trichopoulos D. Textbook of Cancer Epidemiology, 2nd Ed. Oxford: Oxford University Press, 2008.

Ambrosone CB. The promise and limitations of genome-wide association studies to elucidate the causes of breast cancer. Breast Cancer Res. 2007;9(6):114.

Antoniou A, Pharoah PD, Narod S, Risch HA, Eyfjord JE, Hopper JL, Loman N, Olsson H, Johannsson O, Borg A et al. Average risks of breast and ovarian cancer associated with

BRCA1 or BRCA2 mutations detected in case series unselected for family history: a combined analysis of 22 studies. Am J Hum Genet. 2003;72(5):1117–1130.

Bach PB, Schrag D, Brawley OW, Galaznik A, Yakren S, Begg CB. Survival of blacks and whites after a cancer diagnosis. JAMA. 2002;287(16):2106–2113.

Barbeau EM, Leavy-Sperounis A, Balbach ED. Smoking, social class, and gender: what can public health learn from the tobacco industry about disparities in smoking? Tob Control. 2004;13(2):115–120.

Barreiro LB, Laval G, Quach H, Patin E, Quintana-Murci L. Natural selection has driven population differentiation in modern humans. Nat Genet. 2008;40(3):340–345.

Berger M, Lund MJ, Brawley OW. Racial disparities in lung cancer. Curr Probl Cancer. 2007;31(3):202–210.

Blanck HM, Gillespie C, Kimmons JE, Seymour JD, Serdula MK. Trends in fruit and vegetable consumption among U.S. men and women, 1994–2005. Prev Chronic Dis. 2008;5(2):A35.

Boccia S, Sayed-Tabatabaei FA, Persiani R, Gianfagna F, Rausei S, Arzani D, La Greca A, D'Ugo D, La Torre G, van Duijn CM et al. Polymorphisms in metabolic genes, their combination and interaction with tobacco smoke and alcohol consumption and risk of gastric cancer: a case-control study in an Italian population. BMC Cancer. 2007;7:206.

Boffetta P, Trichopoulos D. Cancer of the Lung, Larynx, and Pleura. In: Adami H-O, Hunter D, Trichopoulos D, eds. Textbook of Cancer Epidemiology, 2nd Ed. Oxford: Oxford University Press, 2008, pp. 349–377.

Bradley PK. Racial and ethnic disparities in cancer care and survivorship. Cancer Nurs. 2006;29(2 Suppl):22–23.

Chang JH, Gertig DM, Chen X, Dite GS, Jenkins MA, Milne RL, Southey MC, McCredie MR, Giles GG, Chenevix-Trench G et al. CYP17 genetic polymorphism, breast cancer, and breast cancer risk factors: Aust Breast Cancer Family Study. Breast Cancer Res. 2005;7(4):R513–521.

Chao C, Zhang ZF, Berthiller J, Boffetta P, Hashibe M. NAD(P)H:quinone oxidoreductase 1 (NQO1) Pro187Ser polymorphism and the risk of lung, bladder, and colorectal cancers: a meta-analysis. Cancer Epidemiol Biomarkers Prev. 2006;15(5):979–987.

Chen J, Giovannucci EL, Hunter DJ. MTHFR polymorphism, methyl-replete diets and the risk of colorectal carcinoma and adenoma among U.S. men and women: an example of gene-environment interactions in colorectal tumorigenesis. J Nutr. 1999;129 (2S Suppl):560S–564S.

Chen J, Stampfer MJ, Hough HL, Garcia-Closas M, Willett WC, Hennekens CH, Kelsey KT, Hunter DJ. A prospective study of N-acetyltransferase genotype, red meat intake, and risk of colorectal cancer. Cancer Res. 1998;58(15):3307–3311.

Chu KC, Miller BA, Springfield SA. Measures of racial/ethnic health disparities in cancer mortality rates and the influence of socioeconomic status. J Natl Med Assoc. 2007;99(10):1092–1100, 1102–1104.

Clapp R. Environment and health:4. Cancer. CMAJ. 2000;163(8):1009–1012.

Clavel J. Progress in the epidemiological understanding of gene-environment interactions in major diseases: cancer. C R Biol. 2007;330(4):306–317.

Cooper RS, Kaufman JS, Ward R. Race and genomics. N Engl J Med. 2003;348(12):1166–1170.

Couch FJ. Genetic epidemiology of BRCA1. Cancer Biol Ther. 2004;3(6):509–514.

Curtis E, Quale C, Haggstrom D, Smith-Bindman R. Racial and ethnic differences in breast cancer survival: how much is explained by screening, tumor severity, biology, treatment, comorbidities, and demographics? Cancer. 2008;112(1):171–180.

Dong LM, Potter JD, White E, Ulrich CM, Cardon LR, Peters U. Genetic susceptibility to cancer: the role of polymorphisms in candidate genes. JAMA. 2008;299(20):2423–2436.

Fan C, Jin M, Chen K, Zhang Y, Zhang S, Liu B. Case-only study of interactions between metabolic enzymes and smoking in colorectal cancer. BMC Cancer. 2007;7:115.

Fearon ER. Human cancer syndromes: clues to the origin and nature of cancer. Science. 1997;278(5340):1043–1050.

Freeman HP, Chu KC. Determinants of cancer disparities: barriers to cancer screening, diagnosis, and treatment. Surg Oncol Clin N Am. 2005;14(4):655–669, v.

Garber JE, Offit K. Hereditary cancer predisposition syndromes. J Clin Oncol. 2005; 23(2):276–292.

Garrod A. The incidence of alkaptonuria: a study in chemical individuality. Lancet. 1902;2:1616–1620.

Ghoussaini M, Song H, Koessler T, Al Olama AA, Kote-Jarai Z, Driver KE, Pooley KA, Ramus SJ, Kjaer SK, Hogdall E et al. Multiple loci with different cancer specificities within the 8q24 gene desert. J Natl Cancer Inst. 2008;100(13):962–966.

Gudmundsson J, Sulem P, Rafnar T, Bergthorsson JT, Manolescu A, Gudbjartsson D, Agnarsson BA, Sigurdsson A, Benediktsdottir KR, Blondal T et al. Common sequence variants on 2p15 and Xp11.22 confer susceptibility to prostate cancer. Nat Genet. 2008;40(3):281–283.

Haga SB, Khoury MJ, Burke W. Genomic profiling to promote a healthy lifestyle: not ready for prime time. Nat Genet. 2003;34(4):347–351.

Haiman CA, Patterson N, Freedman ML, Myers SR, Pike MC, Waliszewska A, Neubauer J, Tandon A, Schirmer C, McDonald GJ et al. Multiple regions within 8q24 independently affect risk for prostate cancer. Nat Genet. 2007;39(5):638–44.

Haldane JBS. The interaction of nature and nurture. Ann Eugen. 1946;13:197–205.

Han J, Hankinson SE, De Vivo I, Spiegelman D, Tamimi RM, Mohrenweiser HW, Colditz GA, Hunter DJ. A prospective study of XRCC1 haplotypes and their interaction with plasma carotenoids on breast cancer risk. Cancer Res. 2003;63(23):8536–41.

Hankinson S, Tamimi R, Hunter D. Breast cancer. In: Textbook of Cancer Epidemiology, 2nd Ed. Adami H-O, Hunter DJ, Trichopoulos D, eds. Oxford: Oxford University Press, 2008, pp 403–445.

He C, Tamimi RM, Hankinson SE, Hunter DJ, Han J. A prospective study of genetic polymorphism in MPO, antioxidant status, and breast cancer risk. Breast Cancer Res Treat. 2009;113(3):585–594.

Hemminki K, Forsti A, Lorenzo Bermejo J. Etiologic impact of known cancer susceptibility genes. Mutat Res. 2008;658(1–2):42–54.

Hung RJ, McKay JD, Gaborieau V, Boffetta P, Hashibe M, Zaridze D, Mukeria A, Szeszenia-Dabrowska N, Lissowska J, Rudnai P et al. A susceptibility locus for lung cancer maps to nicotinic acetylcholine receptor subunit genes on 15q25. Nature. 2008;452(7187): 633–637.

Hunter DJ. Gene-environment interactions in human diseases. Nat Rev Genet. 2005; 6:287–298.

Institute of Medicine. Crossing the Quality Chasm: A New Health System for the 21st Century. Washington DC: National Academy Press, 2001.

Institute of Medicine. Unequal Treatment: Confronting Racial and Ethnic Disparities in Health Care. Smedley BD, Stith AY, Nelson AR, eds. Washington, DC: The National Academies Press, 2002.

Institute of Medicine. The Future of the Public's Health. Washington, DC: National Academy Press, 2003a.

Institute of Medicine. Who Will Keep the Public Healthy: Educating Public Helath Professionals for the 21st Century. Washington, DC: National Academy Press, 2003b.

Institute of Medicine. Genes, Behavior, and the Social Environment: Moving Beyond the Nature/Nurture Debate. Washington, DC: The National Academies Press, 2006.

International HapMap Consortium. A haplotype map of the human genome. Nature. 2005;437(7063):1299–1320.

Ioannidis JP, Ntzani EE, Trikalinos TA. 'Racial' differences in genetic effects for complex diseases. Nat Genet. 2004;36(12):1312–1318.

Ishibe N, Hankinson SE, Colditz GA, Spiegelman D, Willett WC, Speizer FE, Kelsey KT, Hunter DJ. Cigarette smoking, cytochrome P450 1A1 polymorphisms, and breast cancer risk in the Nurses' Health Study. Cancer Res. 1998;58(4):667–671.

Ishibe N, Wiencke JK, Zuo ZF, McMillan A, Spitz M, Kelsey KT. Susceptibility to lung cancer in light smokers associated with CYP1A1 polymorphisms in Mexican- and African-Americans. Cancer Epidemiol Biomarkers Prev. 1997;6(12):1075–1080.

Ito H, Matsuo K, Hamajima N, Mitsudomi T, Sugiura T, Saito T, Yasue T, Lee KM, Kang D, Yoo KY et al. Gene-environment interactions between the smoking habit and polymorphisms in the DNA repair genes, APE1 Asp148Glu and XRCC1 Arg399Gln, in Japanese lung cancer risk. Carcinogenesis. 2004;25(8):1395–1401.

Jemal A, Tiwari RC, Murray T, Ghafoor A, Samuels A, Ward E, Feuer EJ, Thun MJ. Cancer Stat. CA Cancer J Clin. 2004;54(1):8–29.

Kaiser Commission on Medicaid and the Uninsured. Access to Care for the Uninsured: An Update. The Henry J. Kaiser Family Foundation, 2003.

Khoury MJ, Little J, Burke W. Human genome epidemiology: scope and strategies. In: Khoury MJ, Little J, Burke W, eds. Human genome epidemiology: A Scientific Foundation for Using Genetic Information to Improve Health and Prevent Disease. New York: Oxford University Press, 2004.

Kiyohara C, Wakai K, Mikami H, Sido K, Ando M, Ohno Y. Risk modification by CYP1A1 and GSTM1 polymorphisms in the association of environmental tobacco smoke and lung cancer: a case-control study in Japanese nonsmoking women. Int J Cancer. 2003;107(1):139–144.

Kiyohara C, Yoshimasu K, Takayama K, Nakanishi Y. NQO1, MPO, and the risk of lung cancer: a HuGE review. Genet Med. 2005;7(7):463–478.

Krieger N. Stormy weather: race, gene expression, and the science of health disparities. Am J Public Health. 2005;95(12):2155–2160.

Krieger N, Quesenberry C, Jr., Peng T, Horn-Ross P, Stewart S, Brown S, Swallen K, Guillermo T, Suh D, Alvarez-Martinez L et al. Social class, race/ethnicity, and incidence of breast, cervix, colon, lung, and prostate cancer among Asian, Black, Hispanic, and White residents of the San Francisco Bay Area, 1988–92 (United States). Cancer Causes Control. 1999;10(6):525–37.

Laso N, Lafuente MJ, Mas S, Trias M, Ascaso C, Molina R, Ballesta A, Rodriguez F, Lafuente A. Glutathione S-transferase (GSTM1 and GSTT1)-dependent risk for colorectal cancer. Anticancer Res. 2002;22(6A):3399–3403.

Lee SS, Mountain J, Koenig B, Altman R, Brown M, Camarillo A, Cavalli-Sforza L, Cho M, Eberhardt J, Feldman M et al. The ethics of characterizing difference: guiding principles on using racial categories in human genetics. Genome Biol. 2008;9(7):404.

Lin WY, Chou YC, Wu MH, Jeng YL, Huang HB, You SL, Chu TY, Chen CJ, Sun CA. Polymorphic catechol-O-methyltransferase gene, duration of estrogen exposure, and breast cancer risk: a nested case-control study in Taiwan. Cancer Detect Prev. 2005;29(5):427–432.

Lucci-Cordisco E, Zito I, Gensini F, Genuardi M. Hereditary nonpolyposis colorectal cancer and related conditions. Am J Med Genet A. 2003;122A(4):325–334.

Lynch HT, de la Chapelle A. Genetic susceptibility to non-polyposis colorectal cancer. J Med Genet. 1999;36(11):801–818.

Manolio TA, Brooks LD, Collins FS. A HapMap harvest of insights into the genetics of common disease. J Clin Invest. 2008;118(5):1590–1605.

Matsuo K, Ito H, Wakai K, Hirose K, Saito T, Suzuki T, Kato T, Hirai T, Kanemitsu Y, Hamajima H et al. One-carbon metabolism related gene polymorphisms interact with alcohol drinking to influence the risk of colorectal cancer in Japan. Carcinogenesis. 2005;26(12):2164–2171.

Mayberry RM, Mill F, Ofilil E. Racial and ethnic differences in access to medical care. Medical Care Res Rev. 2000;57(suppl 1):108–145.

Mittal RD, Srivastava DL. Cytochrome P4501A1 and microsomal epoxide hydrolase gene polymorphisms: gene-environment interaction and risk of prostate cancer. DNA Cell Biol. 2007;26(11):791–798.

Moolchan ET, Fagan P, Fernander AF, Velicer WF, Hayward MD, King G, Clayton RR. Addressing tobacco-related health disparities. Addiction. 2007;102(Suppl 2):30–42.

Mucci LA, Signorello LB, Adami H-O. 2008. Prostate cancer. In: Adami H-O, Hunter DJ, Trichopoulos D, eds. Textbook of Cancer Epidemiology. 2nd Ed. Oxford: Oxford University Press, 2008, pp 517–554.

Mucci LA, Wedren S, Tamimi RM, Trichopoulos D, Adami HO. The role of gene-environment interaction in the aetiology of human cancer: examples from cancers of the large bowel, lung and breast. J Intern Med. 2001;249(6):477–493.

Narod SA, Foulkes WD. BRCA1 and BRCA2: 1994 and beyond. Nat Rev Cancer. 2004;4(9):665–676.

Nelson HD, Huffman LH, Fu R, Harris EL. Genetic risk assessment and BRCA mutation testing for breast and ovarian cancer susceptibility: systematic evidence review for the U.S. Preventive Services Task Force. Ann Intern Med. 2005;143(5):362–379.

Newman LA, Martin IK. Disparities in breast cancer. Curr Probl Cancer. 2007;31(3): 134–156.

Office of Budget and Management. Recommendations from the Interagency Committee for the Review of the Racial and Ethnic Standards to the Office of Management and Budget Concerning Changes to the Standards for the Classification of Federal Data on Race and Ethnicity. Washington DC, 1997.

Olden K. Opportunities in environmental health science research. Environ Health Perspect. 1993;101(1):6–7.

Olden K. Thinking big: four ways to advance environmental health research to answer the needs of public policy. Environ Health Perspect. 1997;105(5):464–5.

Olden K, Guthrie J, Newton S. A bold new direction for environmental health research. Am J Public Health. 2001;91(12):1964–1977.

Pachkowski BF, Winkel S, Kubota Y, Swenberg JA, Millikan RC, Nakamura J. 2006. XRCC1 genotype and breast cancer: functional studies and epidemiologic data show interactions between XRCC1 codon 280 His and smoking. Cancer Res. 2006;66(5): 2860–2868.

Park SK, Yoo KY, Lee SJ, Kim SU, Ahn SH, Noh DY, Choe KJ, Strickland PT, Hirvonen A, Kang D. Alcohol consumption, glutathione S-transferase M1 and T1 genetic polymorphisms and breast cancer risk. Pharmacogenetics. 2000;10(4):301–309.

Peto J. Cancer epidemiology in the last century and the next decade. Nature. 2001;411(6835):390–395.

Phillips JM, Williams-Brown S. Cancer prevention among racial ethnic minorities. Semin Oncol Nurs. 2005;21(4):278–285.

Powers M, Faden R. Social Justice: The Moral Foundations of Public Health and Health Policy, Oxford: Oxford: University Press, 2006.

Raaschou-Nielsen O, Sorensen M, Overvad K, Tjonneland A, Vogel U. Polymorphisms in nucleotide excision repair genes, smoking and intake of fruit and vegetables in relation to lung cancer. Lung Cancer. 2008;59(2):171–179.

Raghavan D. Disparities in cancer care: challenges and solutions. Oncology (Williston Park). 2007;21(4):493–496,499,503,506.

Ratnasinghe DL, Yao SX, Forman M, Qiao YL, Andersen MR, Giffen CA, Erozan Y, Tockman MS, Taylor PR. Gene-environment interactions between the codon 194 polymorphism of XRCC1 and antioxidants influence lung cancer risk. Anticancer Res. 2003;23(1B):627–632.

Reddy S, Shapiro M, Morton R, Jr., Brawley OW. Prostate cancer in black and white Americans. Cancer Metastasis Rev. 2003;22(1):83–86.

Risch N. Dissecting racial and ethnic differences. N Engl J Med. 2006;354(4):408–411.

Russo D, Purohit V, Foudin L, Salin M. Workshop on Alcohol Use and Health Disparities 2002: a call to arms. Alcohol. 2004;32(1):37–43.

Rybicki BA, Neslund-Dudas C, Nock NL, Schultz LR, Eklund L, Rosbolt J, Bock CH, Monaghan KG. Prostate cancer risk from occupational exposure to polycyclic aromatic hydrocarbons interacting with the GSTP1 Ile105Val polymorphism. Cancer Detect Prev. 2006;30(5):412–422.

Sakamoto H, Yoshimura K, Saeki N, Katai H, Shimoda T, Matsuno Y, Saito D, Sugimura H, Tanioka F, Kato S et al. Genetic variation in PSCA is associated with susceptibility to diffuse-type gastric cancer. Nat Genet. 2008;40(6):730–740.

Sankar P, Cho MK, Condit CM, Hunt LM, Koenig B, Marshall P, Lee SS, Spicer P. Genetic research and health disparities. JAMA. 2004;291(24):2985–2989.

Sarin R. A decade of discovery of BRCA1 and BRCA2: are we turning the tide against hereditary breast cancers? J Cancer Res Ther. 2006;2(4):157–158.

Schwartz D, Collins F. Medicine. Environmental biology and human disease. Science. 2007;316(5825):695–696.

Schwartz KL, Crossley-May H, Vigneau FD, Brown K, Banerjee M. Race, socioeconomic status and stage at diagnosis for five common malignancies. Cancer Causes Control. 2003;14(8):761–766.

Shields AE, Fortun M, Hammonds E, King PA, Lerman C, Rapp R, Sullivan PF. The use of race variables in genetic studies of complex traits and the goal of reducing health disparities: a transdisciplinary perspective. Am Psychol. 2005;60(1):77–103.

Shriver MD, Parra EJ, Dios S, Bonilla C, Norton H, Jovel C, Pfaff C, Jones C, Massac A, Cameron N et al. Skin pigmentation, biogeographical ancestry and admixture mapping. Hum Genet. 2003;112(4):387–399.

Sorensen M, Raaschou-Nielsen O, Brasch-Andersen C, Tjonneland A, Overvad K, Autrup H. Interactions between GSTM1, GSTT1 and GSTP1 polymorphisms and smoking and intake of fruit and vegetables in relation to lung cancer. Lung Cancer. 2007;55(2):137–144.

Stacey SN, Manolescu A, Sulem P, Thorlacius S, Gudjonsson SA, Jonsson GF, Jakobsdottir M, Bergthorsson JT, Gudmundsson J, Aben KK et al. Common variants on chromosome 5p12 confer susceptibility to estrogen receptor-positive breast cancer. Nat Genet. 2008;40(6):703–706.

Stokols D, Fuqua J, Gress J, Harvey R, Phillips K, Baezconde-Garbanati L, Unger J, Palmer P, Clark MA, Colby SM et al. Evaluating transdisciplinary science. Nicotine Tob Res. 2003;5(supp 1):S21–S39.

Stokols D, Harvey R, Gress J, Fuqua J, Phillips K. In vivo studies of transdisciplinary scientific collaboration: lessons learned and implication for active living research. Am J Prev Med. 2005;28(2S2):202–213.

Strate LL, Syngal S. Hereditary colorectal cancer syndromes. Cancer Causes Control. 2005;16(3):201–213.

Subar AF, Heimendinger J, Patterson BH, Krebs-Smith SM, Pivonka E, Kessler R. Fruit and vegetable intake in the United States: the baseline survey of the Five A Day for Better Health Program. Am J Health Promot. 1995;9(5):352–360.

Suzuki T, Matsuo K, Hirose K, Hiraki A, Kawase T, Watanabe M, Yamashita T, Iwata H, Tajima K. One-carbon metabolism-related gene polymorphisms and risk of breast cancer. Carcinogenesis. 2008;29(2):356–362.

Tan XL, Nieters A, Hoffmeister M, Beckmann L, Brenner H, Chang-Claude J. Genetic polymorphisms in TP53, nonsteroidal anti-inflammatory drugs and the risk of colorectal cancer: evidence for gene-environment interaction? Pharmacogenet Genomics. 2007;17(8):639–645.

Tenesa A, Farrington SM, Prendergast JG, Porteous ME, Walker M, Haq N, Barnetson RA, Theodoratou E, Cetnarskyj R, Cartwright N et al. Genome-wide association scan identifies a colorectal cancer susceptibility locus on 11q23 and replicates risk loci at 8q24 and 18q21. Nat Genet. 2008;40(5):631–637.

Thorgeirsson TE, Geller F, Sulem P, Rafnar T, Wiste A, Magnusson KP, Manolescu A, Thorleifsson G, Stefansson H, Ingason A et al. A variant associated with nicotine dependence, lung cancer and peripheral arterial disease. Nature. 2008;452(7187):638–642.

Tishkoff SA, Verrelli BC. Patterns of human genetic diversity: implications for human evolutionary history and disease. Annu Rev Genomics Hum Genet. 2003;4:293–340.

U.S. Department of Health and Human Services. Healthy People 2010: Understanding and Improving Health. Washington, DC: U.S. Government Printing Office, 2000.

Wright S. Isolation by distance. Genetics. 1942;28:114–138.

Yin J, Li J, Ma Y, Guo L, Wang H, Vogel U. The DNA repair gene ERCC2/XPD polymorphism Arg 156Arg (A22541C) and risk of lung cancer in a Chinese population. Cancer Lett. 2005; 223(2):219–226.

Zhang Y, Wise JP, Holford TR, Xie H, Boyle P, Zahm SH, Rusiecki J, Zou K, Zhang B, Zhu Y et al. Serum polychlorinated biphenyls, cytochrome P-450 1A1 polymorphisms, and risk of breast cancer in Connecticut women. Am J Epidemiol. 2004;160(12):1177–1183.

Zheng T, Holford TR, Zahm SH, Owens PH, Boyle P, Zhang Y, Wise JP, Sr., Stephenson LP, Ali-Osman F. Cigarette smoking, glutathione-s-transferase M1 and t1 genetic polymorphisms, and breast cancer risk (United States). Cancer Causes Control. 2002;13(7):637–645.

Zhou W, Liu G, Miller DP, Thurston SW, Xu LL, Wain JC, Lynch TJ, Su L, Christiani DC. Polymorphisms in the DNA repair genes XRCC1 and ERCC2, smoking, and lung cancer risk. Cancer Epidemiol Biomarkers Prev. 2003;12(4):359–365.

Zhou W, Liu G, Thurston SW, Xu LL, Miller DP, Wain JC, Lynch TJ, Su L, Christiani DC. Genetic polymorphisms in N-acetyltransferase-2 and microsomal epoxide hydrolase, cumulative cigarette smoking, and lung cancer. Cancer Epidemiol Biomarkers Prev. 2002;11(1):15–21.

Zhou W, Thurston SW, Liu G, Xu LL, Miller DP, Wain JC, Lynch TJ, Su L, Christiani DC. The interaction between microsomal epoxide hydrolase polymorphisms and cumulative cigarette smoking in different histological subtypes of lung cancer. Cancer Epidemiol Biomarkers Prev. 2001;10(5):461–466.

Chapter 4
Work and Occupation: Important Indicators of Socioeconomic Position and Life Experiences Influencing Cancer Disparities

Glorian Sorensen, Grace Sembajwe, Amy Harley, and Lisa Quintiliani

Introduction

A growing literature documents persistent disparities by socioeconomic position (SEP) and race/ethnicity across the cancer control continuum, with higher risk and worse outcomes observed for lower socioeconomic groups and those representing some ethnic/racial minorities (Institute of Medicine 1999, Lantz et al. 1998, Levy et al. 2006, Schwartz et al. 2003, Sorensen et al. 1995). These disparities are evident for cancer risk-related behaviors, including tobacco use, diet, and physical activity; risk factors such as overweight and obesity; cancer screening for early detection; diagnosis and treatment; and quality of life associated with survivorship and treatment at the end of life (Christian et al. 2006, Institute of Medicine 1999, 2003, Sequist and Schneider 2006); as well as for morbidity and mortality rates (Bouchardy et al. 2002, Melchior et al. 2007, Menvielle et al. 2005, Rosengren and Wilhelmsen 2004, Rosvall et al. 2006). Redressing these disparities is a central goal of public health practice (US Department of Health and Human Services 2000) and cancer research efforts (National Cancer Institute 2005).

The most commonly used measures of SEP include education, income, and occupation (Fox 1989, Lahelman 2001, Marmot and Wilkinson 1999, Siegrist and Marmot 2004). In this chapter, we focus on occupation to illustrate some of the mechanisms through which SEP may influence cancer outcomes, and highlight implications for interventions. Although occupation can only be assessed for the proportion of the population currently employed, focusing on it has several advantages. Occupation indicates both qualifications and social status

This paper draws in part from a prior paper: G. Sorensen and E. Barbeau, "Steps to a Healthier US Workforce: Integrating Occupational Health and Safety and Worksite Health Promotion: State of the Science," Commissioned paper for NIOSH *Steps to a Healthier US Workforce* Symposium, October 26–28, 2004, Washington, DC.

G. Sorensen (✉)
Harvard School of Public Health, Department of Society, Human Development and Health, Dana-Farber Cancer Institute, Center for Community-Based Research, Boston, MA, USA

H.K. Koh (ed.), *Toward the Elimination of Cancer Disparities*,
DOI 10.1007/978-0-387-89443-0_4, © Springer Science+Business Media, LLC 2009

at the time of data collection, and links well to education and income, given that increasing education generally facilitates employment in higher paying occupations. In addition to providing income and social status, moreover, occupation can contribute independently to health outcomes (Barbeau et al. 2004, Berkman and Kawachi 2000, Berkman and MacIntyre 1997, Krieger et al. 1997, Marmot and Wilkinson 1999, Menvielle et al. 2005), including serving as a means to build social networks, social support, and self-esteem (LaMontagne and Keegel 2008, Siegrist and Marmot 2004, World Health Organization 2007). At the same time, occupation can present certain health risks, whether directly through hazardous exposures and deleterious psychosocial experiences on the job, or indirectly by affecting health behaviors (Eakin 1997, Green and Johnson 1990, Johansson et al. 1991, LaMontagne and Keegel 2008, Landsbergis et al. 1998, Levy and Wegman 2000, Mullen 1992, Sorensen et al. 2002).

This chapter examines disparities in cancer outcomes by occupation as one important indicator of SEP. Specifically, we describe the occupational gradient in cancer morbidity and mortality, and in cancer risk-related behaviors. We examine the roles of the work environment in influencing cancer outcomes to understand possible mechanisms through which occupation may influence disparities in these outcomes. We also briefly describe the evidence for a comprehensive workplace intervention to reduce cancer risk, particularly for those in working-class or low-wage occupations, by targeting health behaviors, work experiences, and hazardous occupational exposures.

Occupational Disparities in Cancer Morbidity and Mortality

Disparities in cancer morbidity and mortality rates have been documented by occupational class, particularly among men (Bouchardy et al. 2002, Melchior et al. 2005, Menvielle et al. 2005, Rosengren and Wilhelmsen 2004, Rosvall et al. 2006). Studies have documented socioeconomic gradients in all-cause cancer mortality, with higher death rates among unskilled, manual laborers than in higher income office workers (Menvielle et al. 2005, Rosengren and Wilhelmsen 2004, Rosvall et al. 2006).

Similar studies, notably from working populations in the European Union, have shown elevated risks for alcohol- and tobacco-related cancers among low-income, blue-collar workers (Bouchardy et al. 2002, Melchior et al. 2005). For example, Bourchardy et al. (2002) examined Swiss cancer registries and noted that among occupation-specific cancers, incidence rates of lung cancer and mesothelioma were elevated for construction workers (stone and earth trades), machinists, and professional drivers compared to white collar workers, even after adjusting for other indicators of socioeconomic class. Melchior et al. (2005) reported a socioeconomic gradient in the incidence of smoking- and alcohol-related cancers among French men, with clerks and manual workers at highest risk. Similarly, several studies have demonstrated an occupational gradient in respiratory cancer mortality, even controlling for tobacco use, with death rates highest for those in manual occupations (Lee et al. 2006, Rosengren and Wilhelmsen 2004, Rosvall et al. 2006). This evidence is consistent with similar studies documenting disparities in cancer morbidity and mortality for other indicators of SEP (Borrell et al. 2003, Bucher and Ragland 1995, Doornbos and Kromhout 1990, Faggiano et al. 1997, Mackenbach et al. 1999, Puigpinos et al. 2000, Steenland et al. 2002).

Occupational Disparities in Cancer Risk-Related Behaviors

Consistent evidence also points to disparities by occupation in cancer risk-related behaviors, including tobacco use, diet, and physical activity. Positive changes in these behaviors can reduce a substantial proportion of the national cancer burden (Byers et al. 1999, Colditz et al. 2000, 1997). Importantly, these health risk behaviors may cluster by occupational group. In an analysis of over 11,000 adults in England, more multiple-risk behaviors (smoking, heavy drinking, lack of fruit/vegetables, lack of physical activity) were found among skilled non-manual, skilled manual, and partly and unskilled manual workers compared to professional and intermediate workers (Poortinga 2007). We discuss the individual contribution of each of these risk behaviors below.

Tobacco

Tobacco use causes cancers of the lung, oropharynx, larynx, esophagus, bladder, and kidney, and is a probable cause of leukemia as well as cancers of the colon, stomach, cervix, and liver (US Department of Health and Human Services 1989). Cessation of use reduces the excess risk of nearly all of these cancers (US Department of Health and Human Services 1990). The evidence has consistently documented a strong social gradient in tobacco use that holds for occupational class, even when education, income, sex, and age are controlled (Barbeau et al. 2004, Barbeau et al. 2004, Covey et al. 1992, Giovino et al. 2000, Nelson et al. 1994). In 2000, 35% of blue-collar workers were smokers, for example, compared to 20% of white-collar workers. Furthermore, blue-collar workers smoke more heavily and are less successful in quitting than other workers despite a similar rate of quit attempts, (Barbeau et al. 2004, Giovino et al. 2000), and rates of smoking are declining more slowly among these workers (Lee et al. 2007, Nelson et al. 1994). Please see Chapter 5 for a more detailed analysis of disparities in tobacco use.

Diet

An estimated 30% of cancer deaths can be attributed to adult diet. Diet can affect risk of cancer either directly, through intake of folate and red meat, and food preservation methods, or indirectly by contributing to overweight and obesity (American Institute for Cancer Research 2007). Convincing evidence links high folate intake with a lower risk of colon cancer (Giovannucci et al. 1998, World Cancer Research Fund 1997). High intake of red meat has been associated with increased risk of colon cancer (Gerhardsson et al. 1991, Giovannucci et al. 1994, Sandhu et al. 2001, Willett et al. 1990) and linked to prostate cancer (Michaud et al. 2001). Food preservation, processing, and preparation methods that include salted foods and aflatoxins are probable risk factors for stomach and liver cancer (American Institute for Cancer Research 2007). Others studies suggest that limiting saturated fat, increasing fruit and vegetable intake, and moderating alcoholic drinks help reduce cancer risk (Glanz and Kristal 2002).

Although there is a paucity of literature examining diet quality by occupational group, baseline data from the Working Well trial (Heimendinger et al. 1995) showed that blue-collar workers consumed less fiber, fruits, and vegetables than other workers. A sample of approximately 1000 households in Australia also reported that food-purchasing behavior differed by occupation, with blue-collar workers purchasing fewer healthful grocery store food items, including fewer fruits and vegetables, than white-collar, manager, and professional occupation groups (Turrell et al. 2002). Additional evidence suggests that diet quality varies by SEP (Beydoun and Wang 2008, Serdula et al. 2004). For example, using the Continuing Survey of Food Intakes by Individuals and Diet and Health Knowledge Survey 1994–1996, Beydoun and Wang (2008) showed significant positive associations between SEP and diet quality, with persons from high-SEP groups consuming less total fat, saturated fat, and cholesterol, and more fiber, fruits, ands vegetables than those in low-SEP groups. These relationships varied somewhat by racial/ethnic group and gender in the subgroup analyses. Similarly, others have shown that fruit and vegetable consumption increases with education and income (Serdula et al. 2004, US Department of Agriculture, US Department of Health and Human Services 2000).

Physical Activity

Regular physical activity lowers the risk of cancers of the colon, breast, and, possibly, prostate (American Institute for Cancer Research 2007, Colditz et al. 1997, Friedenreich and Rohan 1995, Marrett et al. 2000). Analyses of 1997–2004 NHIS data showed that roughly 31% of the male and 36% of the female US workers surveyed met Healthy People 2010 guidelines for leisure-time physical activity (Caban-Martinez et al. 2007). By occupational category, however, the estimated pooled annual proportion of female workers meeting guidelines ranged from 16 to 46%, with the five groups reporting the lowest proportions (16–20%) classified as blue-collar (e.g., machine operators, fabricators, assemblers, material moving equipment operators, cleaning and building service workers, and freight, stock, and material handlers). The lowest proportions of workers meeting guidelines among males (25–27%) were also from blue-collar occupations (e.g., farm workers, construction laborers, cleaning and building service workers, and forestry and fishing workers). These findings are consistent with other examinations of leisure-time physical activity levels by occupational group (Burton and Turrell 2000, Salmon et al. 2000).

One hypothesis explaining lower participation in leisure-time physical activity among blue-collar workers is that these workers participate in higher levels of physical labor associated with work ("occupational activity"). Indeed, King and colleagues (King et al. 2001) showed that individuals with high occupational activity, even with no leisure-time physical activity, were 42% less likely to be obese than their counterparts in low occupational activity professions with no leisure-time physical activity. However, the shift in percentage of the US workforce engaged in high versus low activity occupations from 1950 to 2000 due to the mechanization of many processes was dramatic, with 30% more workers in high- than in low-activity occupations in 1950 and roughly twice as many people employed in low- versus high-activity jobs in 2000 (Brownson et al. 2005). As such, it is important to examine further techniques to remedy the disparity in leisure-time physical activity between white- and blue-collar workers whose jobs may be declining in activity level.

Overweight and Obesity

One major contributor to mortality in the US is overweight/obesity (Mokdad et al. 2004). Associated with both physical inactivity and diet, obesity increases the risk of cancers of the breast, endometrium, colon and rectum, kidney, gall bladder, and possibly of the prostate and pancreas (Colditz et al. 2000). A landmark review published in 1997 by the World Cancer Research Fund and the American Institute for Cancer Research reported that healthy diets, regular physical activity, and maintaining a normal weight over time could reduce new cancer cases by approximately 30–40% globally. The number of overweight individuals is projected to increase from 1 billion in 2005 to 1.5 billion in 2015, across all income groups globally (World Health Organization 2008). In addition, both the American Cancer Society (Kushi et al. 2006) and the American Institute for Cancer Research (2007) have identified reducing overweight and obesity as a primary goal for cancer prevention.

Caban et al. (2005) examined the prevalence of obesity among 41 occupational groups, as well as in 17-year trends using 1986–2002 National Health Interview Survey (NHIS) data. During the period from 1997 to 2002, the highest pooled obesity rates among males (28–32%) were for those employed as motor vehicle and other transportation operators, police and firefighters, and material moving equipment operators. Among women, the highest rates (25–31%) were among motor vehicle operators, other protective service workers, material moving equipment workers, and cleaning and building service workers. No downward trends in obesity were seen for any occupational group for the entire study period (1987–2002). Similar associations between higher BMI and blue-collar or manual occupational groups have been reported in general (Sarlio-Lahteenkorva et al. 2004) and among women (Galobardes et al. 2000). Similarly, overweight status is inversely associated with education level (Everson et al. 2002, Galobardes et al. 2000, Mokdad et al. 2003, Sarlio-Lahteenkorva et al. 2004) and occupation (Galobardes et al. 2000, Sarlio-Lahteenkorva et al. 2004).

Contributions of the Work Environment to Cancer Disparities

We employed a social contextual framework, illustrated in Fig. 4.1 (Sorensen et al. 2003, 2004, 2007), to explore the pathways through which occupation influences cancer outcomes. This model is designed to illuminate the social context that may influence health behaviors as well as cancer morbidity and mortality. Social contextual factors may function as either modifying conditions or mediating mechanisms, depending on their location within or outside the causal pathway between the intervention and the outcomes. Modifying conditions independently influence health behaviors but are not amenable to change, while mediating mechanisms are potentially amenable to change. By allowing us to identify these factors, this model facilitates intervention design and development. Modifying conditions, as illustrated in the figure, are outside the pathway of the intervention, whereas it may be possible to design interventions to influence the mediating mechanisms.

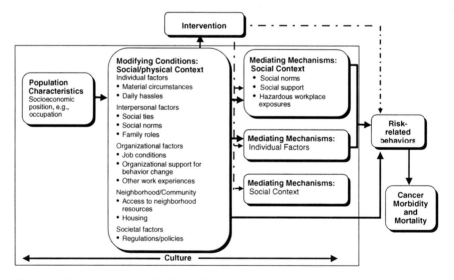

Fig. 4.1 Social contextual model for health behavior change (Sorensen et al. 2004, 2003)

In this section, we explore core components of the context of the work environment influencing cancer outcomes, including exposures to hazardous substances and the psychosocial work experiences. We examine the associations of these work conditions to cancer outcomes, occupational disparities in these conditions of work, and the ways in which these work experiences may contribute to cancer risk-related behaviors.

Hazardous Occupational Exposures

Cancer is the leading cause of workplace fatalities worldwide, accounting for 32% of them in contrast to 26% from circulatory diseases and 17% from workplace accidents (Hamalainen et al. 2007, World Health Organization 2006). The World Health Organization (WHO) and others have estimated that 8–16% of all cancers are caused by preventable occupational exposures (Gennaro and Tomatis 2005, Hamalainen et al. 2007, International Agency for Research on Cancer 1987, Landrigan and Baker 1995, World Health Organization 2006). The International Labor Organization (ILO) conservatively estimates that occupational cancers cause 600,000 deaths per year (about 10% of all cancer deaths) in industrialized countries. The WHO has reported that lung cancer, mesothelioma, and bladder cancer are among the most common types of occupational cancers and that over 90,000 deaths per year can be attributed to asbestos-related diseases alone with an additional tens of thousands of deaths due to benzene compound exposures (Johnson 2003, Levy et al. 2006).

A considerable literature spanning several centuries directly links a number of occupations with cancer. The first association between cancer and occupation was reported by Percival Pott, a London physician, who (in 1775) connected soot exposure and scrotal cancer in chimney sweeps. Later, several other compounds within manufacturing and mining occupations were identified as human carcinogens (Johnson 2003, Levy et al. 2006). The International Agency for Research on Cancer (IARC) has definitively linked a number of workplace chemicals with cancer. Asbestos exposure, for example, is responsible for the highest number of worker deaths annually, about 10,000 per year (LaDou 2004). (A detailed list of definite and probable carcinogens and related occupations and industries can be found at IARC, ILO, and WHO websites (International Agency for Research on Cancer 1987, World Health Organization 2006, 2007, World Health Organization IAfRoC 1993).) Significantly, of the more than one million pounds of chemicals produced in the US, fewer than 10% to date have complete profiles for carcinogenicity (Johnson 2003, Levy et al. 2006).

These risks are not evenly distributed across workers. Blue-collar workers, such as those in manufacturing, mining, construction, and insulation installation, are at the highest risk for exposures to carcinogens on the job (Infante 1995, Sorensen et al. 1995, World Health Organization IAfRoC 1993). Studies conducted in the European Union have estimated that blue-collar workers are eight times more likely than their white-collar counterparts to be at risk for all types of cancer due to occupational exposures (Kauppinen et al. 2001, 2000, Ministere de l'Emploi de la Cohesion Sociale et du Logement 2004).

Psychosocial Work Environment

The psychosocial work environment refers to the "socio-structural range of opportunities that is available to an individual person to meet his or her needs for well being, productivity, and positive self-experience" (Siegrist and Marmot 2004). Work may contribute to self-efficacy and self-esteem (Bandura 1986, Rolls 2000, Siegrist and Marmot 2004) and provide important opportunities for garnering social support and positive social networks (McLeroy et al, 2002), all of which contribute to health outcomes. Conversely, exposure to an adverse psychosocial environment at work similarly has important consequences for workers' health outcomes which can impact cancer (Karasek and Theorell 1990, Racial 1990, LaMontagne and Keegel 2008, Piotrkowski 1998, Siegrist and Marmot 2004, Straif et al. 2007, Toscano et al. 1998).

Two complementary models provide useful frameworks for these relationships (Siegrist and Marmot 2004). According to Karasek's and Theorell's demand/control model, "job strain" occurs when workers experience high psychological workload demands combined with low control or decision-making latitude in meeting those demands; its effects may be compounded by a lack of social support (Karasek and Theorell 1990). Strong evidence exists that job strain, independent of physical exposures, is a risk factor for increased systolic blood pressure, smoking, and musculoskeletal disease (Bongers et al. 1993, Brulin et al. 2000, Dyrehag et al. 1998, Houtman et al. 1994, Leino and Magni 1993, Lundberg 1999, Thorbjornsson et al. 1999). Conversely, job tasks that involve high psychological demands along with high decision levels may contribute to enhanced mastery and self-efficacy, thereby buffering stress and contributing to improved health (Karasek and Theorell 1990, Siegrist and Marmot 2004).

Second, the effort-reward imbalance model developed by Siegrist (Siegrist 1996) focuses on assumptions of social reciprocity within work contracts. Accordingly, ongoing imbalance between the costs of doing work and the resulting gains, including both financial and social rewards, may make workers feel that they are being treated unfairly, contributing to reduced self-esteem, emotional distress, and a stress response. The effort-reward imbalance model has been associated with increased risk of cardiovascular disease, alcohol dependence, and other poor health outcomes which can impact cancer (Perrewe and Ganster 2002, Schnall et al. 2000, Siegrist and Marmot 2004, Stansfield and Marmot 2002).

In addition to these associations with the psychosocial work environment, the IARC recently cited evidence that shift work involving circadian disruption is a probable carcinogen in humans (Straif et al. 2007). IARC cited evidence from studies among health care workers and flight attendants of an increased risk of breast cancer among long-term night workers, also noting that up to 30% of health care workers and 15–20% of all workers in the US and Europe are involved in night work. The roles of other work experiences with respect to cancer are also being explored. For example, in the Black Women's Health Study, perceived racial discrimination on the job was significantly associated with increased breast cancer incidence (Taylor et al. 2007).

Psychosocial exposures generally follow an occupational gradient. Both low control at work and low reward at work are more prevalent among workers of low SEP compared to high-SEP workers (Bosma et al. 1998, Lundberg 1999, Niedhammer et al. 2000, Siegrist et al. 2004). Although similar evidence is not available for cancer outcomes, studies have indicated a stronger effect of job strain and high effort and low reward for risk of coronary heart disease among workers in low status and low-wage jobs (Hallqvist et al. 1998, Kuper et al. 2002). The impact of these conditions may be greater among these workers due to their heightened vulnerability (Siegrist and Marmot 2004). For example, Kristenson et al. (2004) observed that lower SEP workers have less successful coping abilities, as well as associated feelings of helplessness that may contribute to psychobiologic responses that, in combination with behavioral choices, lead to poor health outcomes. Adverse psychosocial work environments are likely to have important implications for observed disparities in cancer and other health outcomes (Cardano et al. 2004).

Additional Links to Risk-Related Behaviors

Work experiences play important roles in cancer risk-related behaviors and the ability to make changes in those behaviors. For example, smoking and difficulty in quitting smoking have been associated with job strain, increased work hours, and shift work (Albertsen et al. 2006, Eriksen 2005, Janzon et al. 2005, Sanderson et al. 2005). Boring, repetitive, and monotonous jobs are also positively related to amount smoked (Albertsen et al. 2006, Hennrikus et al. 1996, Rose et al. 1983). Conversely, resources in the work environment, such as emotional support and job decision latitude, appear to facilitate smoking cessation and are also associated with smoking fewer cigarettes and lower relapse rates (Albertsen et al. 2006, Eakin 1997, Janzon et al. 2005). Social norms supporting non-smoking and smoking cessation have been shown to be more prevalent among white-collar than blue-collar workers (Sorensen et al. 2002), just as fruit and vegetable consumption appear to increase in people with good social support at work (Sorensen et al. 2007, Steptoe et al. 2004) and other supportive social norms (Sorensen et al. 2007). Evidence is mixed, however, regarding the relationship between improvements in job organization and increased physical activity (Johansson et al. 1991, Landsbergis et al. 1998).

A number of studies have also highlighted associations between risk-related behaviors and exposures to job hazards (Johansson et al. 1991, Landsbergis et al. 1998,

Levy and Wegman 2000, Levy et al. 2006, Sorensen et al. 1996). One study reported that blue-collar workers exposed to hazards on the job were more likely to smoke than unexposed cohorts (Sorensen et al. 1996). Exposure to hazards on the job also has been linked with unhealthy dietary habits among blue-collar workers (Kant et al. 1991, Patterson and Block 1988). In addition, hazardous exposures on the job may increase the risks associated with some health behaviors (Walsh et al. 1995). Tobacco, for example, contains some of the same toxic agents (e.g., benzene) present in some worksites, thereby increasing overall exposure of workers who also happen to be smokers (Stokols et al. 1996). In addition, tobacco smoke and some workplace hazards (e.g., asbestos) may interact synergistically, multiplying the impact of the exposure. Smoking can also transform certain workplace chemicals into more harmful agents in various ways; for example, some chemicals may interact with the heat generated by a burning cigarette (Karasek et al. 1987, Marmot and Theorell 1991).

Implications for Interventions

Given the strong associations among work experiences, cancer risk-related behaviors, and disparities in cancer outcomes, it is imperative that worksite cancer prevention efforts address the full spectrum of potential work experiences and exposures. Workers' health traditionally has been the central concern of two parallel functions within worksites: (1) occupational safety and health (OSH) and (2) worksite health promotion (WHP). OSH interventions are designed to minimize workers' exposures to job-related risks, including exposures to physical, biological, chemical, ergonomic, and psychosocial hazards (Levy and Wegman 2000). WHP has focused primarily on workers' individual health behaviors. In this section, we briefly describe the efforts of each and turn to the potential advantages accrued from integrated and coordinated efforts across these functions.

Occupational Health and Safety

Occupational safety and health programs have traditionally been concerned with reducing hazardous exposures that can lead to work-related injury, illness, and disability, including exposures to dusts, mists, and fumes (LaMontagne and Keegel 2008, Taylor 1996). They may include changes in the organization and environment, such as substituting products, instituting engineering controls, and redesigning jobs, as well as individual efforts, generally viewed as supplemental measures, such as using personal protective equipment. These interventions are predominantly within the domain of management decisions rather than individual worker's actions (DeJoy and Southern 1993, Green and Johnson 1990), and may also be the subject of joint decision-making by labor and management through collective bargaining or less formal means. Work organization and staffing decisions also directly influence workplace injury and illness rates (Levy et al. 2006).

The Occupational Safety and Health Administration (OSHA) has outlined four program elements essential to OSH:

(1) *Management commitment to and employee participation in OSH activities.* A company with this commitment regularly sets health and safety goals and allocates money specifically for health and safety, with managers directly accountable for health and safety in their areas. Employees also participate in health and safety committees, and resources are made available for employees to report health and safety hazards and concerns.

(2) *Workplace analysis.* This element involves reviewing new processes, machinery, methods, and materials for health and safety before they are introduced into the work environment, as well as health and safety audits, and investigations of injuries, property damage, and near misses.

(3) *Hazard prevention and control.* Companies set specific time deadlines to correct identified hazards and make follow-up inspections for corrective action. While adopting personal protective equipment or administrative controls, they also establish engineering controls designed to eliminate or substitute hazards.

(4) *Education and training.* This element involves providing health and safety training to all employees, as well as additional training to contract or part-time employees and to those who might encounter new hazards when changing jobs within the company.

Worksite Health Promotion

Worksite health promotion efforts have traditionally focused on promoting workers' health by changing individual health behaviors, including those related to cancer (Lamontagne 2004, O'Donnell 2002). Although many studies have looked at the impact of WHP programs targeting single health behaviors, increasingly the emphasis is on a more comprehensive approach, as recommended by the Centers for Disease Control and Prevention (CDC), which suggests programs built around five elements: (1) health education, including a focus on skill development for health behavior change, and information dissemination and awareness building, preferably tailored to employees' interests and needs; (2) supportive social and physical environments, including implementation of policies that promote health and reduce risk of disease; (3) integration of the program into the worksite's organizational structure; (4) linkage to related programs, such as employee assistance programs and programs to help employees balance work and family; and (5) worksite screening programs, ideally linked to medical care to ensure appropriate follow-up and treatment (Business for Social Responsibility, Corporate Social Responsibility 2004). Comprehensive, multi-component WHP programs have been demonstrated to have beneficial effects across a variety of outcomes, including health behaviors, health indicators such as cholesterol and blood pressure, and organizational outcomes such as absenteeism and return on investment (Heaney and Goetzel 1997, Pelletier, 1991, 1996, 1999, 2001, 2005).

There are distinct disparities, however, in the availability of these programs. Compared to other workers, low-wage, blue-collar, non-professional, black, and/ or part-time workers have less access to WHP programs (Grosch et al. 1998, Stoltzfus 2006). Even when programs are available, participation rates follow a similar social gradient, with participants more likely to be salaried, white-collar employees (Conrad 1987, Erfurt 1995, Gebhardt and Crump 1990, Glasgow et al. 1993, Linnan et al. 2001, Morris et al. 1999, Sorensen et al. 1996, US Department of Health and Human Services 2000). Low participation also is associated with lack of access to and extent of health insurance coverage (Association for Worksite Health Promotion 1999, US Department of Health and Human Services 2000). Low participation may be in part a consequence of ineffective "marketing" of programs to these workers (Association for Worksite Health Promotion 1999, US Department of Health and Human Services 2000) as well as structural barriers to participation. For example, supervisors may function as gatekeepers controlling worker access to WHP activities and may be reluctant to allow workers to attend programs on work time, thus presenting the greatest barriers for those workers with the least amount of discretion over their time (Linnan et al. 1999, Morris et al. 1999). In a cross-sectional survey of 24 US manufacturing worksites, line supervisors were more likely than senior managers to report production conflicts, cost, and space as barriers to offering health-promotion programs in the worksite, perhaps because they are more in tune to the day-to-day realities of managing work productivity (Linnan et al. 2007). Other structural barriers may include working overtime, shift work, or second jobs; long commute times; and competing home responsibilities (Alexy 1990).

Integrated Approaches to Cancer Prevention Using a Social Contextual Framework

Applying the social contextual model focuses our attention on addressing work experiences and working conditions relevant within a particular work setting. As we discussed previously, blue-collar workers experience a high prevalence of hazardous exposures on the job and deleterious psychosocial conditions, such as job strain. These workers are also are more likely to engage in cancer risk-related behaviors than other workers. To redress cancer disparities through worksite interventions, we must attend to all of these factors—through interventions not only aimed at changing work conditions, but also by addressing negative day-to-day work experiences and risk-related behaviors.

Worksite health promotion and OSH provide two parallel pathways for addressing these disparities by promoting workers' health. These parallel efforts may be strengthened, however, when they are coordinated and integrated—and this integration has particular impact for workers exposed to hazardous work conditions or poor psychosocial work experiences. As documented by a report of the Institute of Medicine, *Integrating Employee Health: A Model Program for NASA,* integrating and coordinating occupational health, health promotion, and related functions supporting employee health can significantly improve workers' health (Institute of Medicine 2005). This report highlights the work of a growing number of vanguard companies using coordinated systems to integrate such functions as occupational health and safety, fitness programs, health promotion, employee assistance programs, and case management.

In support of this trend, the National Institute of Occupational Safety and Health established its WorkLife Initiative, which aims to promote healthy workplaces that are free from recognized hazards and that assure workers ready access to effective policies, programs, and services to protect and promote their health, safety, and well-being (National Institute for Occupational Safety and Health 2008). WHO has proposed similar frameworks to achieve integrated WHP programs (World Health Organization 2007). In addition, some experts have posited coordinating—rather than competing for—resources may enhance an organization's overall success (Chu et al. 1997, DeJoy and Southern 1993, LaMontagne 2004, World Health Organization 1999). The WHO's Regional Guidelines for the Development of Healthy Workplaces, for example, underscore the benefits of coordinated efforts to create a healthy workplace, which they define as one that aims to create a healthy and safe work environment, ensure that WHP and occupational health and safety are an integral part of management practices, foster work styles and lifestyles conducive to health, ensure total organizational participation, and extend the positive impacts to the surrounding community and environment (World Health Organization 1999). Benefits of such coordinated efforts, they maintain, include contributing to a positive and caring image for the company, improving staff morale, reducing turnover and absenteeism, and boosting productivity (World Health Organization 1999).

With the clear rationale for integrating and coordinating WHP and OSH and increasing discussions of the benefits of integrated OSH/WHP interventions (Baker et al. 1996, Blewett and Shaw 1995, Chu et al. 1997, Corneil and Yassi 1998, DeJoy and Southern 1993, Dryson 1995, Eakin 1997, Israel et al. 1996, LaMontagne 2004, Shain and Kramer 2004), there is a growing literature systematically assessing the efficacy of these integrated interventions. The strongest available evidence supports the efficacy of the intervention model in promoting smoking cessation, particularly among blue-collar workers (Sorensen et al. 2007, Sorensen et al. 1998, 2002). Additional evidence indicates significant effects on increasing physical activity, as well as the consumption of fruits and vegetables (Sorensen et al. 2003). Of central importance, these studies document that the integrated OSH/WHP model has particular relevance for positive health behavior changes and program participation by blue-collar workers (Sorensen et al. 1996). Little evidence is available to date, however, documenting the impact of these programs on occupational health and safety outcomes.

Best practices and processes of integrated OSH/WHP programs are already well documented. As part of its WorkLife Initiative, for example, NIOSH has outlined a set of essential elements to guide program planning (National Institute for Occupational Safety and Health 2008). The IOM similarly delineated core approaches to assure program effectiveness (Institute of Medicine 2005). The aim across these recommendations is to link the full range of programs supporting workers' health—including WHP and OSH, as well as medical benefits design, disability programs, workers' compensation, and disease management programs—into a single coordinated effort (Institute of Medicine 2005). Integrated efforts are likely to require a change from traditional organizational structures that place these functions in separate silos with little cross-communication. Careful program planning is central, however, to ensure fit with the worksite and its employees. Worker participation in program planning, with special attention to including employee representatives across racial, ethnic, age, and work shift groups, helps set priorities and establish the basis for broad participation. Formative research may guide program planning and help to adapt programs to meet the needs of specific types of workers. Best-practice interventions are aimed at multiple levels of influence, including interventions designed to educate individual workers and build social norms supportive of health, as well as efforts aimed at promoting health by changing the work or organizational environment (McLeroy et al. 1988, Stokols et al. 1996). Organizational support is necessary to maintain a connection between programmatic efforts and the organization's core mission and values and to provide ongoing resources to maintain successful programs.

Summary and Conclusion

This chapter has documented persistent social disparities in cancer morbidity and mortality, as well as cancer risk-related behaviors. We have focused particular attention on disparities by occupation to explore the possible pathways through which SEP may operate to influence cancer outcomes. Work experiences not only provide opportunities to build social support, self-esteem, and other benefits to health, but also pose health threats related to hazardous exposures and poor psychosocial working conditions. Of particular concern, deleterious work experiences are not only especially common among blue-collar workers, but also particularly likely to have greater health consequences due to a combination of more risk behaviors and heightened vulnerability within this population.

Effective worksite cancer prevention interventions are especially needed for blue-collar, low-wage workers. Coordinated programs that address cancer risk-related behaviors, occupational hazards, and psychosocial conditions at work hold considerable promise for redressing occupational disparities in cancer, as well as related health outcomes. However, more research is still needed to explore further the characteristics of worksite programs, policies, and practices most effective in reducing disparities in cancer risk and risk-related behaviors, and to assure that evidence-based best practices are broadly applied across a range of work settings.

Acknowledgments This work has been funded in part by the National Cancer Institute (1K05 CA108663 and 2R25 057711) and through the support of a grant from Liberty Mutual, Inc.

References

Albertsen K, Borg V, Oldenburg B. A systematic review of the impact of work environment on smoking cessation, relapse and amount smoked. Preventive Medicine 2006;43:291–305.

Alexy B. Workplace health promotion and the blue-collar worker. American Association of Occupational Health Nurses Journal 1990;38:12–16.

American Institute for Cancer Research. Food, nutrition and the prevention of cancer: A global perspective. Washington, DC: World Cancer Research Fund, American Institute for Cancer Research, 2007.

Anonymous. Harvard report on cancer prevention, volume 1: Causes of human cancer. Cancer Causes and Control 1996;7:S3–S9.

Association for Worksite Health Promotion. 1999 National Worksite Health Promotion Survey. Northbrook, IL: Association for Worksite Health Promotion, 1999.

Baker E, Israel B, Schurman S. The integrated model: Implications for worksite health promotion and occupational health and safety practice. Health Education Quarterly 1996;23:175–188.

Bandura A. Social foundations of thought and action: A social cognitive theory. Englewood Cliffs, NJ: Prentice Hall, 1986.

Barbeau E, Krieger N, Soobader M. Working class matters: Socioeconomic disadvantage, race/ethnicity, gender and smoking in the National Health Interview Survey, 2000. American Journal of Public Health 2004;94:269–278.

Barbeau E, McLellan D, Levenstein C, Delaurier G, Kelder G, Sorensen G. Reducing occupation-based disparities related to tobacco: Roles for occupational health and organized labor. American Journal of Industrial Medicine 2004;46:170–179.

Berkman LF, Kawachi I. Social epidemiology. New York, NY: Oxford University Press, 2000.

Berkman LF, MacIntyre S. The measurement of social class in health studies: Old measures and new formulations. In: Kogevinas M, Pearce N, Susser M, Boeffetta P, eds. Social inequalities and cancer. Lyon, France: International Agency for Research on Cancer Scientific Publications, 1997, pp. 51–64.

Beydoun MA, Wang Y. How do socioeconomic status, perceived economic barriers and nutritional benefits affect quality of dietary intake among US adults? European Journal of Clinical Nutrition 2008;62(3):303–313.

Blewett V, Shaw A. Health promotion, handle with care: Issues for health promotion in the workplace. Journal of Occupational Health Safety 1995;11:461–465.

Bongers PM, deWinter CR, Kompier MA, Hildebrandt VH. Psychosocial factors at work and musculoskeletal disease. Scandinavian Journal of Work Environment and Health 1993;19:297–312.

Borrell C, Cortes I, Artazcoz L, Molinero E, Moncada S. Social inequalities in mortality in a retrospective cohort of civil servants in Barcelona. International Journal of Epidemiology 2003;32:386–389.

Bosma H, Peter R, Siegrist J, Marmot M. Two alternative job stress models and the risk of coronary heart disease. American Journal of Public Health 1998;88:68–74.

Bouchardy C, Schuler G, Minder C, et al. Cancer risk by occupation and socioeconomic group among men—a study by the Association of Swiss Cancer Registries. Scandinavian Journal of Work, Environment & Health 2002;28(Suppl 1):1–88.

Brownson RC, Boehmer TK, Luke DA. Declining rates of physical activity in the United States: what are the contributors? Annual Review of Public Health 2005;26:421–443.

Brulin C, Winkvist A, Langendoen S. Stress from working conditions among home care personnel with musculoskeletal symptoms. Journal of Advanced Nursing 2000;31: 181–189.

Bucher HC, Ragland DR. Socioeconomic indicators and mortality from coronary heart disease and cancer: a 22-year follow-up of middle-aged men. American Journal of Public Health 1995;85:1231–1236.

Burton NW, Turrell G. Occupation, hours worked, and leisure-time physical activity. Preventive Medicine 2000;31:673–681.

Business for Social Responsibility, Corporate Social Responsibility. Issue Brief: Health and Wellness: Business for Social Responsibility, 2004.

Byers T, Mouchawar J, Marks J, et al. The American Cancer Society challenge goals: How far can cancer rates decline in the US by the year 2015? Cancer 1999;86:715–727.

Caban-Martinez AJ, Lee DJ, Fleming LE, et al. Leisure-time physical activity levels of the US workforce. Preventive Medicine 2007;44(5):432–436.

Caban AJ, Lee DJ, Fleming LE, Gomez-Marin O, LeBlanc W, Pitman T. Obesity in US workers: The National Health Interview Survey, 1986 to 2002. American Journal of Public Health 2005;95:1614–1622.

Cardano M, Costa G, Demaria M. Social mobility and health in the Turin longitudinal study. Social Science & Medicine 2004;58:1563–1574.

Christian CK, Niland J, Edge SB, et al. A multi-institutional analysis of the socioeconomic determinants of breast reconstruction: a study of the National Comprehensive Cancer Network. Annals of Surgery 2006;243:241–249.

Chu C, Driscoll T, Dwyer S. The health-promoting workplace: An integrative perspective. The Australian and New Zealand Journal of Public Health 1997;21:377–385.

Colditz G, Atwood K, Emmons K, Willett W, Trichopoulos D, Hunter DJ. Harvard report on cancer prevention: Harvard cancer risk index, volume 4. Cancer Causes and Control 2000;11:477–488.

Colditz G, DeJong D, Emmons K, Hunter D, Mueller N, Sorensen G. Harvard report on cancer prevention: Prevention of human cancer, volume 2. Cancer Causes and Control 1997;8.

Colditz GA, Cannuscio C, Frazier A. Physical activity and reduced risk of colon cancer: Implications for prevention. Cancer Causes and Control 1997;8:649–667.

Conrad P. Wellness in the work place: Potentials and pitfalls of work-site health promotion. Milbank Quarterly 1987;65:255–275.

Corneil DW, Yassi A. Ethics in Health Protection and Health Promotion. Encyclopedia of Occupational Health and Safety 1998;19:18–23.

Covey LS, Zang SA, Wydner EL. Cigarette smoking and occupational status: 1977 to 1990. American Journal of Public Health 1992;82:1230–1234.

DeJoy D, Southern D. An integrative perspective on worksite health promotion. Journal of Medicine 1993;35:1221–1230.

Doornbos G, Kromhout D. Educational level and mortality in a 32-year follow-up study of 18-year-old men in The Netherlands. International Journal of Epidemiology 1990;19:374–379.

Dryson EW. Preferred components of an occupational health service for small industry in New Zealand: Health protection or health promotion? Occupational and Environmental Medicine 1995;45:31–34.

Dyrehag LE, Widerstrom-Noga EG, Carlsson SG, et al. Relations between self-rated musculoskeletal symptoms and signs and psychological distress in chronic neck and shoulder pain. Scandanavian Journal of Rehabilitation Medicine 1998;30:235–242.

Eakin JM. Work-related determinants of health behavior. In: Gochman DS, ed. Handbook of health behavior research I: Personal and social determinants. New York, NY: Plenum Press, 1997, pp. 337–357.

Erfurt J. The Wellness Outreach at Work program: A step-by-step guide. Washington, DC: National Institutes of Health, 1995.

Eriksen W. Work factors and smoking cessation in nurses' aides: a prospective cohort study. BMC Public Health 2005;5:p142.

Everson SA, Siobhan CM, Lynch JW, Kaplan GA. Epidemiologic evidence for the relation between socioeconomic status and depression, obesity, and diabetes. Journal of Psychosomatic Research 2002;53:891–895.

Faggiano F, Partanen T, Kogevinas M, Boffetta P. Socioeconomic differences in cancer incidence and mortality. IARC Scientific Publications 1997:65–176.

Fox J. Health inequalities in European countries. Aldershot: Gower, 1989.

Friedenreich CM, Rohan TE. Physical activity and risk of breast cancer. European Journal of Cancer Prevention 1995;4:145–151.

Galobardes B, Morabia A, Bernstein MS. The differential effect of education and occupation on body mass and overweight in a sample of working people of the general population. Annals of Epidemiology 2000;10:532–537.

Gebhardt DL, Crump C. Employee fitness and wellness programs in the workplace. American Psychology 1990:262–272.

Gennaro V, Tomatis L. Business bias: how epidemiologic studies may underestimate or fail to detect increased risks of cancer and other diseases. International Journal of Occupational and Environmental Health 2005;11:356–359.

Gerhardsson M, Hagman U, Peters RK, Steineck G, Overvik E. Meat, cooking methods and colorectal cancer: A case-referent study in Stockholm. International Journal of Cancer 1991;49:520–525.

Giovannucci E, Rimm EB, Stampfer MJ, Colditz GA, Ascherio A, Willett WC. Intake of fat, meat, and fiber in relation to risk of colon cancer in men. Cancer Research 1994;54:2390–2397.

Giovannucci E, Stampfer M, Colditz G, et al. Multivitamin use, folate and colon cancer in women in the Nurses' Health Study. Annals of Internal Medicine 1998;129:517–524.

Giovino G, Pederson L, Trosclair A. The prevalence of selected cigarette smoking behaviors by occupation in the United States. Work, Smoking and Health: A NIOSH Scientific Workshop. Washington, DC, 2000.

Glanz K, Kristal AR. Worksite nutrition programs. In: O'Donnell MP, ed. Health promotion in the workplace, 3rd edition. Toronto, ON: Delmar Thompson Learning, 2002, pp. 274–292.

Glasgow RE, McCaul KD, Fisher KJ. Participation in worksite health promotion: A critique of the literature and recommendations for future practice. Health Education Quarterly 1993;20:391–408.

Green KL, Johnson JV. The effect of psychological work organization on patterns of cigarette smoking among male chemical plant employees. American Journal of Public Health 1990;80:1368–1371.

Grosch J, Alterman T, Petersen M, Murphy L. Worksite health promotion programs in the US: Factors associated with availability and participation. American Journal of Health Promotion 1998;13:36–45.

Hallqvist J, Diderichsen F, Theorell T, Reuterwall C, Ahlbom A. Is the effect of job strain on myocardial infarction risk due to interaction between high psychological demands and low decision latitude? Results from Stockholm Heart Epidemiology Program (SHEEP). Social, Science & Medicine 1998;46:1405–1415.

Hamalainen P, Takala J, Saarela KL. Global estimates of fatal work-related diseases. American Journal of Industrial Medicine 2007;50:28–41.

Heaney CA, Goetzel RZ. A review of health-related outcomes of multi-component worksite health promotion programs. American Journal of Public Health 1997;11:290–308.

Heimendinger J, Feng Z, Emmons K, et al. The Working Well trial: Baseline dietary and smoking behaviors of employees and related worksite characteristics. Preventive Medicine 1995;24:180–193.

Hennrikus DJ, Jeffrey RW, Lando HA. Occasional smoking in a Minnesota working population. American Journal of Public Health 1996;86:1260–1266.

Houtman IL, Bongers PM, Smulders PG, Kompier MA. Psychosocial stressors at work and musculoskeletal problems. Scandanavian Journal of Work Environment and Health 1994;20:139–145.

Infante P. Cancer and blue-collar workers: Who cares? New Solutions 1995;5:52–57.

Institute of Medicine. The unequal burden of cancer. Washington, DC: National Academy Press, 1999.

Institute of Medicine. Fulfilling the potential of cancer prevention and early detection. Washington, DC: National Academies Press, 2003.

Institute of Medicine, Committee to Assess Worksite Preventive Health Program Needs for NASA Employees, Food and Nutrition Board. Integrating employee health: A model program for NASA. Washington, DC: Institute of Medicine, National Academies Press, 2005.

International Agency for Research on Cancer. IARC Monographs on the evaluation of carcinogenic risks to humans: Overall evaluation of carcinogenicity, supplement 7. Lyon, France: IARC, 1987.

Israel B, Baker E, Goldenhar L, Heaney C, Schurman S. Occupational stress, safety, and health: Conceptual framework and principals for effective prevention interventions. Journal of Occupational Health Psychology 1996;1:261–286.

Janzon E, Engstrom G, Lindstrom M, Berglund G, Hedblad B, Janzon L. Who are the "quitters"? A cross-sectional study of circumstances associated with women giving up smoking. Scandinavian Journal of Public Health 2005;33:175–182.

Johansson G, Johnson JV, Hall EM. Smoking and sedentary behavior as related to work organization. Social Science & Medicine 1991;32:837–846.

Johnson FM. How many high production chemicals are rodent carcinogens? Why should we care? What do we need to do about it? Mutation Research 2003;543:201–215.

Kant AK, Schatzkin A, Block G, Ziegler RG, Nestle M. Food group intake patterns and associated nutrient profiles of the US population. Journal of the American Dietetic Association 1991;91:1532–1537.

Karasek R, Gardell B, Lindell J. Work and non-work correlates of illness and behaviour in male and female Swedish white-collar workers. Journal of Occupational Behaviour 1987;8:187–207.

Karasek R, Theorell T. Healthy work: Stress, productivity, and the reconstruction of working life. New York, NY: Basic Books, 1990.

Kauppinen T, Pajarskiene B, Podniece Z, et al. Occupational exposure to carcinogens in Estonia, Latvia, Lithuania and the Czech Republic in 1997. Scandinavian Journal of Work, Environment & Health 2001;27:343–345.

Kauppinen T, Toikkanen J, Pedersen D, et al. Occupational exposure to carcinogens in the European Union. Occupational and Environmental Medicine 2000;57:10–18.

King GA, Fitzhugh EC, Bassett DR, et al. Relationship of leisure-time physical activity and occupational activity to the prevalence of obesity. International Journal of Obesity 2001;25:606–612.

Krieger N. Racial and gender discrimination: Risk factors for high blood pressure? Social Science and Medicine 1990;30:1273–1281.

Krieger N, Williams DR, Moss NE. Measuring social class in US public health research: Concepts, methodologies, and guidelines. Annual Review of Public Health 1997;18: 341–378.

Kristenson M, Eriksen HR, Sluiter JK, Starke D, Ursin H. Psychobiological mechanisms of socioeconomic differences in health. Social, Science & Medicine 2004;58:1511–1522.

Kuper H, Singh-Manoux A, Siegrist J, Marmot M. When reciprocity fails: effort-reward imbalance in relation to coronary heart disease and health functioning within the Whitehall II study. Occupational and Environmental Medicine 2002;59:777–784.

Kushi LH, Byers T, Doyle C, et al. American Cancer Society guidelines on nutrition and physical activity for cancer prevention: Reducing the risk of cancer with healthy food choices and physical activity. CA A Cancer Journal for Clinicians 2006;56:254–281.

LaDou J. The asbestos cancer epidemic. Environmental Health Perspectives 2004;112:285–290.

Lahelman E. Health and social stratification. In: Cockerham WC, ed. The Blackwell companion to medical sociology. Oxford, UK: Blackwell Publishers, 2001, pp. 64–93.

LaMontagne AD. Integrating health promotion and health protection in the workplace. In: Moodie R, Hulme A, eds. Hands-on health promotion. Melbourne, VIC: IP Communications, 2004, pp. 285–298.

LaMontagne AD, Keegel T. Work environments as a determinant of health. In: Keleher H, MacDougall C, eds. Understanding health: A determinants approach, 2nd edition. Oxford, UK: Oxford University Press, 2008, pp. 210–217.

Landrigan PJ, Baker DB. Clinical recognition of occupational and environmental disease. The Mount Sinai Journal of Medicine 1995;62:406–411.

Landsbergis PA, Schnall PL, Deitz DK, Warren K, Pickering TG, Schwartz JE. Job strain and health behaviors: Results of a prospective study. American Journal of Health Promotion 1998;12:237–245.

Lantz PM, House JS, Lepkowski JM, Williams DR, Mero RP, Chen J. Socioeconomic factors, health behaviors, and mortality: Results from a nationally representative prospective study of US adults. Journal of the American Medical Association 1998;279:1703–1708.

Lee DJ, Fleming LE, Arheart KL, et al. Smoking rate trends in US occupational groups: the 1987 to 2004 National Health Interview Survey. Journal of Occupational and Environmental Medicine 2007;49:75–81.

Lee DJ, Fleming LE, Leblanc WG, et al. Occupation and lung cancer mortality in a nationally representative US Cohort: The National Health Interview Survey (NHIS). Journal of Occupational and Environmental Medicine 2006;48:823–832.

Leino P, Magni G. Depressive and distress symptoms as predictors of low back pain, neck-shoulder pain, and other musculoskeletal morbidity: A 10-year follow-up of metal industry employees. Pain 1993;53:89–94.

Levy BS, Wegman DH. Occupational health: Recognizing and preventing work-related disease and injury. Philadelphia, PA: Lippincott, Williams and Wilkins, 2000.

Levy BS, Wegman DH, Baron SL, Sokas RK. Occupational and environmental health: Recognizing and preventing disease and injury, 5th edition. Philadelphia, PA: Lippincott Williams & Wilkins, 2006.

Linnan L, Fava JL, Thompson B, et al. Measuring participatory strategies: Instrument development for worksite populations. Health Education Research 1999;14:371–386.

Linnan L, Weiner B, Graham A, Emmons K. Manager beliefs regarding worksite health promotion: Results from the Working Healthy Project 2. American Journal of Health Promotion 2007;21:521–528.

Linnan LA, Sorensen G, Colditz G, Klar N, Emmons K. Using theory to understand the multiple determinants of low participation in worksite health promotion programs. Health Education and Behavior 2001;28:591–607.

Lundberg U. Stress responses in low-status jobs and their relationship to health risks: Musculoskeletal disorders. Annals of the New York Academy of Science 1999;896:162–172.

Mackenbach JP, Kunst AE, Groenhof F, et al. Socioeconomic inequalities in mortality among women and among men: an international study. American Journal of Public Health 1999;89:1800–1806.

Marmot M, Theorell T. Social class and cardiovascular disease: The contribution of work. In: Johnson J, Johansson G, eds. The psychosocial work environment: Work organization, democratization and health. Amityville, NY: Baywood, 1991, pp. 21–48.

Marmot M, Wilkinson R. Social determinants of health. Oxford, UK: Oxford University Press, 1999.

Marrett L, Thesis B, Ashbury F, and an expert panel. Workshop report: Physical activity and cancer prevention. Chronic Diseases in Canada 2000;21:1–11.

McLeroy K, Bibeau D, Steckler A, Glanz K. An ecological perspective on health promotion programs. Health Education Quarterly 1988;15:351–77.

McLeroy KR, Gottlieb NH, Nad Heaney CA. Chapter 17: Social health in the workplace. In: O'Donnell MP, ed. Health Promotion in the Workplace, 3rd edition. Albany, NY: Delmar, 2002.

Melchior M, Berkman L F, Niedhammer I, Zins M, Goldberg M. The mental health effects of multiple work and family demands. A prospective study of psychiatric sickness absence in the French GAZEL study. Social Psychiatry and Psychiatric Epidemiology 2007;42(7):573–582.

Melchior M, Goldberg M, Krieger N, et al. Occupational class, occupational mobility and cancer incidence among middle-aged men and women: a prospective study of the French GAZEL cohort. Cancer Causes Control 2005;16:515–524.

Menvielle G, Luce D, Geoffroy-Perez B, Chastang JF, Leclerc A. Social inequalities and cancer mortality in France, 1975–1990. Cancer Causes Control 2005;16:501–513.

Michaud DS, Augustsson K, Rimm EB, Stampfer MJ, Willett WC, Giovannucci E. A prospective study on intake of animal products and risk of prostate cancer. Cancer Causes and Control 2001;12:557–67.

Ministere de l'emploi de la cohesion sociale et du logement. Les expositions aux produits cancerogenes. Premiere Syntheses Informations DARES 2005;28:Annexe.

Mokdad AH, Ford ES, Bowman BA, et al. Prevalence of obesity, diabetes, and obesity-related health risk factors, 2001. Journal of the American Medical Association 2003;289:76–79.

Mokdad AH, Marks JS, Stroup DF, Gerberding JL. Actual causes of death in the United States, 2000. Journal of the American Medical Association 2004;291:1238–1245.

Morris W, Conrad K, Marcantonio R, Marks B, Ribisl K. Do blue-collar workers perceive the worksite health climate differently than white-collar workers? Journal of Health Promotion 1999;13:319–324.

Mullen K. A question of balance: Health behaviour and work context among male Glaswegians. Sociology of Health and Illness 1992;14:73–97.

National Cancer Institute. The nation's investment in cancer research: A plan and budget proposal for fiscal year 2007. Bethesda, MD: US Department of Health and Human Services, National Institutes of Health, 2005.

National Institute for Occupational Safety and Health. NIOSH WorkLife Initiative. Atlanta, GA: NIOSH, CDC, 2008.

Nelson DE, Emont SL, Brackbill RM, Cameron LL, Peddicord J, Fiore MC. Cigarette smoking prevalence by occupation in the United States. Journal of Occupational and Environmental Medicine 1994;36:516–525.

Niedhammer I, Siegrist J, Landre MF, Goldberg M, Leclerc A. Psychometric properties of the French version of the Effort-Reward Imbalance model. Rev Epidemiol Sante Publique 2000;48:419–437.

O'Donnell MP. Health promotion in the workplace, 3rd edition. Toronto, ON: Delmar Thomson Learning, 2002.

Patterson B, Block G. Food choices and the cancer guidelines. American Journal of Public Health 1988;78:282–286.

Pelletier KR. A review and analysis of the clinical and cost-effectiveness studies of comprehensive health promotion and disease management programs at the worksite: 1993–1995 Update. American Journal of Health Promotion 1996;10:380–388.

Pelletier KR. A review and analysis of the clinical and cost-effectiveness studies of comprehensive health promotion and disease management programs at the worksite: 1995–1998 Update (IV). American Journal of Health Promotion 1999;13:333–345.

Pelletier KR. A review and analysis of the clinical and cost-effectiveness studies of comprehensive health promotion and disease management programs at the worksite: 1998–2000 update. American Journal of Health Promotion 2001;16:107–116.

Pelletier KR. A review and analysis of the clinical and cost-effectiveness studies of comprehensive health promotion and disease management programs at the worksite: update VI 2000–2004. Journal of Occupational and Environmental Medicine 2005;47:1051–1058.

Pelletier KRe. A Review and Analysis of the Health and Cost-Effective Outcome Studies of Comprehensive Health Promotion and Disease Prevention Programs. American Journal of Health Promotion 1991;5:311–313.

Perrewe P, Ganster D. Research in occupational stress and well being: Historical and current perspectives on stress and health, volume 2. Amsterdam, Netherlands: JAI, 2002.

Piotrkowski CS. Gender harassment, job satisfaction, and distress among employed white and minority women. Journal of Occupational Health Psychology 1998;3:33–43.

Poortinga W. The prevalence and clustering of four major lifestyle risk factors in an English adult population. Preventive Medicine 2007;44:124–128.

Puigpinos R, Borrell C, Pasarin MI, et al. Inequalities in mortality by social class in men in Barcelona, Spain. European Journal of Epidemiology 2000;16:751–756.

Rolls ET. The orbitofrontal cortex and reward. Cerebral Cortex 2000;10:284–294.

Rose JE, Ananda S, Jarvik ME. Cigarette smoking during anxiety-provoking and monotonous tasks. Addictive Behaviors 1983;8:353–359.

Rosengren A, Wilhelmsen L. Cancer incidence, mortality from cancer and survival in men of different occupational classes. European Journal of Epidemiology 2004;19:533–540.

Rosvall M, Chaix B, Lynch J, Lindstrom M, Merlo J. Contribution of main causes of death to social inequalities in mortality in the whole population of Scania, Sweden. BMC Public Health 2006;6:79.

Salmon J, Bauman A, Crawford D, Timperio A, Owen N. The association between television viewing and overweight among Australian adults participating in varying levels of leisure-time physical activity. International Journal of Obesity and Related Metabolic Disorders 2000;24:600–606.

Sanderson DM, Ekholm O, Hundrup YA, Rasmussen NK. Influence of lifestyle, health, and work environment on smoking cessation among Danish nurses followed over 6 years. Preventive Medicine 2005;41:757–760.

Sandhu MS, White IR, McPherson K. Systematic review of the prospective cohort studies on meat consumption and colorectal cancer risk: A meta-analytical approach. Cancer Epidemiology, Biomarkers and Prevention 2001;10:439–446.

Sarlio-Lahteenkorva S, Silventoinen K, Lahelma E. Relative weight and income at different levels of socioeconomic status. American Journal of Public Health 2004;94:468–472.

Schnall PL, Belkic K, Landsbergis P, Baker D. The workplace and cardiovascular disease. Occupational Medicine: State of the Art Reviews 2000;15:1–334.

Schwartz KL, Crossley-May H, Vigneau FD, Brown K, Banerjee M. Race, socioeconomic status and stage at diagnosis for five common malignancies. Cancer Causes Control 2003;14:761–766.

Sequist TD, Schneider EC. Addressing racial and ethnic disparities in health care: using federal data to support local programs to eliminate disparities. Health Service Research 2006;41:1451–1468.

Serdula MK, Gillespie MS, Kettel-Khan L, Farris R, Syemour J, Denny C. Trends in fruit and vegetable consumption among adults in the United States: Behavioral risk factor surveillance system, 1994–2000. American Journal of Public Health 2004;94:1014–1018.

Shain M, Kramer DM. Health promotion in the workplace: Framing the concept, reviewing the evidence. Occupational and Environmental Medicine 2004;61:643–648.

Siegrist J. Adverse health effects of high-effort/low-reward conditions. Journal of Occupational Health Psychology 1996;1:27–41.

Siegrist J, Marmot M. Health inequalities and the psychosocial environment-two scientific challenges. Social, Science & Medicine 2004;58:1463–1473.

Siegrist J, Starke D, Chandola T, et al. The measurement of effort-reward imbalance at work: European comparisons. Social, Science & Medicine 2004;58:1483–1499.

Sorensen G, Barbeau E, Hunt MK, Emmons K. Reducing social disparities in tobacco use: A social contextual model for reducing tobacco use among blue-collar workers. American Journal of Public Health 2004;94:230–239.

Sorensen G, Barbeau E, Stoddard A, Hunt MK, Kaphingst K, Wallace L. Promoting behavior change among working-class, multi-ethnic workers: Results of the Healthy Directions Small Business Study. American Journal of Public Health 2005;95:1389–1395.

Sorensen G, Barbeau E, Stoddard AM, et al. Tools for Health: The efficacy of a tailored intervention targeted for construction laborers. Cancer Causes and Control 2007;18:51–59.

Sorensen G, Emmons K, Hunt MK, et al. Model for incorporating social context in health behavior interventions: Applications for cancer prevention for working-class, multiethnic populations. Preventive Medicine 2003;37:188–197.

Sorensen G, Emmons K, Stoddard AM, Linnan L, Avrunin J. Do social influences contribute to occupational differences in smoking behaviors? American Journal of Health Promotion 2002;16:135–141.

Sorensen G, Himmelstein JS, Hunt MK, et al. A model for worksite cancer prevention: Integration of health protection and health promotion in the WellWorks project. American Journal of Health Promotion 1995;10:55–62.

Sorensen G, Stoddard A, Dubowitz T, Barbeau EM, Berkman LF, Peterson KE. The influence of social context on changes in fruit and vegetable consumption: Results of the Healthy Directions Studies. American Journal of Public Health 2007;97:1216–1227.

Sorensen G, Stoddard A, Hammond SK, Hebert JR, Ocklene JK. Double jeopardy: Job and personal risks for craftspersons and laborers. American Journal of Health Promotion 1996;10:355–363.

Sorensen G, Stoddard A, Hunt MK, et al. The effects of a health promotion-health protection intervention on behavior change: The WellWorks Study. American Journal of Public Health 1998;88:1685–1690.

Sorensen G, Stoddard A, LaMontagne A, et al. A comprehensive worksite cancer prevention intervention: Behavior change results from a randomized controlled trial in manufacturing worksites (United States). Cancer Causes and Control 2002;13:493–502.

Sorensen G, Stoddard A, Ockene JK, Hunt MK, Youngstrom R. Worker participation in an integrated health promotion/health protection program: Results from the WellWorks Project. Health Education Quarterly 1996;23:191–203.

Stansfield S, Marmot M. Stress and the heart: Psychosocial pathways to coronary heart disease. London, UK: BMJ Books, 2002.

Steenland K, Henley J, Thun M. All-cause and cause-specific death rates by educational status for two million people in two American Cancer Society cohorts, 1959–1996. American Journal of Epidemiology 2002;156:11–21.

Steptoe A, Siegrist J, Kirschbaum C, Marmot M. Effort-reward imbalance, overcommitment, and measures of cortisol and blood pressure over the working day. Psychosomatic Medicine 2004;66:323–329.

Stokols D, Pelletier K, Fielding J. The ecology of work and health: Research and policy directions for the promotion of employee health. Health Education Quarterly 1996;23:137–158.

Stoltzfus E. Emerging benefits: Access to health promotion benefits in the United States, private industry, 1999 and 2005. Washington, DC: US Department of Labor, Bureau of Labor Statistics, 2006.

Straif K, Baan R, Grosse Y, et al. Carcinogenicity of shift-work, painting, and fire-fighting. Lancet Oncology 2007;8:1065–1066.

Taylor CA. The corporate response to rising health care costs. Ottawa, ON: The Conference Board of Canada, 1996.

Taylor TR, Williams CD, Makambi KH, et al. Racial discrimination and breast cancer incidence in US Black women: the Black Women's Health Study. American Journal of Epidemiology 2007;166:46–54.

Thorbjornsson CB, Michelsen H, Kilbom A. Method for retrospective collection of work-related psychosocial risk factors for musculoskeletal disorders: Reliability and aggregation. Journal of Occupational Health Psychology 1999;4:193–206.

Toscano GA, Windau JA, Knestaut A. Work Injuries and Illnesses Occurring to Women. Compensation and Working Conditions 1998;3:16–23.

Turrell G, Hewitt B, Patterson C, Oldenburg B, Gould T. Socioeconomic differences in food purchasing behaviour and suggested implications for diet-related health promotion. Journal of Human Nutrition and Dietetics 2002;15:355–364.

US Department of Agriculture, US Department of Health and Human Services. Nutrition and your health: Dietary guidelines for Americans, 5th edition. Washington, DC: US Government Printing Office, 2000.

US Department of Health and Human Services. Reducing the health consequences of smoking: 25 years of progress, A report of the Surgeon General. Rockville, MD: US Department of Health and Human Services, Public Health Service, Centers for Disease Control, Center for Chronic Disease Prevention and Health Promotion, Office on Smoking and Health, 1989.

US Department of Health and Human Services. Health benefits of smoking cessation: A report of the Surgeon General: Public Health Service, Centers for Disease Control, Center for Chronic Disease Prevention and Health Promotion, Office on Smoking and Health, 1990.

US Department of Health and Human Services. Healthy People 2010: Understanding and improving health and objectives for health, 2nd edition. Washington, DC: US Government Printing Office, 2000.

Walsh DC, Sorensen G, Leonard L. Gender, health, and cigarette smoking. In: Amick BCI, Levine S, Tarlov AR, Walsh DC, eds. Society and health. New York, NY: Oxford University Press, 1995, pp. 131–171.

Willett WC, Stampfer MJ, Colditz GA, Rosner BA, Speizer FE. Relation of meat, fat and fiber intake to the risk of colon cancer in a prospective study among women. New England Journal of Medicine 1990;323:1664–1672.

World Cancer Research Fund. Food, nutrition and the prevention of cancer: A global perspective. Washington, D.C.: American Insitute for Cancer Research, 1997.

World Health Organization. Regional guidelines for the development of healthy workplaces. Shanghai: World Health Organization, Western Pacific Regional Office, 1999, p. 66.

World Health Organization. Prevention of occupational cancer. World Health Organisation (WHO) GOHNET newsletter 2006, p. 11.

World Health Organization. Employment conditions and health inequalities: Final report of the WHO Commission on Social Determinants of Health (CSDH). Geneva, Switzerland: WHO, 2007.

World Health Organization. WHO calls for prevention of cancer through healthy workplaces. Geneva, Switzerland: WHO, 2007.

World Health Organization. Preventing chronic diseases: A vital investment. Geneva, Switzerland: WHO, 2008.

World Health Organization IAfRoC. Lists of IARC evaluations according to IARC monographs. Geneva, Switzerland and Lyon, France: WHO, IARC, 1993.

Part II
Specific Challenges in Cancer Disparities

Chapter 5
Disparities in Tobacco Use and Lung Cancer

Howard K. Koh, Loris Elqura, and Sarah Massin Short

Introduction

The burden of tobacco use is not distributed equally throughout the population. Striking disparities exist in tobacco use around the world and in the US, not only across dimensions such as race/ethnicity and socioeconomic position but also across the continuum of tobacco use from initiation to cessation (See Fig. 5.1). Diseases caused by tobacco use, especially lung cancer, reflect and perpetuate these disparities and contribute to economic costs of smoking in the US estimated to be $167B/year (CDC 2007a). This chapter reviews these disparities, focusing particularly on the US, and offers some strategies to reduce them.

Data Sources and Scope

We reviewed the literature using PubMed and other sources, including national reports such as the US Surgeon General Reports on Tobacco Use Among Racial/Ethnic Minority Groups (1998) and Reducing Tobacco Use (2000), the 2007 Institute of Medicine (IOM) Report (Ending the Tobacco Problem: A Blueprint for the Nation), the Public Health Services Clinical Practice Guidelines Treating Tobacco Use and Dependence: 2008 Update (Fiore et al. 2008), and Healthy People 2010. We also examined national datasets including the following: (1) the Behavioral Risk Factor Surveillance Survey (BRFSS), a state-based random telephone survey conducted by state health departments in collaboration with the Centers for Disease Control and Prevention (CDC); (2) the National Health Interview Survey (NHIS), a cross-sectional household interview survey conducted by the National Center for Health Statistics; (3) the National Survey on Drug Use and Health (NSDUH), an in-person interview among a sample of

H.K. Koh (✉)
Harvey V. Fineberg Professor of the Practice of Public Health, Associate Dean for Public Health Practice, Director, Division of Public Health Practice, Harvard School of Public Health, Boston, MA, USA
e-mail: hkoh@hsph.harvard.edu

H.K. Koh (ed.), *Toward the Elimination of Cancer Disparities*,
DOI 10.1007/978-0-387-89443-0_5, © Springer Science+Business Media, LLC 2009

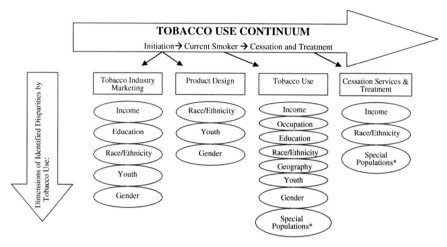

*Special populations can include those with mental illness, disability, as well as Lesbian, Gay,
Bisexual, and Transgender, and military populations

Fig. 5.1 Disparities along the tobacco use continuum

individuals in their residence, conducted by the Research Triangle Institute;
(4) the National Program of Cancer Registries (NPCR), which funds state
cancer registries to collect population-based cancer incidence data administered by the CDC; and (5) Surveillance, Epidemiology and End Results
(SEER), conducted by the National Cancer Institute (NCI), which collects
and publishes data from population-based cancer registries as well as the CDC
Wonder Data 2010 database.

Throughout this chapter, we employ the NHIS definition for a current
smoker, as those who had smoked at least 100 cigarettes in their lifetime and
who, at the time of the interview, reported smoking every day or some days
(CDC 2007a). The chapter restricts analyses to cigarette smoking in the US
while acknowledging the rising worldwide importance of other smoked-tobacco
products (such as bidis, kreteks, and shisha) as well as smokeless tobacco use.

Current Status of Disparities in Tobacco Use, Especially
Socioeconomic Status

Tobacco use, the single greatest risk factor for preventable death in the world,
accounted for 100 million deaths in the twentieth century and is predicted to
cause an estimated one billion deaths in the next century (WHO 2008). Developing countries suffer a disproportionate burden of these deaths, in part because of
a global disparity in usage: about 35% of males in developed countries smoke
tobacco, compared to 50% of males in developing countries (Mackay et al. 2006).
Heavy targeting by the tobacco industry, among other factors, is expected to

heighten striking disparities in mortality, with 80% of tobacco-related deaths predicted to occur in the developing world by 2030 (WHO 2008).

Even within the US, however,—where the US Department of Health and Human Services' (US DHHS) agenda for healthy promotion and disease prevention, Healthy People 2010, sets a national objective to reduce adult smoking prevalence to $\leq 12\%$ (27-1a) by the year 2010—smoking remains a significant health burden, particularly among certain populations. While US adult smoking prevalence has declined from 25.5% in 1990 (CDC 1992) to 20.8% in 2006 (CDC 2007a), few states or populations have been able to meet this objective. In fact, from a population-based perspective, in 2006, only Utah (9.8%) and the US Virgin Islands (9.1%) have yet been successful in this regard (CDC 2007b). Furthermore, only certain subsets of the US population have achieved this objective: Hispanic and Asian women (10.1% and 4.6%, respectively), men and women with undergraduate degrees (10.8% and 8.4%, respectively), men and women with graduate degrees (7.3% and 5.8% respectively), and women ≥ 65 years old (8.3%) (CDC 2007a). Most other subgroups in the country have much higher smoking rates (Table 5.1).

Socioeconomic Status

Of all the disparities in smoking prevalence, socioeconomic status (SES) (as measured by income, occupation, and education) appears to be among the most striking. For example, in 2006, 30.6% of individuals with incomes below the Federal Poverty Level (FPL) were current smokers, compared to 20.4% of adults at or above that level (CDC 2007a). Moreover, smoking prevalence follows a distinct trend along income subcategories. Smoking rates are highest among the poor (34.7%), followed by the near-poor (34.2%), and then middle-income (200–299% of FPL) (31.4%); rates are lowest among high-income individuals ($\geq 300\%$ of FPL) (20.7%) (Barbeau et al. 2004; IOM 2007).

In addition, individuals in working class professions, identified as either service or blue-collar workers, also have higher smoking prevalence rates than the general population. Moolchan et al. (2007), for example, found that one in three blue-collar and service workers are smokers, compared to one in five white-collar workers. An analysis of 2000 NHIS data also found current smoking rates highest in both blacks and whites who reported being in such occupations (Barbeau et al. 2004). Similarly, there are a disproportionately higher number of smokers among Medicaid enrollees (35% in 2006) (CDC 2008a) than among the general population (20.8% in 2006) (CDC 2007a).

Educational attainment is another strong predictor of smoking status. Individuals with less than a high-school education are two times more likely to be smokers than the general population (Fagan et al. 2004). Among adults with a General Education Development (GED) diploma (the equivalent of a high-school diploma), cigarette smoking estimates are the highest (46%), followed by adults with 9–11 years of education (35.4%); estimates are lowest

Table 5.1 NHIS data for smoking prevalence from 1998 to 2006*

Objective	Baseline/ 1998	2000	2002	2004	2006	Target/ 2010
Family Income Level						
Poor[1]	33%	32%	31%	28%	30%	12%
Near Poor[2]	30%	30%	28%	26%	26%	12%
Middle/High income[3]	21%	20%	20%	19%	18%	12%
Education Level (persons aged 25 years and over)						
Less than 9 years	27%	23%	23%	20%	19%	12%
9–11 years,	38%	36%	35%	34%	34%	12%
High School graduate	29%	29%	28%	26%	26%	12%
At least some college	17%	16%	16%	16%	15%	12%
16 years or more	11%	11%	10%	10%	8%	12%
Race/Ethnicity						
American Indian or Alaskan Native only	35%	31%	34%	28%	27%	12%
Asian only	13%	14%	12%	11%	11%	12%
Native Hawaiian or Other Pacific Islander only	–	–	–	30%	–	12%
Hispanic or Latino	19%	18%	16%	14%	15%	12%
non-Hispanic black	25%	23%	22%	20%	22%	12%
non-Hispanic white	25%	24%	24%	23%	23%	12%
Gender						
Female	22%	21%	20%	19%	18%	12%
Male	26%	25%	25%	23%	24%	12%
Disability Status						
Persons with disabilities	32%	31%	32%	28%	30%	12%
Persons without disabilities	23%	22%	21%	20%	20%	12%

*Data from CDC Wonder: Data 2010
[1]Poor < 100% of Federal Poverty Level (FPL) [2] Near Poor 100–199% of FPL [3] Middle High income > 200% of FPL
–N/A

among adults with undergraduate college degrees (9.6%) or graduate degrees (6.6%) (CDC 2007a).

Race/Ethnicity

The United States smoking prevalence, as well as morbidity and mortality, varies by racial and ethnic group. American Indian and Alaska Natives have the highest use rates of any racial/ethnic group in the US, followed by non-Hispanic whites, non-Hispanic blacks, Hispanic Americans, and, lastly, Asian Americans. Rates vary within these populations by age, gender, location, place of origin, and education level as well. Within and between these groups, too, there are significant disparities in smoking topography and patterns of smoking initiation.

American Indian and Alaskan Natives

American Indian and Alaskan Natives have the highest tobacco use rates of any racial/ethnic group in the US, with a 2006 smoking prevalence rate among adults of 32.4% (CDC 2007a). According to 2004 NHIS data, smoking rates were higher among men (37.3%) than women (28.5%). Smoking rates varied by location, with the highest rates in the Northern Plains (44.5%) and Alaska (39.9%) and the lowest in the Southwest (21.5%) (CDC 2000).

Non-Hispanic White Americans

Non-Hispanic whites typically have the second (sometimes third) highest smoking prevalence rate in the US (21.9% in 2006, third highest) (CDC 2007a). In addition, non-Hispanic white smokers tend to be heavy smokers; the Multi-ethnic Cohort study found that 19.2% of men and 9.4% of women smoked more than 31 cigarettes per day (cpd) (Haiman et al. 2006). Among high-school students, non-Hispanic whites report a younger age of smoking initiation than their peers (CDC 2007c) and have a higher smoking prevalence rate (23.2%) than Hispanics (16.7%) and African Americans (11.6%) (CDC 2008b).

Non-Hispanic Black Americans

With 2006 data exempted, non-Hispanic blacks rank third in smoking prevalence. However, fewer black Americans appear to be heavy smokers, e.g., only 5.8% of black men and 2.6% of black women ($\geq$ 31 cpd) (compared to 19.2% of white men and 9.4% of white women) (Haiman et al. 2006). African American adolescents also have a delayed onset of smoking compared with their white peers (Fagan et al. 2007). Despite these patterns and despite the fact that both adolescent and adult African Americans smoke fewer cigarettes per day than their white counterparts (2007), they have a higher incidence and mortality from lung cancer (See Table 5.2 later in this chapter) (Fagan et al. 2007). These trends are confounded by socioeconomic status as, among racial and ethnic groups, blacks/African Americans have the highest poverty rates (24.3%) and lowest household median income ($31,969) (DeNavas-Walt, Proctor and Smith 2007).

Of note, American-born blacks have a relatively higher smoking prevalence rate than immigrants from Haiti and the Caribbean. For example, Fagan et al. (2007) reported that Haitian-born immigrants and Caribbean-born blacks had a smoking prevalence of 9.7% and 7.1%, respectively, vs. 23.4% among American-born blacks.

Early research suggests differences in the smoking topography of African Americans, i.e., the way an individual smokes, including frequency of puffs, duration of puffs, time between puffs and cigarette duration, and puff volume. African Americans more frequently smoke mentholated cigarettes (Muscat et al. 2002). Of African American smokers, 68.9% of them smoke menthol compared to only 29.2% of Hispanic and 22.4% of white smokers (Giovino et al. 2004). Mentholated cigarettes may influence inhalation patterns by encouraging deeper inhalation (Fernander et al. 2007), may increase nicotine consumption per cigarette as well as cover up symptoms of disease, thereby delaying medical care and thus contributing to a relatively late stage of diagnosis (Garten and Falkner 2003). Such factors may contribute to the clinical outcomes noted above.

Hispanic Americans

Hispanic Americans have an adult smoking prevalence rate of 15.2% (CDC 2007a), with an estimated 21.1% in men and 11.1% in women (CDC 2006a). These numbers are significantly lower than in all other subgroups except Asian Americans. In addition, Hispanics tend to be light smokers (Fagan et al. 2007). The Multiethnic Cohort Study reported that of current smokers 59% of Hispanic men and 74.9% of woman smoked fewer than ten cigarettes per day (Haiman et al. 2006; Fagan et al. 2007).

Asian Americans

Asian Americans born in the US have the lowest adult smoking prevalence rate (10.4%) among the five racial and ethnic groups highlighted here (CDC 2007a; IOM 2007). However, Asian immigrant groups (including both men and women) have among the highest prevalence rates of all Americans, ranging from 34–43% among immigrants from Vietnam, Cambodia, and Laos (Fagan et al. 2007). In California, similar rates are found among Vietnamese men (35–57%) and Korean men (38.7%) (Fagan et al. 2007).

Although small sample sizes make it difficult to identify national ethnic specific data on Asian Americans, some data show variation by ethnicity. For example, a recent California study found that the Korean population had a smoking prevalence rate of 15.3%, but the rate among men was 27.9%, greater than that of California men in general (19.1%) and more than five times higher than that of Korean women (4.3%). Chinese and Asian Indian Americans, on the other hand, had smoking prevalence rates that were much lower than California's overall prevalence rate (7.7% and 5.5%, respectively) (Carrs et al. 2005).

Youth

Youth represent potentially new smokers, and each day 4,000 young people smoke their first cigarette (SAMHSA 2006). The Healthy People 2010 national objectives (27-2b) include reducing current cigarette use among high-school students to ≤ 16%. Current cigarette use among high-school students increased from 27.5% in 1991 to 36.4% in 1997. This rate then decreased to 21.9% in 2003 but has since stalled (CDC 2008b). The NSDUH showed the highest youth (12–17 years) smoking prevalence among American Indians/Alaska Natives (23.1%), followed by non-Hispanic whites (14.9%), Hispanics (9.3%), non-Hispanic blacks (6.5%), and Asians (4.3%) (CDC 2006b). Such youth trends mirror the racial/ethnic patterns noted above in adults (with the exception of Hispanic youth).

Geography

Recent regional data noted the highest smoking prevalence rates in the Midwest, followed by the South, the Northeast, and, finally, the West. Smoking prevalence in 2006 was highest in Kentucky (28.6%) and West Virginia (25.7%) and lowest in Utah (9.8%) and the US Virgin Islands (9.1%) (CDC 2007b). These rates appear to be affected by factors such as the magnitude of state cigarette excise taxes, the level of funding for statewide tobacco control programs, and socioeconomic characteristics of the specific population (CDC 2007b).

Gender

In the past decades, male smoking rates greatly exceeded those for women. For example, in 1965, the US rate was 51.9% for men and 33.9% for women. By 1990, this discrepancy had narrowed to 28.4% and 22.8% respectively (Giovino 2002), although, even today, the percentage of male smokers (23.9%) remains higher than that for women (18.0%) (CDC 2007a; CDC Wonder: Data 2010). Men are also more likely to be heavy smokers and to smoke more cigarettes per day than their female counterparts (IOM 2007). However, smoking rates of high-school males (21.3%) and females (18.7%) are almost identical (CDC 2008b).

Special Populations

Disparities also exist among special populations, including people with mental illness or other disabilities, gays and lesbians, and military personnel. The smoking prevalence among individuals with disabilities, for example, is considerably higher than among those without (29.9% vs. 19.8%). A population-based study by Lasser et al. (2000) found differences in smoking prevalence between individuals without mental illness (22.5%), with lifetime history of mental illness (34.8%), and with past-month mental illness (41.0%). In fact, persons with mental illness are twice as likely to smoke as those without, and they consume more than 44% of the cigarettes in the US (Lasser et al. 2000).

Sexual orientation is also associated with tobacco disparities. One study of Californians, for example, showed a higher smoking prevalence rate among lesbians (25.3%) than heterosexual women (14.9%), and a higher prevalence among gay men (33.2%) than heterosexual men (21.3%). This study also found even higher smoking prevalence for each of these subgroups among those with lower educational attainment and among those with lower household income (Tang et al. 2004).

The Department of Defense (DoD) has focused increasing attention on tobacco dependence too, as it now spends an estimated $1.6 B on medical care and lost productivity associated with regular tobacco use (Trent et al. 2007). Smoking among military populations dramatically increased during WWI with the inclusion of cigarettes in soldier rations (Giovino 2002; Nelson and Penderson 2008). Traditionally, cigarette smoking among military populations has exceeded that of the general population, specifically among military men and women aged 18–25 (men 42.4% vs. 37.6%; women 29.2% vs. 25.8%) (RTI-DoD 2006). A recent study looked at smoking rates among Marine Corps military recruits and found that, prior to boot camp, 41% were smokers, 26% used smokeless tobacco, and many used both. Trent et al. (2007) concluded that of these recruits, 57% were at risk for continued tobacco use following boot camp even though tobacco use is prohibited during this time. Of concern, the military environment may encourage tobacco use. A study conducted in 1999 found that high-school smokers who entered the military following high school were 2.5 times more likely to smoke a half-pack of cigarettes per day than those entering college (Bachman et al. 1999; Nelson and Penderson 2008).

Disparities in Secondhand Smoke Exposure

Secondhand smoke (SHS), also known as environmental tobacco smoke (ETS), is a known carcinogen that increases lung cancer risk by 20–30% in nonsmokers and causes about 3,000 annual lung cancer deaths in US adult nonsmokers (US DHHS 2006). In 2005, the Society of Actuaries estimated that exposure to SHS cost the US $10 B per year (CDC 2007d).

Children of smoking parents are the most vulnerable to SHS. Smoke-free home policies offer a viable way to protect them from exposure. The percentage of smoke-free homes within the US ranges from 53.4% in Kentucky to 88.8% in Utah, with an overall US average of 72.2% (CDC 2007e). Disparities exist by occupational status as well. Despite smoking bans in workplaces, including an increasing number of smoking bans designed to protect hospitality industry employees, a 2002 study showed that workers in bars and restaurants were exposed to SHS at levels 2–6 times higher than those in office workplaces (US DHHS 2002).

Factors Contributing to Tobacco Disparities

A framework that investigates the tobacco use continuum from initiation to cessation can be useful in explaining tobacco disparities (Moolchan et al. 2007). Using this lens, research suggests that the risk of tobacco use over the life cycle may be lowered by factors including education on the dangers of smoking, acculturation, and access to cessation services. However, the most powerful element in driving disparities may well be tobacco industry marketing.

Tobacco Industry Marketing

The tobacco industry spent roughly $15.2 B for cigarette marketing in 2003 alone, nearly tripling their spending from 1996 (Federal Trade Commission 2005; CDC 2006c). This spending increase may seem paradoxical in that it correlates with significant decreases in adult smoking prevalence and parallels the relatively stable prevalence rates since 2004 (CDC 2007a). However, these efforts fueled disparities, particularly given the tobacco company history of strategically targeting lower SES and racial and ethnic minority communities (Ward et al. 2004). In fact, internal documents (made available to the public by the Master Settlement Agreement in 1998) show that the tobacco industry used tactics including media campaigns, special products, and promotional offers to reach female, minority, and youth markets with specific products. For example, Philip Morris introduced the "Virginia Slims" brand in the 1960s with the motto, "You've come a long way baby," celebrating the women's liberation movement and implying female smoking as a marker of an empowered woman (IOM 2007). Also, packaging and advertising appealed to women's psychological and social needs of the time period, e.g., the brand "Satin" was linked to relaxation for the busy career woman of the 1980s, while the Virginia Slims slogan "It's a woman thing" was used to build female camaraderie in the 1990s (Anderson et al. 2005; Carpenter et al. 2005). After the introduction of Virginia Slims, smoking initiation increased by 110% among 12-year-old girls (Pierce et al. 1994; Gallogly 2007). The most recent example of such direct targeting of women is the brand "Camel No. 9," with a hot pink and black logo mimicking the perfume Chanel No. 9. Similarly, cigarette brand names such as "Rio" and "Dorado" were designed to appeal to the growing Hispanic market.

The tobacco industry has also targeted the African American population. For example, it is 1.7 times more likely that any given billboard in an African American neighborhood will be smoking-related than one in a Caucasian market (Primack et al. 2007). In addition, the density of smoking-related billboards in these neighborhoods is 2.6 times higher than in Caucasian markets (Primack et al. 2007).

Tobacco companies have also frequently contributed to schools, scholarship funds, and cultural events in an attempt to increase support among marginalized local communities (US DHHS 1998). For example, the Brown and Williamson's Kool Music campaigns, which stemmed from the 1970s "Kool Jazz Festivals," used music festivals and music-themed advertisements to appeal to the young adult African American male population (Hafez and Ling 2006). These efforts later evolved into the Kool Mixx promotional campaign, which began in 2004 and included limited edition cigarette packs featuring artwork reflecting the hip-hop element, as well as youth-geared promotional offers such as magazine subscriptions. The promotional cigarette packs were eventually recalled when the New York Supreme Court ruled that the campaign with its overt appeal to youth violated the Master Settlement Agreement (MSA), in which major tobacco companies agreed to not target their products at youth (Hafez and Ling 2006).

Price promotions are yet another strategy for targeting vulnerable groups. Low-income populations are the most sensitive to price increases and taxation (Chaloupka 1999). To counteract price hikes through tax increases, the tobacco industry has increased promotional marketing for cigarettes. In 2002, the tobacco industry spent 72% ($8.9 B) of the total budget on promotional offers, such as "dollar off" coupons and multi-pack discounts (White et al. 2006). One study reports that use of promotional offers by non-daily smokers was highest among 18- to 24-year-olds and a high proportion of moderate-to-heavy smokers in this age group took advantage of these offers (White et al. 2006). The study also found that women, African Americans, and heavy smokers, along with menthol smokers, are segments of the populations most likely to take advantage of promotional offers (White et al. 2006).

Young adults represent a new and growing generation of smokers as well, and the tobacco industry has strategized on how to best target this population. Through marketing analysis, the tobacco industry found that menthol, because of its ability to mask the harshness of smoking, was found to be popular among new smokers. The tobacco industry thus manipulated the menthol content of its cigarettes and increased menthol content of brands smoked by current smokers (Kreslake et al. 2008).

Disparities in Cessation Services

Not only are racial and ethnic minorities targeted more frequently by tobacco advertisements, but they may experience more difficulty accessing smoking cessation programs than their Caucasian counterparts (Fu et al. 2007; Fiore et al. 2008). Of the 20.9% of US adults who are current smokers, 69.5% want to quit (CDC 2007c), a figure that varies somewhat between different racial and ethnic groups (61.5% of Hispanic smokers vs. 68.8% of Asian Americans, 70.3% of whites, and 70.7% of African Americans). However, all may not have equal access to the cessation benefits recommended by the Clinical Practice Guideline: Treating Tobacco Use and Dependence Update 2008 (Fiore et al. 2008). For example, in one study of an equal access system (Veterans Affairs medical and ambulatory care centers), 50% of white smokers said they have ever used nicotine replacement therapy (NRT), compared to only 34% of African Americans and 26% of Hispanic smokers. In the past year, moreover, the study found that 20% of African Americans, 22% of Hispanics, and 34% of white smokers used NRT in a quit attempt (Fu et al. 2005).

These disparities may be attributable to numerous barriers including under-utilization of cessation methods (in turn, related to non-existent or inadequate insurance, as well as lack of awareness regarding cessation benefits or Medicaid programs) (Moolchan et al. 2007), inadequate access to primary care, and mis-conceptions about treatments. Other factors may include suboptimal social sup-port and lack of use of available tobacco dependence treatments (TDTs), as well as differences in access to cessation services (including counseling and pharmacother-apy) and in receipt of stop-smoking advice from physicians (Fu et al. 2007).

Disparate Perceptions About Cessation Methods

In 2008 the US Public Health Service (PHS) released the updated version of the Clinical Practice Guidelines for Treating Tobacco Use and Dependence for smoking cessation (Fiore et al. 2008), recommending full health insurance coverage for treatments demonstrated to be effective, including NRT in the form of gum, lozenge, patch, nasal spray, and the inhaler/puffer, Varenicline (Chantix) or Bupropion SR (Zyban or Wellbutrin), and counseling services (including individual, group, and proactive telephone counseling) (McMenamin et al. 2004; Fiore et al. 2008). However, Medicaid coverage for these TDTs varies by state. A 2002 survey found that only 21 state Medicaid programs covered pharmacotherapy recommended by the PHS guidelines (McMenamin et al. 2006). Furthermore, in 2006 only 39 (76.5%) state Medicaid programs reported covering at least one type of TDT as an optional benefit while four covered cessation treatments exclusively for pregnant women (CDC 2008a). Little research has been done to determine the effectiveness of these programs and interventions in a culturally appropriate context (Fu et al. 2007).

Misconceptions about TDTs are also prevalent among lower income (Medicaid) groups as well as among racial and ethnic minorities (McMenamin et al. 2006; Fiore et al. 2008) and may help to explain usage disparities as well. For example, McMenamin et al. (2006) found that fewer than half of Medicaid smokers thought the NRT patch (44%) and individual or group counseling (46%) were effective.

Level of awareness regarding Medicaid coverage for TDTs

Many studies have determined that knowledge of Medicaid coverage for TDTs is generally low among Medicaid recipients, and lower income individuals are relatively less likely to use them, which undoubtedly perpetuates the tobacco disparity (Murphy et al. 2005; Fiore et al. 2008). Indeed, awareness of TDTs by Medicaid enrollees is critical, given the high number of smokers in this popula-tion (36%) compared to the general population (23%) (McMenamin et al. 2006).

One survey of two states with comprehensive TDT Medicaid coverage indicated that only 36% of Medicaid-enrolled smokers and 60% of Medicaid physicians knew that the Medicaid program covered any TDTs (McMenamin et al. 2004). Similarly, Murphy et al. (2005) found that most Medicaid smokers in Western New York (54%) were unaware of smoking cessation pharmacotherapy benefits. Outreach programs may help improve awareness as well as utilization. The McMenamin et al. (2006) study of three states conducting a TDT outreach program for Medicaid enrollees, for example, found an improved but still significant knowledge gap, with 41% of enrolled smokers or recent quitters aware of the pharmacotherapy benefit and 46% aware that their state covered at least one TDT.

Other groups may face a knowledge gap as well. One study of smokers with a disability, for example, found that 70% who reported having seen a medical provider in the past 12 months had been advised to quit, but only 40% of those were told about specific available smoking cessation programs (Armour et al. 2007).

Clinical Disparities and Lung Cancer

Lung Cancer Incidence, Mortality, and Survival

Of all the clinical outcomes caused by tobacco use, lung cancer has the most striking medical and public health impact. Lung cancer, the most commonly diagnosed cancer and leading cause of cancer death in the US, accounts for 12% of all cancer deaths worldwide (Abidoye et al. 2007) and has a 5-year survival rate of 14% in the US (Du et al. 2006). It was estimated that in 2007, 213,380 people (114,760 men and 98,620 women) would be diagnosed with lung and bronchus cancer and that 160,390 men and women would die of these diseases (Ries et al. 2007).

There are approximately 438,000 deaths from tobacco-related illness in the US each year (Fagan et al. 2007), lung cancer comprises 80% of smoking attributable cancers. Cigarette smoking accounts for 88% of male and 72% of female lung cancer deaths (Thun and Jemal 2006). The highest lung cancer incidence and mortality rates are found among black men followed by white men, white women, and, lastly, black women.

Disparities in Lung Cancer Incidence and Mortality

Overall, male lung cancer mortality rates increased sharply from 1950–1975, and then more gradually before leveling off in the 1990s. Meanwhile, lung cancer death rates among women increased most steeply from 1975–1990 and have leveled off but have not yet begun to decrease. From 1991–2003, lung cancer death rates decreased by 20% among men, but increased by 9.6% among women (Thun and Jemal 2006). Since 1987, lung cancer has been the leading cancer killer among women (Patel 2005). Whether the increased risk of developing lung cancer among women is due to an increased susceptibility to the carcinogenic effects of cigarette smoke remains controversial. A review

Table **5.2** Age-adjusted SEER incidence and mortality rates (per 100,000), and 5-year survival rates (percentages).*

Lung & Bronchus Cancer	Incidence (2000–2004)			Mortality (2000–2004)			Survival (1996–2003)[1]		
	Total	Male	Female	Total	Male	Female	Total	Male	Female
All Races	64.5	81.2	52.3	54.7	73.4	41.1	15.0%	13.0%	17.4%
Whites[2]	65.7	81.0	54.6	55.0	72.6	42.1	15.3%	13.2%	17.6%
Blacks	76.6	110.6	53.7	62.0	95.8	39.8	12.0%	10.2%	14.6%
Asian/Pacific Islander	39.4	55.1	27.7	26.9	38.3	18.5	–	–	–
American Indian/ Alaska Native	44.0	53.7	36.7	39.9	49.6	32.7	–	–	–
Hispanic	33.3	44.7	25.2	23.6	36.0	14.6	–	–	–

* Ries et al. 2007

– N/A

[1] Survival for all stages at diagnosis

[2] Whites includes both Hispanic and non-Hispanic whites, this category is not mutually exclusive

conducted by Patel (2005) found contradictory evidence surrounding the relationship between gender and lung cancer risk. However, the type of lung cancer found in women is different than that in men, and never-smokers diagnosed with adenocarcinoma lung cancer are 2.5 times more likely to be women than men (Patel 2005).

Lung cancer incidence and mortality also vary between racial and ethnic groups (Haiman et al. 2006). Lung cancer incidence rates are second only to prostate cancer incidence among white, black, Asian/Pacific Islander, and American Indian/Alaska Native men. Among Hispanic men, lung cancer incidence is the third most common following prostate and colorectal cancer. However, lung cancer is the leading cause of cancer death among men of all races and Hispanic ethnicity. Among women, lung cancer incidence is the second most common cancer among whites and American Indian/Alaska Natives and third among black, Asian/Pacific Islander, and Hispanic women. Lung cancer is the leading cause of cancer death among whites, blacks, Asian/Pacific Islanders, and American Indian/Alaska Natives and second among Hispanic women (United States Cancer Statistics 2007).

There are disparities by socioeconomic status and geography as well. In general, poorer counties (i.e., those with 20% of the population below the FPL) have a 13% higher death rate from lung cancer among men, and a 3% higher rate among women than higher income counties. Furthermore, stratifying 5-year survival data by race and income level reveals that for non-Hispanic whites, African Americans, Asian/Pacific Islanders, and Hispanic-Latinos in the US, survival rates decrease as poverty levels increase. Only American Indian/Alaska Natives, groups with high smoking prevalence, were exempt from this trend (Ward et al. 2004) and, surprisingly, also have the second lowest lung cancer incidence of the five racial and ethnic groups compared among men.

The 5-year survival rate may serve as a quality measure for cancer treatment as it compares patient survival given the same stage at diagnosis. African Americans have a lower stage-specific survival rate than whites, perhaps attributable in part to disparities in access to care and quality of cancer treatment. They are less likely to receive the recommended treatment of surgery than whites for stage I and II non-small cell lung cancer (NSCLC), for example, even if they have insurance and are at the same income level (Ward et al. 2004).

Geographic variations of note include highest lung cancer mortality and incidence rates in the Southern US, followed by the Midwest, the Northeast, and, lastly, the West (United States Cancer Statistics 2007).

Racial and Ethnic Disparities in the Smoking-Related Risk of Lung Cancer

The risk of lung cancer does not necessarily mirror variations in smoking behavior among racial and ethnic groups. It is well known, for example, that blacks have a lower rate of heavy smoking and overall smoking prevalence but a higher incidence of lung cancer than other racial and ethnic groups (See Table 5.2) (Ries et al. 2007). The variation in lung cancer incidence among racial and ethnic groups led to an 8-year Multiethnic Cohort Study (Haiman et al. 2006) that followed five self-reported racial and ethnic populations (African Americans, Japanese Americans, Latinos, Native Hawaiians, and whites) accounting for factors such as smoking variations, occupation, level of education, and intake of fruits and vegetables. Variations in smoking topography and lung cancer incidence among the five groups appeared related to an unexplored difference in nicotine metabolism, which, in turn, may underlie differences in susceptibility to smoking-related lung cancer (Haiman et al. 2006).

Other studies also suggest that comparing cigarette consumption among racial and ethnic groups alone is insufficient in explaining lung cancer disparities. Susceptibility to the carcinogenic effects of cigarette smoke may be greater, for example, among African Americans and Native Hawaiians than among Latinos and Japanese Americans (Risch 2006). Differences have been found between racial and ethnic groups in ability to metabolize nicotine into the byproduct cotinine. In fact, some studies have found ethnic variation in blood levels of nicotine and cotinine (Risch 2006). Blacks tend to have higher cotinine levels than white or Hispanic smokers even after smoking the same number of cigarettes (Haiman et al. 2006).

Racial and Ethnic Disparities in Cancer Treatment

Multiple barriers may affect the equitable receipt of appropriate lung cancer treatment and underlie disparities in the treatment of lung cancer (Fig. 5.2).

Types of Lung Cancer Treatment

Surgical Lung Resection. Experts traditionally divide lung cancer into small cell lung cancer (SCLC, also known as oat cell cancer), an aggressive form that accounts for 10%–15% of lung cancers, and non-small cell lung cancer (NSCLC) which accounts for 85%–90% (American Cancer Institute 2008). Typically, small-cell lung cancer is usually not surgically resected, whereas one-third of NSCLCs can be if diagnosed early (Shavers and Brown 2002). The most effective treatment for stage I NSCLC is surgical lung resection. Patients who receive a lung resection for a stage I NSCLC diagnoses have a 65% probability of surviving five or more years, compared to a survival rate of less than 2 years for those who do not undergo lung resection at this stage (Wisnivesky et al. 2005). However, various studies show disparities in the receipt of lung resection along socioeconomic and racial/ethnic lines, attributable in part to issues of insurance coverage and access to care, as well as patient-provider relationships and, sometimes, a history of mistrust between these parties (Wisnivesky et al. 2005).

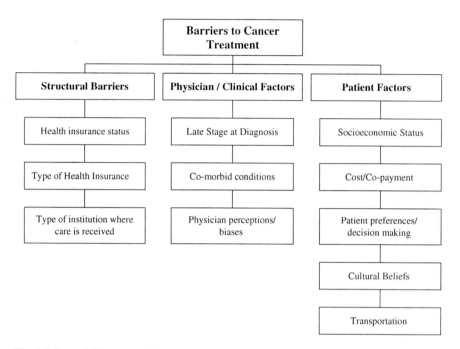

Fig. 5.2 Potential barriers to lung cancer treatment

Previous studies have indicated that lower rates of surgical resection among black patients may account for their decreased rate of lung cancer survival (Bach et al. 1999; McCann et al. 2005). Hispanic patients, who have a significantly lower lung cancer survival rate than whites (54.2% vs. 62.2%), are also less likely to receive surgical resection and more likely to be diagnosed with stage IB than stage IA lung cancer (Wisnivesky et al. 2005). African Americans are also less likely to have surgical lung resection than their white counterparts (Bach et al. 1999; Lathan et al. 2006; Gross et al. 2008). For example, Bach et al. (1999) found that the surgical resection rates (in the SEER-Medicare database) for black patients were 64% vs. 76.7% among white patients; these results were similar to those found in Gross's 10-year study (2007) (64.0% among black patients vs. 78.5% among white patients) (SEER-Medicare database). The 5-year survival rate in the Bach et al. (1999) study was also lower for blacks (26.4% vs. 34.1% among whites). Of note, 5-year survival rates are similar both among black and white patients who have undergone lung resection (Bach et al. 1999; Lathan et al. 2006) and among black and white patients who have not had lung resection (Lathan et al. 2006). Unfortunately, Gross et al. (2008) showed not only a downward trend in resection rates over time for both white and black patients, but also indicated that the relative disparities between these rates actually widened. Specifically, the initial period from 1992–1994 showed an adjusted rate of early stage lung resection (stages I and II) among whites to be

84.9% and 73.1% among blacks. These rates of lung resection were actually lower in 2000–2002 (79.3% and 64.9%, respectively). However, other factors may be involved since black cancer patients in this study were significantly more likely than their white counterparts to live in areas with the lowest quintile for median income, have state-sponsored health insurance such as Medicare, and not to have seen a physician before their cancer diagnosis. In addition, these patients were more likely to have comorbid conditions that could complicate cancer diagnosis and treatment (Gross et al. 2008).

Why surgical lung resection is performed less often on black patients remains unclear. Differences could be due to a variety of factors, including the likelihood of accepting surgical treatment. A study conducted by McCann et al. (2005) in a tertiary-referral hospital in Detroit found that black patients were three times as likely as their white counterparts to decline lung resection (18% vs. 5%). Additionally, the significantly lower surgical rate among black vs. white patients (58% vs. 74%) occurred even though surgical resection was offered at similar rates (McCann et al. 2005).

Lathan et al. (2006) conducted a study to determine the relationship between willingness to undergo invasive surgical staging for early stage lung cancer diagnosis as an indicator of willingness to accept surgical lung resection. Black patients obtained NSCLC staging less often than white patients. Moreover, even black patients who received staging had surgical lung resections at a lower rate than white patients, suggesting that both physician behavior and patient attitudes may play a role. Physician bias and training may also underlie disparities in resection rates. Physicians who care for black patients are also less likely to be board certified. Furthermore, primary care physicians have a harder time obtaining access for black patients to high quality physicians and hospitals, and few providers are "culturally competent" (Bach et al. 2004).

Patient-provider trust and communication, as well as patient beliefs, are probably key factors as well. Trust in one's physician was lower among black patients visiting a Southern VA hospital for suspicious pulmonary nodules or lung cancer treatment recommendations than among their white counterparts. Specific findings indicate that communication is an important barrier to patient trust in their physician. Black patients viewed their physicians as being less supportive, less partnering, and less informative than did white patients (Gordon et al. 2006). The misconception that air exposure causes a tumor to spread, for example, is pervasive, particularly among African Americans surveyed at pulmonary and lung cancer clinics (61% vs. 29% of whites—$p < 0.001$) and may contribute to the disparity in surgical lung resection between white and black patients. A bigger concern is that 5% of white and 19% of African American patients ($p = 0.001$) would decline lung resection surgery based on this idea, and 5% of white and 14% of African American patients ($p = 0.001$) would not believe their doctor on this issue (Margolis et al. 2003).

Additional factors that may underlie disparities include the type of facility in which the surgery is performed. Hospitals that perform few resections ("low-volume" hospitals), for example, not only have lower 5-year survival rates (low volume 37.5% vs. high volume hospitals 43.5%) (Birkmeyer et al. 2007) but also are more likely to have patients who are uninsured, Medicaid recipients, and/or members of racial and ethnic minorities (Liu et al. 2006; Neighbors et al. 2007). Liu et al. (2006) found that blacks, Asians, Hispanics, uninsured patients, and those with Medicaid were generally less likely to go to a high-volume facility for lung cancer resection than whites and those with Medicare. Medicaid and uninsured patients were also much more likely to receive surgical care from a low-volume hospital, whereas privately insured patients were much more likely to receive care from a high-volume hospital.

Radiation Therapy and Chemotherapy. Radiation therapy and chemotherapy are other treatment options—often palliative—for lung cancer. African Americans are less likely to receive radiation therapy, chemotherapy, or any other definitive treatment (including surgical resection) for lung cancer (Shavers and Brown 2002). In fact, not only are African Americans the least likely of all racial/ethnic groups not to receive chemotherapy for NSCLC, but they are also 30% less likely than whites to receive palliative chemotherapy even when they had the same insurance. In addition to race, lower SES and treatment in a non-teaching hospital were also associated with lower chances of receiving chemotherapy (Shavers and Brown 2002).

Access to Clinical Trials

Surprisingly, only 5% of newly diagnosed cancer adult patients participate in clinical studies (Du et al. 2006). Currently, racial and ethnic minorities, women, elderly, and rural residents tend to be under-represented (Murthy et al. 2004; Du et al. 2006; Ford et al. 2007), which threatens the generalizability of results (Giuliano et al. 2000). Ford et al. (2007) systematically reviewed the literature on clinical trial participation and highlighted numerous barriers to recruitment and participation by under-represented populations. They classified these barriers into three groups with respect to (1) awareness, including lack of culturally appropriate information and cancer knowledge, as well as inadequate education about clinical trials and physician awareness of trials; (2) opportunity, including older age, lower SES, racial/ethnic minority status, inadequate or non-existent health insurance, comorbid conditions, and under-referral; and (3) acceptance of enrollment, including perceived harm, time commitment, loss of income, availability of transportation, and general mistrust of research and the medical system. Age, SES, racial/ethnic minority status, and comorbid conditions were the most common factors associated with reduced participation.

Other structural, cultural, and linguistic factors may influence minority participation, including study duration, time, cost, follow-up, side effects, and a focus on economic survival over health or well-being. The latter is especially an issue for lower SES individuals, who often receive only limited prevention and diagnostic procedures and who are more likely to have Medicaid or Medicare, which often does not cover costs associated with participation in a clinical trial (Giuliano et al. 2000). Furthermore, limited English abilities among certain minority populations may impede provider-patient communication, as well as recruitment practices. Historical experience—such as memories of the Tuskegee Syphilis Study—may also lead certain groups to mistrust the health system and thus create another barrier to participation in clinical research (Giuliano et al. 2000; Du et al. 2006).

Interventions and Recommendations

From a global perspective, reducing tobacco consumption by half would prevent 20–30 million people from dying from all tobacco-related diseases, including lung cancer, before 2025 (WHO 2005a). Attempts at intervention thus far repeatedly suggest that achieving this goal and, more specifically, reducing tobacco usage and associated lung cancer disparities will require broad societal approaches. A comprehensive, multi-level strategy is essential, including legal, regulatory, policy and health system interventions, patient education and empowerment, cultural competence training among health professionals, and a focus on data collection and monitoring of racial and ethnic data.

While the evidence for racial and ethnic disparities is already well documented, narrowing disparities will require further research to better understand the sources of disparities and effective ways to eliminate them. Gross et al. (2008), for example, found that regardless of the increased attention and investment in identifying and reducing racial disparities along the cancer continuum, these disparities in cancer care had not decreased in the past 10 years. They also suggest that, in addressing disparities in cancer treatment, a focus on quality improvement is necessary to increase attention to measuring and improving quality of cancer care and eventually reducing health disparities (Gross et al. 2008). Of note, only recently have disparities in cancer treatment evolved from documenting disparities to assessing actual interventions.

WHO Framework Convention for Tobacco Control

The World Health Organization (WHO) Framework Convention for Tobacco Control (FCTC), the world's first public health treaty adopted in 2003, aims to "protect present and future generations from the devastating health, social, environmental, and economic consequences of tobacco consumption and exposure to tobacco smoke (WHO 2005b)." The treaty, legally binding for nations that sign and ratify it, delineates measures to establish comprehensive tobacco control programs. These include implementing bans on advertising and misleading marketing terms (e.g., "light"), protecting the public from exposure to SHS in workplaces and other indoor environments, increasing tobacco taxes, placing warning labels that cover at least 30% of the packaging on tobacco products, and combating smuggling of tobacco products (WHO 2005b). Societies that seek to implement the FCTC need to create broad popular support and build broad coalitions across multiple sectors of society (WHO 2005b). While these are surely daunting tasks, to date, 163 countries have ratified the FCTC, with the US being an exception (WHO 2009). The treaty's articles relating to large warning labels on the package, clean indoor air provisions, and banning of misleading terms such as "light" and "mild" would be particularly relevant in the US.

CDC Best Practices

In 2007, the CDC published "Best Practices for Comprehensive Tobacco Control Programs" to advise state-level policy makers about strengthening and implementing tobacco control programs. The report stresses investing in a multi-pronged approach targeting many aspects of the tobacco use continuum, from prevention to cessation as well as using a mix of educational, clinical, economic, and social strategies (CDC 2007d). The recommendations call for the following components: state and community interventions (e.g., supporting and/or facilitating tobacco control coalitions between state and local entities); health communication interventions (e.g., traditional mass media-based anti-tobacco ad campaigns and newly innovative approaches like text messaging); cessation interventions (e.g., health care system-based cessation counseling and NRT services and population-based services like toll-free "quit-lines"); surveillance and evaluation; and administration and management (CDC 2007d).

2007 IOM Report on Tobacco Control

The IOM recently published a national blueprint to "reduce tobacco use so that it is no longer a significant health problem for the nation" by (1) strengthening traditional tobacco control measures and (2) creating measures that change the retail environment of tobacco products (IOM 2007). Among the recommendations for strengthening traditional tobacco control programs are supporting comprehensive state tobacco control programs, increasing excise taxes, strengthening smoking restrictions, limiting youth access to tobacco products, intensifying prevention efforts (such as youth-directed education campaigns), and increasing smoking cessation interventions. The IOM Report states that these recommendations would help reach the Healthy People 2010 targets of 12% smoking prevalence rate in 2020 and 10% prevalence in 2025 (IOM 2007).

The IOM committee also recommends policy initiatives to change the environment in which tobacco is commercially distributed and thus help reduce tobacco use nationally. Among the recommendations is national and state legislation regulating point of sale of tobacco products (such as requiring all retail outlets that carry tobacco products to be licensed and monitored).

Further, the committee recommends encouraging Congress to enact a National Tobacco Control Funding Plan (if states fail to raise tobacco excise taxes) to fund a national tobacco control program and to give low-tax states incentives to increase state spending on tobacco control and raise taxes. Finally, in response to scientific evidence recognizing the causal relationship between tobacco advertising and increased tobacco consumption, the committee recommends legislation limiting advertising in mass media and reducing advertising at point of sale to a text-only format.

Specific Interventions

Statewide Efforts: California, Massachusetts, and Florida

States that have invested in sustained, comprehensive tobacco control programs have already seen great reductions in smoking rates among both youth and adult populations, as well as declines in cigarette sales. The longer states invest in such programs, the higher rate of return. For example, as a result of California's program, which began in 1989, smoking rates have declined from 22.7% to 13.3% in 2006 (California Dept of Health Services 2007). Furthermore, the US has witnessed the efficacy of comprehensive statewide tobacco control programs (Farrelly et al. 2003; IOM 2007; Farrelly et al. 2008), defined as "a coordinated effort to establish smoke-free policies and social norms, to promote and assist tobacco users to quit, and to prevent initiation of tobacco use that combines educational, clinical, regulatory, economic, and social strategies" (CDC 2007d). States such as California, Massachusetts, and others have created successful state-based comprehensive tobacco control programs that have successfully driven down consumption at rates several times greater than the national average (Koh et al. 2005).

An examination of several specific comprehensive state programs underscores the efficacy and history of such approaches. California, Massachusetts, and Florida have run longstanding, well-funded media campaigns focusing on counter-industry messages, such as the manipulation and population targeting of the tobacco industry. These states had larger declines in youth smoking rates than states without such campaigns (Hersey et al. 2005).

In particular, California's Tobacco Control Program, which began in 1989 after passage of a historic tobacco tax initiative petition, served as a landmark program. Funds generated from Proposition 99, the California Tobacco Tax and Health Promotion Act, led to a 25-cent/pack increase on cigarettes, with 20% of the revenues earmarked for a health education campaign (Hu et al. 1994). Included were an anti-smoking multimedia campaign (Hu et al. 1994), which contributed to reducing cigarette sales by 232 million packs from the end of 1990 to 1992 (Hu et al. 1994). Additionally, during the first decade, the program resulted in a 6% decline in lung cancer incidence, equating to 11,000 fewer cases of lung cancer (Barnoya and Glantz 2004). Furthermore, specific messages targeted minority populations and free tobacco quit-lines featured services in multiple languages (California Department of Health Services, 1998).

The Massachusetts Tobacco Control Program (MTCP) used a multi-pronged approach to preventing tobacco use among youth specifically, although it also impacted adult smokers. The program, which included a strong education and anti-tobacco media component, had broad reach as 88% of adults and 94% of adolescents reported seeing the anti-smoking advertisements that involved highly effective true stories as the basis for the advertisements. In addition to television, radio, and print ads, school-based programs helped disseminate positive health behavior messages. The media campaign, together with other components of the MTCP's youth restriction laws and smoke-free policies, helped decrease both youth and adult smoking rates (Koh et al. 2005). Florida's tobacco control program also heavily focused on a youth-directed anti-tobacco media campaign, the "Truth" campaign, which reduced high school student smoking rates by 35% (Bauer et al. 2000; CDC 2007d). Because of its success, the "Truth" campaign was later adopted and expanded by the American Legacy Foundation and used as a national media campaign.

Targeted Efforts

While the above broad tobacco control measures should reduce all disparities, other efforts have aimed specifically at reducing tobacco-related disparities among target populations such as low SES women and girls. For example, the Low SES Women's and Girl's Project, part of the Tobacco Research Network on Health Disparities (TReND)—formed in 2004 by the NCI and the American Legacy Foundation—resulted in new research examining best practices for tobacco control (McLellan and Kaufman 2006). Media campaigns and tax increases were found to have significantly more impact on less-educated women than on better educated women (Levy et al. 2006).

WellWorks, an integrated health promotion–health protection worksite intervention on individual behaviors, including smoking, conducted by Sorensen et al. (1998), suggested effective approaches to reaching blue-collar workers in particular. The primary outcome for smoking was 6-month abstinence rates, which, among the intervention work sites, was 15% compared to 9% among the control work sites. While these results were not statistically significant, they do suggest that this integrated intervention could be effective on a population level (Sorensen et al. 1998). Furthermore, in WellWorks 2—a randomized control design to compare an intervention combining health promotion and occupational health and safety to one only focusing on health promotion—smoking quit rates among blue-collar smokers in the integrated intervention group were double those receiving the health promotion intervention only. The successful smoking quitting rates among those in the integrated intervention group were comparable to white-collar workers, indicating the efficacy of this program with this particular population (Sorensen et al. 2002).

Future intervention efforts will need to expand the reach of these programs even further to target other specific groups facing disparities. The smoking prevalence rate is highest among non-Hispanic whites, for example, and their lung cancer rate, while second to non-Hispanic blacks, remains quite high. Even so, most of the lung cancer literature addresses racial/ethnic disparities without special attention to high-risk non-Hispanic whites. To address this particular disparity, we need to develop programs that focus on individuals who are near poor (i.e., ineligible for Medicaid or otherwise lacking TDT coverage) and who work in the service industry or are blue-collar workers. This overlooked population spans race and ethnicity and would benefit from programs that target them specifically.

Other chapters in this book (specifically Chapter 14 by Gottlieb) address potential tobacco control interventions to reduce disparities using a workplace, community-based, and broad population-based approach. As mentioned in Chapter 14, the National Conference on Tobacco and Health Disparities (NCTHD) identified the best practices to combat tobacco-related disparities (Fagan et al. 2004). The focus of the NCTHD's recommendations is on the individual, rather than the community. However, a more comprehensive approach to eliminating disparities must involve the intricacy of individual and community-level factors that influence the various stages of the tobacco use continuum (Fagan et al. 2004). An additional recommendation was the use of community-based participatory research (CBPR), which can serve as a tool to engage the community in taking an active role in eliminating tobacco-related disparities.

The extraordinary level of addiction caused by the tobacco industry on global populations and the disproportionate weight of this burden and related lung cancer on lower socioeconomic populations remains one of the great public health challenges of our time. Preventing tobacco use, related cancer, and the associated disparities must remain one of our highest societal priorities.

Acknowledgments This publication was supported in part by MassCONECT funded under Grant Number 5 U01 CA114644 from the National Cancer Institute. Its contents are solely the responsibility of the authors and do not necessarily represent the official views of the National Cancer Institute's Center to Reduce Cancer Health Disparities.

References

Abidoye O, Ferguson MK, Salgia R. Lung carcinoma in African Americans. Nat Clin Pract Oncol 2007;4(2):118–29.

American Cancer Society. What is Small Cell Lung Cancer? October 2008. Available at http://www.cancer.org/docroot/CRI/content/CRI_2_4_IX_What_is_small_cell_lung_cancer.asp Accessed on 25 February 2009.

Anderson SJ, Glantz SA, Ling PM. Emotions for sale: cigarette advertising and women's psychosocial needs. Tob Control 2005;14(2):127–35.

Armour B, Campbell V, Crews J, Malarcher A, Maurice E, Richard R. State-Level Prevalence of Cigarette Smoking and Treatment Advice, by Disability Status, United States, 2004. Prev Chronic Dis 2007 October;4(4). Published online 15 September 2007.

Bach PB, Cramer LD, Warren JL, Begg CB. Racial differences in the treatment of early-stage lung cancer. N Engl J Med 1999;341(16):1198–205.

Bach PB, Pham HH, Schrag D, Tate RC, Hargraves JL. Primary care physicians who treat blacks and whites. N Engl J Med 2004;351(6):575–84.

Bachman JG, Freedman-Doan P, O'Malley PM, Johnston LD, Segal DR. Changing patterns of drug use among US military recruits before and after enlistment. Am J Public Health 1999;89(5):672–7.

Barbeau EM, Krieger N, Soobader MJ. Working class matters: socioeconomic disadvantage, race/ethnicity, gender, and smoking in NHIS 2000. Am J Public Health 2004a;94(2):269–78.

Barnoya J, Glantz S. Association of the California tobacco control program with declines in lung cancer incidence. Cancer Causes Control 2004;15(7):689–95.

Bauer UE, Johnson TM, Hopkins RS, Brooks RG. Changes in Youth Cigarette Use and Intentions Following Implementation of a Tobacco Control Program: Findings from the Florida Youth Tobacco Survey, 1998–2000. JAMA 2000;284(6):723–8.

Birkmeyer JD, Sun Y, Wong SL, Stukel TA. Hospital volume and late survival after cancer surgery. Ann Surg 2007;245(5):777–83.

California Department of Health Services. A Model for Change: The California Experience in Tobacco Control. Sacramento, CA; 1998

California Department of Health Services. News Release No. 07–37: New data show 91 percent of California women don't smoke; 2007. http://www.dhs.ca.gov/tobacco/documents/press/2007Releaseof2006PrevData.pdf

Carpenter CM, Wayne GF, Connolly GN. Designing cigarettes for women: new findings from the tobacco industry documents. Addiction 2005;100(6):837–51.

Carrs K, Beers M, Kassebaum T, Chen M. California Korean American Tobacco Use Survey–2004. Sacramento, CA: California Department of Health Services; 2005.

CDC. Cigarette Smoking Among Adults – United States, 1990. MMWR 1992;41(20):354–355.

CDC. Prevalence of Selected Risk Factors for Chronic Disease and Injury Among American Indians and Alaska Natives – United States, 1995–1998. MMWR 2000;49(04): 79–82,91.

CDC. CDC Wonder: Data 2010. CDC; Atlanta, GA, 2008. http://wonder.cdc.gov/data2010/

CDC. State-Specific Prevalence of Current Cigarette Smoking Among Adults and Second-hand Smoke Rules and Policies in Homes and Workplaces – UNited States, 2005. MMWR 2006a;55(42):1148–1151.

CDC. Racial/Ethnic Differences Among Youths in Cigarette Smoking and Susceptibility to Start Smoking – United States, 2002–2004. MMWR 2006b;55(47):1275–1277.

CDC. Tobacco Use Among Adults – United States, 2005. MMWR 2006c;55(42):1145–1148.

CDC. Cigarette Smoking Among Adults – United States, 2006. MMWR 2007a;56(44):1157–1161.

CDC. State-Specific Prevalence of Cigarette Smoking Among Adults and Quitting Among Persons Aged 18–35 Years – United States, 2006 MMWR 2007b;56(38):993–996.

CDC. Smoking & Tobacco Use: Fact Sheet Hispanics and Tobacco. 2007c 10/17/2007; Available from: http://www.cdc.gov/tobacco/data_statistics/Factsheets/hispanics_tobacco.htm

CDC. Best Practices for Comprehensive Tobacco Control Programs-2007. Atlanta: U.S. Department of Health and Human Services. Centers for Disease Control and Prevention. National Center for Chronic Disease Prevention and Health Promotion. Office on Smoking and Health; 2007d.

CDC. State-Specific Prevalence of Smoke-Free Home Rules – United States, 1992–2003. MMWR 2007e;56(20):501–504.

CDC. State Medicaid Coverage for Tobacco-Dependence Treatments – United States, 2006. MMWR 2008a;57(05):117–122.

CDC. Cigarette Use Among High School Students – United States, 1991–2007. MMWR 2008b;57(25):689–691.

Chaloupka FJ. Macro-social influences: the effects of prices and tobacco-control policies on the demand for tobacco products. Nicotine Tob Res 1999;1 Suppl 1:S105–9.

Denavas-Walt C, Proctor B, Smith J. Income, Poverty, and Health Insurance Coverage in the United States: 2006. Washington, DC: U.S. Census Bureau, Current Population Reports, P60–233; 2007.

Du W, Gadgeel SM, Simon MS. Predictors of enrollment in lung cancer clinical trials. Cancer 2006;106(2):420–5.

Fagan P, King G, Lawrence D, Petrucci SA, Robinson RG, Banks D, et al. Eliminating tobacco-related health disparities: directions for future research. Am J Public Health 2004;94(2):211–7.

Fagan P, Moolchan ET, Lawrence D, Fernander A, Ponder PK. Identifying health disparities across the tobacco continuum. Addiction 2007;102 Suppl 2:5–29.

Farrelly M, Pechacek T, Chaloupka F. The impact of tobacco control program expenditures on aggregate cigarette sales: 1981–2000. J Health Econ 2003;22(5):843–59.

Farrelly M, Pechacek T, Thomas K, Nelson D. The impact of tobacco control programs on adult smoking. Am J Public Health 2008;98(2):304–9.

Federal Trade Commission. Cigarette Report for 2003. Washington DC: Federal Trade Commission; 2005.

Fernander AF, Shavers VL, Hammons GJ. A biopsychosocial approach to examining tobacco-related health disparities among racially classified social groups. Addiction 2007;102 Suppl 2:43–57.

Fiore M, Jaén C, Baker T, et al. Treating Tobacco Use and Dependence: 2008 Update. Rockville, MD: U.S. Department of Health and Human Services. Public Health Service; May 2008.

Ford JG, Howerton MW, Lai GY, Gary TL, Bolen S, Gibbons MC, et al. Barriers to recruiting underrepresented populations to cancer clinical trials: A systematic review. Cancer 2007;112(2):228–42.

Fu SS, Burgess D, van Ryn M, Hatsukami DK, Solomon J, Joseph AM. Views on smoking cessation methods in ethnic minority communities: a qualitative investigation. Prev Med 2007;44(3):235–40.

Fu SS, Sherman SE, Yano EM, van Ryn M, Lanto AB, Joseph AM. Ethnic disparities in the use of nicotine replacement therapy for smoking cessation in an equal access health care system. Am J Health Promot 2005;20(2):108–16.

Gallogly M. Background on Women & Girls and Tobacco. April 6, 2007 (Accessed on November 20, 2007); Available from: http://tobaccofreekids.org/research/factsheets/pdf/0137.pdf

Garten S, Falkner RV. Continual smoking of mentholated cigarettes may mask the early warning symptoms of respiratory disease. Prev Med 2003;37(4):291–6.

Giovino GA. Epidemiology of tobacco use in the United States. Oncogene 2002;21(48):7326–40.

Giovino GA, Sidney S, Gfroerer JC, O'Malley PM, Allen JA, Richter PA, et al. Epidemiology of menthol cigarette use. Nicotine Tob Res 2004;6 Suppl 1:S67–81.

Giuliano AR, Mokuau N, Hughes C, Tortolero-Luna G, Risendal B, Ho RCS, et al. Participation of minorities in cancer research: the influence of structural, cultural, and linguistic factors. Ann Epidemiol 2000;10(8 Suppl):S22–34.

Gordon HS, Street RL, Jr., Sharf BF, Kelly PA, Souchek J. Racial differences in trust and lung cancer patients' perceptions of physician communication. J Clin Oncol 2006;24(6):904–9.

Gross CP, Smith BD, Wolf E, Andersen M. Racial disparities in cancer therapy: did the gap narrow between 1992 and 2002? Cancer 2008; 112(4):900–8.

Hafez N, Ling PM. Finding the Kool Mixx: how Brown & Williamson used music marketing to sell cigarettes. Tob Control 2006;15(5):359–66.

Haiman CA, Stram DO, Wilkens LR, Pike MC, Kolonel LN, Henderson BE, et al. Ethnic and racial differences in the smoking-related risk of lung cancer. N Engl J Med 2006;354(4):-333–42.

Hersey JC, Niederdeppe J, Ng SW, Mowery P, Farrelly M, Messeri P. How state counter-industry campaigns help prime perceptions of tobacco industry practices to promote reductions in youth smoking. Tob Control 2005;14(6):377–83.

Hu TW, Bai J, Keeler TE, Barnett PG, Sung HY. The impact of California Proposition 99, a major anti-smoking law, on cigarette consumption. J Public Health Policy 1994;15(1):26–36.

Institute of Medicine. Ending the Tobacco Problem: A Blueprint for the Nation. Washington, DC: National Academies Press; 2007.

Koh HK, Judge CM, Robbins H, Celebucki CC, Walker DK, Connolly GN. The first decade of the Massachusetts Tobacco Control Program. Public Health Rep 2005;120(5):482–95.

Kreslake JM, Wayne GF, Alpert HR, Koh HK, Connolly GN. Tobacco industry control of menthol in cigarettes and targeting of adolescents and young adults. Am J Public Health 2008;98(9):1685–92.

Lasser K, Boyd JW, Woolhandler S, Himmelstein DU, McCormick D, Bor DH. Smoking and mental illness: A population-based prevalence study. JAMA 2000;284(20):2606–10.

Lathan CS, Neville BA, Earle CC. The effect of race on invasive staging and surgery in non-small-cell lung cancer. J Clin Oncol 2006;24(3):413–8.

Levy DT, Mumford EA, Compton C. Tobacco control policies and smoking in a population of low education women, 1992–2002. J Epidemiol Community Health 2006;60 Suppl 2:20–6.

Liu JH, Zingmond DS, McGory ML, SooHoo NF, Ettner SL, Brook RH, et al. Disparities in the utilization of high-volume hospitals for complex surgery. JAMA 2006;296(16):1973–80.

Mackay J, Eriksen M, Shafey O. The Tobacco Atlas. 2nd ed. Atlanta, GA: Am Cancer Soc; 2006.

Margolis ML, Christie JD, Silvestri GA, Kaiser L, Santiago S, Hansen-Flaschen J. Racial differences pertaining to a belief about lung cancer surgery: results of a multicenter survey. Ann Intern Med 2003;139(7):558–63.

McCann J, Artinian V, Duhaime L, Lewis J, Kvale P, GDiGiovine B. Evaluation of the Causes for Racial Disparity in Surgical Treatment of Early Stage Lung Cancer. Chest 2005;128:3440–6.

McLellan DL, Kaufman NJ. Examining the effects of tobacco control policy on low socio-economic status women and girls: an initiative of the Tobacco Research Network on Disparities (TReND). J Epidemiol Community Health 2006;60 Suppl 2:5–6.

McMenamin SB, Halpin HA, Bellows NM. Knowledge of Medicaid coverage and effective-ness of smoking treatments. Am J Prev Med 2006;31(5):369–74.

McMenamin SB, Halpin HA, Ibrahim JK, Orleans CT. Physician and enrollee knowledge of Medicaid coverage for tobacco dependence treatments. Am J Prev Med 2004;26(2):99–104.

Moolchan ET, Fagan P, Fernander AF, Velicer WF, Hayward MD, King G, et al. Addressing tobacco-related health disparities. Addiction 2007;102 Suppl 2:30–42.

Murphy JM, Mahoney MC, Hyland AJ, Higbee C, Cummings KM. Disparity in the use of smoking cessation pharmacotherapy among Medicaid and general population smokers. J Public Health Manag Pract 2005;11(4):341–5.

Murthy VH, Krumholz HM, Gross CP. Participation in cancer clinical trials: race-, sex-, and age-based disparities. JAMA 2004;291(22):2720–6.

Muscat JE, Richie JP, Jr., Stellman SD. Mentholated cigarettes and smoking habits in whites and blacks. Tob Control 2002;11(4):368–71.

Neighbors CJ, Rogers ML, Shenassa ED, Sciamanna CN, Clark MA, Novak SP. Ethnic/racial disparities in hospital procedure volume for lung resection for lung cancer. Med Care 2007;45(7):655–63.

Nelson JP, Pederson LL. Military tobacco use: A synthesis of the literature on prevalence, factors related to use, and cessation interventions. Nicotine Tob Res 2008;10(5):775–90.

Patel JD. Lung cancer in women. J Clin Oncol 2005;23(14):3212–8.

Pierce JP, Lee L, Gilpin EA. Smoking initiation by adolescent girls, 1944 through 1988. An association with targeted advertising. JAMA 1994;271(8):608–11.

Primack BA, Bost JE, Land SR, Fine MJ. Volume of tobacco advertising in African American markets: systematic review and meta-analysis. Public Health Rep 2007;122(5):607–15.

Ries L, Melbert D, Krapcho M. et al. (eds). SEER Cancer Statistics Review, 1975–2004. National Cancer Institute; Bethesda, MD, http://seer.cancer.gov/csr/1975_2004/ based on November 2006 SEER data submission, posted to the SEER web site, 2007.

Risch N. Dissecting racial and ethnic differences. N Engl J Med 2006;354(4):408–11.

RTI. 2005 Department of Defense Survey of Health Related Behaviors Among Active Duty Military Personnel: RTI International, Department of Defense, December 2006.

Shavers VL, Brown ML. Racial and ethnic disparities in the receipt of cancer treatment. J Natl Cancer Inst 2002;94(5):334–57.

Sorensen G, Stoddard A, Hunt MK, Hebert JR, Ockene JK, Avrunin JS, et al. The effects of a health promotion-health protection intervention on behavior change: the WellWorks Study. Am J Public Health 1998;88(11):1685–90.

Sorensen G, Stoddard AM, LaMontagne AD, Emmons K, Hunt MK, Youngstrom R, et al. A comprehensive worksite cancer prevention intervention: behavior change results from a randomized controlled trial (United States). Cancer Causes Control 2002;13(6):493–502.

Substance Abuse and Mental Health Services Administration. Results from the 2005 National Survey on Drugs Use and Health: National findings Rockville, MD: U.S. Department of Health and Human Services Administration, Office of Applied Science; 2006.

Tang H, Greenwood GL, Cowling DW, Lloyd JC, Roeseler AG, Bal DG. Cigarette smoking among lesbians, gays, and bisexuals: how serious a problem? (United States). Cancer Causes Control 2004;15(8):797–803.

Thun MJ, Jemal A. How much of the decrease in cancer death rates in the United States is attributable to reductions in tobacco smoking? Tob Control 2006;15(5):345–7.

Trent LK, Hilton SM, Melcer T. Premilitary tobacco use by male Marine Corps recruits. Mil Med 2007;172(10):1077–83.

U.S. Cancer Statistics Working Group. United States Cancer Statistics: 2004 Incidence and Mortality. Atlanta: U.S. Department of Health and Human Services, Centers for Disease Control and Prevention, National Cancer Institute, 2007.

U.S. Department of Health and Human Services. Report on Carcinogens. U.S. Department of Health and Human Services, National Toxicology Program; 2002.

U.S. Department of Health and Human Services. Tobacco Use Among U.S. Racial/Ethnic Minority Groups: United States Department of Health and Human Services; 1998

U.S. Department of Health and Human Services. The Health Consequence of Involuntary Exposure to Tobacco Smoke: A Report of the Surgeon General. Atlanta: U.S. Department of Disease Control and Prevention, Coordinating Center for Health Promotion, National Center for Chronic Disease Prevention and Health Promotion, Office on Smoking and Health; 2006.

Ward E, Jemal A, Cokkinides V, Singh GK, Cardinez C, Ghafoor A, et al. Cancer disparities by race/ethnicity and socioeconomic status. CA Cancer J Clin 2004;54(2):78–93.

White VM, White MM, Freeman K, Gilpin EA, Pierce JP. Cigarette promotional offers: who takes advantage? Am J Prev Med 2006;30(3):225–31.

WHO. Framework Convention on Tobacco Control. 2009. Available from: http://www.who.int/fctc/en/ Accessed on 24 February 2009.

WHO. Global Action Against Cancer NOW! Geneva: World Health Organization; 2005a.

WHO. WHO Framework Convention on Tobacco Control. Geneva: World Health Organization; 2005b.

WHO. WHO Report on the Global Tobacco Epidemic, 2008: The MPOWER package. Geneva: World Health Organization; 2008.

Wisnivesky JP, McGinn T, Henschke C, Hebert P, Iannuzzi MC, Halm EA. Ethnic disparities in the treatment of stage I non-small cell lung cancer. Am J Respir Crit Care Med 2005;171(10):1158–63.

Chapter 6
Socioeconomic Status and Breast Cancer Disparities

Sherrie Flynt Wallington, Otis W. Brawley, and Michelle D. Holmes

> *"In all societies, health and functioning vary according to socioeconomic position"*
>
> (National Research Council 2001)

This quote by the National Research Council, which captures the long history of related research and robust findings regarding the connection between socioeconomic status (SES) and health, cogently illustrates the central theme of this chapter and, indeed, of this book. The traditional socioeconomic indicators of education, income, occupation, and insurance status have repeatedly been shown to be predictive of health and mortality in the US, Canada, the United Kingdom, and a number of other European countries (Marmot et al. 1995; House et al. 1990; Preston and Taubman 1994). Comparing studies is difficult, however, as SES measures are inconsistent and poorly validated. Futhermore, the prognostic value of SES is confounded by diet, lifestyle, and cultural factors, all of which may have ethnic-based variations (Gordon 2003; Newman 2005). Also, minority racial and ethnic groups in the US tend to be disproportionately weighted with poor or socioeconomically deprived persons. In all cases, however, the poor or more deprived have worse outcomes than their more affluent counterparts (Byers et al. 2008; Kim and Jang 2008).

These relationships are particularly complex when assessing the determinants of breast cancer disparities. The incidence of breast cancer in the US is known to be higher among white than black women and among women of higher SES, but once a woman, whether black or white, has the disease, she is more likely to have recurrence or death from breast cancer if she is of lower SES (Gordon 2003). Explanations for these observed differences, however, are inconsistent and largely unclear. In this chapter, we therefore seek to disentangle the influence of SES on breast cancer disparities as much as possible, building on the breast cancer disparities work of one of our co-authors

S.F. Wallington (✉)
Postdoctoral Fellow, Harvard School of Public Health and Dana Farber Cancer Institute, Boston, MA, USA
e-mail: sherrie_wallington@dfci.harvard.edu

H.K. Koh (ed.), *Toward the Elimination of Cancer Disparities,*
DOI 10.1007/978-0-387-89443-0_6, © Springer Science+Business Media, LLC 2009

(Bigby and Holmes 2005) and others (McCarthy et al. 2006; Newman and Martin 2007; Vainshtein 2008).

Background

The American Cancer Society (ACS) projects that there will be 1,437,180 new cancer cases and 565,650 deaths from cancer in the US in 2008. Breast cancer remains the most common cancer and is the second leading cause of cancer-related death—after lung cancer—among women in the US (ACS 2008). In 2008, breast cancer alone is expected to account for 26% (182,460) of all new cancer cases among women. The ACS also forecasts that about 67,770 new cases of carcinoma in situ or non-invasive breast cancer will be diagnosed in 2008 (ACS 2008).

Despite these sobering figures, over the past few decades our nation has made an unparalleled investment in the fight against breast cancer on many levels. This investment has resulted in substantial and groundbreaking advances in the fields of biomedical sciences, technology, and drug development, and has significantly increased detection and treatment capabilities (Hiatt and Rimer 1999; Institute of Medicine [IOM] 2002; National Cancer Institute [NCI] 2006). Further, there is a growing consensus that some breast cancer risk factors are attributable to lifestyle behaviors that are modifiable, such as birthing habits, diet and nutrition, exercise, proper health care, and health information (Emmons 2000; Linos et al. 2007; Linos and Willett 2007).

Moreover, the energy generated around breast cancer both nationally and locally has generated enormous public support for finding a cure. Because of this, policymakers, academicians and researchers, and health organizations and communities, particularly at the grass-roots level, are joining to foster collaborative partnerships to fight breast cancer (Bigby et al. 2003; Israel et al. 2006; Minkler 2000). Together, these partnerships are developing targeted research and applied approaches within and beyond the clinical setting to translate and disseminate new scientific discoveries and evidenced-based interventions more quickly and efficiently (Kerner et al. 2005). These advances, along with our enhanced and growing understanding of cancer, have contributed to a continuing decline in cancer-related deaths in the US for the first time since the 1930s (NCI 2006). Equally noteworthy are recent drops in the incidence rate of breast cancer (Centers for Disease Control 2007; Jemal et al. 2007), as well as in breast cancer death rates (ACS 2008).

Despite such declines in mortality, some question the overall progress apparent in these national statistics. In particular, emerging research about the social determinants of health has emerged suggesting that SES is a factor in determining a person's health (Krieger et al. 2005; Kawachi and Kennedy 1997; Williams et al. 2003). Several of these studies in particular have underscored the significance of social health determinants, specifically SES, and their implications for breast cancer (Baquet and Commiskey 2000; Bigby and Holmes 2005; Chu et al. 2007). Rising breast cancer incidence rates over the past 30 years, for example, may be due to one or more of a number of social determinants of health. Some researchers have attributed the increase to the rising number of women electing not to have a child or delaying childbirth until after the age of 30, which are risk factors for breast cancer (Britt et al. 2007).

It has also been suggested that the increase in breast cancer incidence rates is related to America's epidemic of obesity and increasing average caloric intake. The consequence of obesity on breast cancer risk depends on a woman's menopausal status (Cui et al. 2002; Huang et al. 1997; Petrelli et al. 2002). Evidence shows that postmenopausal obesity is an established risk factor for breast cancer (Colditz and Rosner 2000; Newman 2005). Other data are also accumulating around the declining use of menopausal hormonal replacement therapy (HRT), which has been linked to an increased risk for breast cancer (Berry and Ravdin 2007; Colditz et al. 1993; Holmberg et al. 2008; Ravdin et al. 2007).

There is evidence of increased breast cancer risk for women working in certain occupations (e.g., professional; managerial, teaching, librarians, clerical) (Rubin et al. 1993; MacArthur et al. 2007;Teitelbaum et al. 2003) and industrial environments (textile, clothing, and night shift work) (Ji et al. 2008; Megdal 2005). All of these factors related to incidence are at least partly influenced by or related to race, ethnicity, culture, and SES.

Breast Cancer Disparities Along the Cancer Continuum

Several studies underscore the significance of SES along with other social determinants of health and their implications for breast cancer. In 1989, Freeman and Wasfie (1989) documented the dominant effects of SES, breast cancer, and race and ethnicity. In a retrospective analysis of 708 patients (94% black) diagnosed, treated, and/or followed at the Harlem Hospital Center in New York between 1964 and 1986, nearly all patients were of low economic status and almost 50% had no medical coverage. Breast cancer survival was low compared to the survival rate of black women nationally and very low compared to white women. These and similar findings called for additional research and policy consideration of the way in which racial/ethnic minority status and socioeconomic characteristics produce disparities in women's experiences with breast cancer (Bradley et al. 2002).

This section briefly describes known disparities between groups along the entire cancer continuum—from incidence and mortality to screening, diagnosis, treatment, and prevention. The section that follows then explores in more depth the ways in which certain often inter-related factors, both socioeconomic and biologic, may underlie these disparities.

Incidence and Mortality/Survival

Table 6.1 lists annualized breast cancer incidence and mortality rates by race/ethnicity. These data are age-adjusted to the year 2000 standard. The NCI Surveillance, Epidemiology and End Results (SEER) program has published black-white data since 1972 and data for blacks, whites, Native Americans, Hispanics, and Asians since 1992. It must be noted that registries with high numbers of Hispanics are generally populated largely with Hispanics of Mexican origin and thus do not adequately reflect data from Hispanics of South and Central American origin. Nor do the registries adequately represent all Native American and Asian populations.

Table 6.1 US breast cancer mortality rates annualized 2000–2005 by race and ethnicity

Race/Ethnicity	Rate per 100,000 Age-adjusted to 2000 standard
White	25.5
Black	33.8
Asian/Pacific Isl.	12.6
Native American	13.9
Hispanic	16.1

NCI SEER

Black and American Indian women have the lowest breast cancer survival rates of all women in the US, while Hispanic and white women have the best survival rates (Chu et al. 2003). The 5-year survival rate for white and black women has narrowed (Table 6.2). It is 90.3% for white and 77.9% for black women. The NCI registry has documented changes in age-adjusted black-white breast cancer incidence and mortality rates over time, as shown in Fig. 6.1. In the US, white women have a higher overall incidence rate of breast cancer than women of any other racial or ethnic group, and yet black American women have the highest breast cancer mortality rates. While white Americans have the

Table 6.2 Breast Cancer 5 Year Survival after Diagnosis (%) By Race

Year of diagnosis	All white females	All black females
1960–1963	63	46
1970–1973	68	51
1975–1977	75.9	62.3
1978–1980	75.6	63.8
1981–1983	77.7	64.1
1984–1986	80.4	65.1
1987–1989	85.3	71.2
1990–1992	86.7	71.7
1993–1995	87.9	72.8
1996–2003	90.3	77.9

NCI SEER

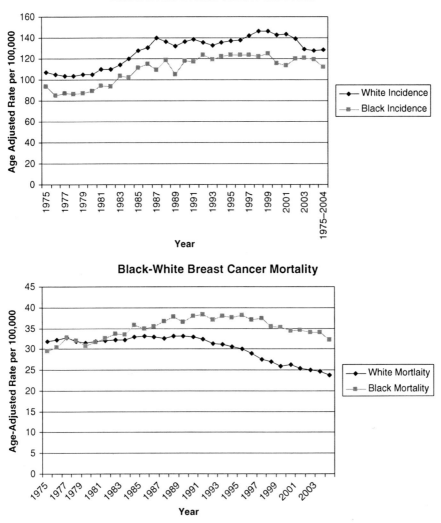

Fig. 6.1 Black-White Breast Cancer Incidence and Mortality

highest overall incidence rates, moreover, black Americans have higher incidence rates among women less than 50 years of age. Age-specific incidence and
mortality rates for blacks and whites are shown in Fig. 6.2. Additionally, black
women diagnosed with breast cancer are two times more likely to die from
breast cancer within 5 years than white women, and Hispanic women are 1.5
times more likely to die within 5 years (Eley 1994). In a meta-analysis, black race
itself was found to be a statistically significant, independent predictor of breast
cancer mortality when various measures of SES are taken into account

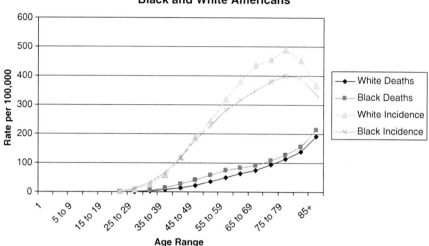

Fig. 6.2 Black-White Breast Cancer Incidence and Mortality

(Newman et al. 2002). Asian Americans, in contrast, have better survival rates than women from all other racial and ethnic groups (Clegg et al. 2002).

The black-white disparity in mortality has also increased significantly over the past three decades. Black-white breast cancer mortality rates were very close in the 1970s, but the gap between the rates has increased annually since 1981. In a Department of Defense population survey, the gap in breast cancer survival rates between white and black women increased for women diagnosed both between the 1980–1984 and the 1985–1990 time periods (Jatoi et al. 2003).

Screening

Differential access to facilities, for example, may account for some disparities in breast cancer screening. The ACS recommends that women follow its current guideline for early detection of breast cancer by beginning a regular program of mammography screening at age 40, followed by mammograms every 1–2 years. However, recently there has been a trend toward fewer mammography facilities. The number of mammography facilities decreased worldwide between 2001 and 2004. This decrease was found to be most often for financial reasons (US Government Accountability Office 2006). Additionally, the number of women getting mammograms increased between 2000 and 2003, while the number of mammography facilities, radiologic technologists, and physicians who could interpret results decreased between 2001 and 2004

(US Government Accountability Office 2006). These declining trends in the number of facilities and technologists could create an access barrier for underserved women, contributing to relatively longer travel distances and wait times and ultimately greater breast cancer disparities.

An early study by McCarthy et al. (1998) gave credence to the notion that the lack of regular mammography screening explains some of the differences in stage at diagnosis between black and white women (see next section). Subsequent research, in fact, has documented lower rates of mammography screening among black women and has spawned targeted efforts to increase mammograms among black women (Bigby and Holmes 2005). Hispanic, American Indian, and Alaska Native women also have lower rates of self-reported mammography screening than white women do. Some evidence reveals group disparities among various racial and ethnic groups, showing significant variations in screening prevalence within groups (Peek and Han 2004). Non-white women are also less likely than white women to follow-up regarding abnormal mammograms (Strzelczyk and Dignan 2002).

Disparate populations can also be described by SES. Both uninsured and less-educated women are less likely to undergo routine breast cancer screening than their insured and/or better educated counterparts (Halpern et al. 2007; Breen 2007). In addition, women with disabilities are likely screened at lower rates. While an earlier study indicated that women with disabilities had similar mammogram screening rates to women without disabilities (Nosek and Howland 1997), this conclusion was based on a relatively small sample. A later study by Schootman and Jeffe (2003), in fact, showed that women with long-term limitations in their activities of daily living (ADLs) or limitations in instrumental activities of daily living (IADLs) were less likely to be screened for breast cancer than those without such limitations.

Breast cancer incidence increases with age and significant age-related disparities also appear to exist for both evidence-based and non-evidence-based cancer-screening interventions (Jerant et al. 2004). Women over the age of 70 have lower breast cancer screening rates than women aged 50–69 years, with 66.7% of women over 70 reporting being screened within the last 2 years versus 77.1% of women 50–69 and 78% of women 50–59 years of age (Peek and Han 2004), although, admittedly, considerable controversy currently exists about whether women over the age of 70 should be screened. Women over the age of 75 are less likely to have regular mammograms and never to have had a mammogram than younger women (Randolph et al. 2002). Women in their forties and those with lower relative incomes were also less likely than older women to undergo screening mammography (Kim and Jang 2008).

Whether or not sexual orientation is linked to screening disparities remains unclear, in part because there is currently little research in this area (Boehmer et al. 2005). In fact, the literature in general clearly indicates a dearth of research about disparities faced by lesbian and bisexual women with regard to breast cancer overall. What we do know is that lesbians and bisexual women have an estimated higher prevalence of risk factors for breast cancer compared with national estimates for women overall, although they report similar rates of mammography as well as rates of breast cancer histories (Cochran et al. 2001). In one study, African American, Hispanic, and Asian American lesbians had similar self-reported mammography screening rates to heterosexual African American, Hispanic, and Asian American women. However, African American and Hispanic lesbians were less likely to report having had a clinical breast exam than African American and Hispanic heterosexual women (Mays et al. 2002).

Although there are scant data about breast cancer disparities between immigrant and non-immigrant populations, it is clear that many immigrant women do not use breast cancer screening services. Specifically, immigrants are less likely than non-immigrants to report having had a mammogram in the past 2 years (Swan et al. 2003) and to having been diagnosed with early stage disease (Heeden and White 2001). Swan et al. (2003) found that immigrant women who had resided in the US for 10 years or more had higher mammography rates than women who had been in the US for less than 10 years. Further, Brown et al. (2006) also found that time spent in the US was associated with a greater number of mammograms and clinical breast exams. In another study using SEER data (1973–1994) to investigate the relationship between survival and place of birth among Asian Americans, Japanese women had significantly better breast cancer survival rates than Chinese, Filipino, or white women.

Diagnosis

In general, women from racial and ethnic minority groups are more likely to be diagnosed with later stage disease and larger tumors than their white counterparts. Studies show that black women are consistently diagnosed with more advanced breast cancer than other women (McCarthy et al. 1998; Strzelczyk and Dignan 2002). Additionally, in managed care and government sponsored settings where women have unrestricted access to care, women from minority groups are still found to have more advanced disease (Royak-Schaler et al. 2003; Li et al. 2003; Jacobellis and Cutter 2002). Uninsured women and women with Medicaid coverage tend to be diagnosed at more advanced stages of disease as well (Roetzheim et al. 1999).

Women with disabilities are also more likely to receive a later stage diagnosis. Specifically, an analysis of the 1991–1993 Medicare-SEER linked dataset found that women who qualified for Social Security Disability Insurance (SSDI) had later stage breast cancer at diagnosis compared with women of the same age who did not qualify for SSDI. Women who qualified for SSDI did not have higher breast cancer specific mortality rates, however, perhaps because they had more comorbidities and died from other causes. Nonetheless, women on SSDI and enrolled in a Medicare HMO were diagnosed at an earlier stage and had better survival than similar women in the Medicare fee-for-service program (Roetzheim and Chirikos 2002).

Education level correlates with the stage of diagnosis. Ward et al. (2008) noted the discrepancies in breast cancer screening behavior apparent both among people of different educational and insurance status. A higher proportion of individuals with less education tend to present with advanced stage compared to those with higher education. The same is true for blacks as well as whites, but the trend toward less distant disease stages associated with increasing levels of education is much more marked for whites than blacks (Merkin et al. 2002).

Treatment

Socioeconomic status, which overlaps with race, may influence quality of breast cancer treatment (Bradley et al. 2002). Researchers have documented, for example, that black women are less likely to receive breast conserving surgery (BCS) than white women (Newman 2005; Griggs et al. 2007), although many of these studies were conducted before BCS was widely practiced. Shavers and Brown (2002) summarize this literature and conclude that after controlling for clinical factors, black women are also less likely than white women to receive BCS and radiation, although rural black and white women have similar rates of BCS. Elderly black women are particularly at risk for not receiving BCS and radiation. After having BCS, black women and women from other racial and ethnic minority groups are less likely than whites to have radiation therapy (Shavers and Brown 2002; Mandelblatt et al. 2002). Black women are also less likely to receive chemotherapy and are more likely to receive lower chemotherapy dosage than their white counterparts (Banerjee et al. 2007; Griggs et al. 2003). Similarly, Asian Pacific Islander women are less likely to have BCS than whites and are less likely to receive radiation, even after controlling for demographics, health insurance, and other socioeconomic factors (Prehan et al. 2002).

In a more recent study, Banerjee et al. (2007) investigated racial disparities in breast cancer treatment by reviewing comprehensive medical records of women diagnosed with breast cancer at the Karmanos Cancer Institute (KCI) in Detroit, Michigan. The study consisted of 651 women who were diagnosed with primary breast cancer between 1990 and 1996. Multivariable logistic regression analysis controlling for sociodemographic factors, tumor characteristics, comorbidities, and health insurance status was used to assess differences between white and black women in their receipt of BCS, radiation, tamoxifen, and chemotherapy. The researchers found no differences in the receipt of BCS versus mastectomy. However, patients with localized disease enrolled in government insurance plans underwent mastectomy more often (versus BCS plus radiation) than did patients enrolled in non-governmental plans. Both white and black women with local-stage disease had similar rates of receipt of tamoxifen and chemotherapy. White women were, however, more likely to receive tamoxifen and/or chemotherapy for regional-stage disease. Further, married women with regional-stage disease were more likely to receive chemotherapy than unmarried women.

Meanwhile, varying research is emerging regarding disparities in breast cancer treatment for women with disabilities. One retrospective review of a relatively small sample of women with breast cancer and physical disabilities found statistically significant differences in prevalence of BCS or adjuvant chemotherapy between disabled and non-disabled women (Caban et al. 2002). Another study by McCarthy et al. (2006) found that women with SSDI and Medicare coverage had lower rates of BCS than other women. Also, among women who have BCS, women with SSDI and Medicare coverage were less likely than other women to receive radiotherapy. Women with SSDI and Medicare coverage, moreover, have lower survival rates than those of other women in all-cause mortality (McCarthy et al. 2006).

These findings have spurred significant research on appropriate treatment which depends on several clinical factors, including menopausal status, tumor size, stage, presence of tumor in auxiliary lymph nodes, and estrogen and progesterone receptor status. In the absence of some of this information, assessing the appropriateness of treatment is impossible, but, at the same time, the absence of this information is itself evidence of inadequate treatment.

Prevention

Awareness of factors related to the use of preventive practices is crucial to identify strategies to decrease cancer incidence and mortality. However, there are still few studies that examine the role of prevention in breast cancer disparities and even fewer studies that examine the influence of SES as it relates to prevention and relieving breast cancer disparities. The few studies that do exist, however, suggest that preventive screening and medical procedures are still associated with SES, including having medical coverage (Cabeza et al. 2007; Segman 1997). Differences in the prevalence of breast cancer risk factors by race or ethnicity raise the possibility of the role of prevention through risk factor modification (Bigby and Holmes 2005).

Reproductive factors such as earlier age at menarche and age at first full term pregnancy, higher parity, and lower rates of breast feeding among black women relative to white women may explain elevated breast cancer rates among black women under age 45 (Berstein et al. 2003). An earlier study by researchers

Forshee et al. (2003) describes the increased risk factors prevalent among black women (e.g., increased Body Mass Index (BMI), less physical activity, poor quality diet, and lower intake of folate and Vitamin A) and suggests interventions to assess primary prevention strategies. An earlier study of natural menopause, oral contraceptive use, and smoking show more complex differences between black and white women that may underlie disparities between them as well (Mayberry and Stoddard-Wright 1992). Moreover, preventing obesity could potentially diminish the tendency for African American women to present at a more advanced stage of breast cancer than white women. The higher prevalence of obesity among black women compared to white women, in fact, appears to explain approximately one-third of the black-white difference in stage at diagnosis (Berstein et al. 2003).

Emerging research has also surfaced regarding the use of tamoxifen and raloxifene in the role of breast cancer prevention (Powles 2008). Tamoxifen is licensed for use as a breast cancer risk reduction agent in the US, and raloxifene has also recently been approved by the FDA for such use. Tamoxifen can reduce the early incidence of breast cancer in pre- and postmenopausal women by about 40%, but causes vasomotor symptoms, thromboembolism, and gynecological toxicity, including uterine polyps, endometrial atypia, and (rarely) cancer. In long follow-up trials, the risk reduction for breast cancer extends beyond the treatment period to at least 15 years, and appears to get larger with time—which indicates a true long-term prevention effect. The toxicity of tamoxifen is confined to the treatment period. Raloxifene has breast cancer risk reduction activity similar to that of tamoxifen but less toxicity and no evidence of an increased risk of endometrial atypia or cancer. Studies document the influence of SES and the use of tamoxifen in treatment (see section on treatment, above), particularly among black and white women, but we still need more research to assess the influence of SES on the ability of these therapies to prevent breast cancer.

Other Factors Linked To Breast Cancer Disparities

Race alone cannot explain breast cancer outcomes, nor can it explain the disparities described above. Factors that contribute to higher death rates among black women, for example, include delayed diagnosis and differences in tumor biology, as well as confounding comorbidities and a variety of other socioeconomic conditions. Trends in incidence and mortality by race/ethnicity and SES suggest that some disparity is also due to differences in extrinsic behavioral influences, such as birthing rates and the use of hormone replacement therapy (Berry and Ravdin 2007). Other data suggest that differences in diet, obesity rates, and BMI influence both incidence and mortality of breast cancer.

Racial/Ethnic Pathological Differences

There are conflicting studies about whether disparities in breast cancer diagnosis might also be related to differences in tumor biology across racial or ethnic groups. Certain racial/ethnic differences in the pathology of breast cancer at diagnosis have been noted, including disproportionately higher grade disease in blacks than in whites with the same size tumor. These differences have been explored primarily among black and white women. Earlier comparative studies have found a higher incidence of poorly differentiated tumors, increased frequency of nuclear atypia, higher mitotic activity, an increased fraction of S-phase cells, and tumor necrosis in the breast cancers of black women (Chen et al. 1994). An earlier study, however, found no histologic differences among a small sample of white, black, and Asian women (Krieger et al. 1997). Among postmenopausal women, variations of standard tumor cell characteristics and breast cancer-specific survival via hormone receptor expression suggest several different phenotypes with overlapping etiologies and distinct clinical features (Anderson et al. 2001).

The proportion of black women with "triple negative" tumors is also higher than in whites. Triple negative tumors are cancers that are estrogen receptor negative (ER–), progesterone receptor negative (PR–), and human epidermal growth factor receptor-2 (her 2 neu) negative. Carey et al. (2006) studied breast cancer subtypes among a group of women diagnosed in the Carolina Breast Cancer Study (Newman et al. 1995) and found that 39% of pre-menopausal African American women had triple negative disease compared to 14% of postmenopausal African American women and 16% of non-African American women of any stage. ER+ and/or progesterone receptor-positive HER2– tumors were also less prevalent among pre-menopausal than in postmenopausal blacks, at 26% and 59%, respectively. This subtype was found in 54% of all non-blacks presenting with breast cancer. On the other hand, there were no racial differences found in the incidences of HER2+ cancers.

It is of note that the overall lower incidence of breast cancer for black women can almost entirely be explained by black women's lower incidence of ER+ tumors. Anderson et al. (2001) plotted incidence rates of breast cancer by race and markers. The incidence rates of triple negative tumors in black and white women are very similar. The incidence rates of ER+ tumors, however, are higher in white Americans. Therefore, the major reason that the proportion of triple negative tumors is lower in white women is because their denominator includes a higher number of ER+ tumors.

The lower proportion of ER– tumors in blacks is somewhat contrary to what would be predicted on the basis of known associations between estrogen and breast cancer risk. This is because elevated endogenous hormone levels— believed to be higher in postmenopausal black women than white American women on the basis of surrogate markers, such as high body mass index/obesity and increased bone mineral density—are associated with increased breast cancer risk and especially increased risk for developing ER+ postmenopausal breast cancer.

Whatever the explanation, the higher prevalence of triple negative tumors contributes to the poorer prognosis of young African American women with breast cancer (Carey et al. 2006). The role of SES in the black-white pathologic disparity has not been fully explored, although there has been some speculation about possible relationships. Middle class and upper middle-class women, for example, tend to have the habits or extrinsic influences associated with the development and diagnosis of less aggressive, better prognosis breast cancers. It may be that these habits portend to ER+, low grade, better prognosis breast cancers. The medical profession has been asking why a higher proportion of black women have more aggressive breast cancers, but the question we should be asking is "Why do white woman have more ER+/less aggressive cancers?"

Discrimination and Racism

There is a fast-growing body of research which suggests that racism and discrimination contributes to negative health outcomes (Clark and Harrell 1992; Harrell et al. 2003; James et al. 1987; Krieger 1990; Mays et al. 2007; Williams et al. 2003). Discrimination and racism influences health indirectly through its impact on social structures such as education, employment, and housing. Racism is itself a significant stressor for black and other women from racial or ethnic minority populations, with psychological, social, and physiological consequences. These psychological, social, and physiological consequences can potentially influence breast cancer risk, treatment outcomes, and survival. Some researchers have begun to explore these consequences of racism on breast cancer (Clark et al. 1999; Moore 2001). A few studies have examined the association of perceived racism on breast cancer treatment outcomes (Dailey et al. 2007; Taylor et al. 2007).

However, research along this vein is difficult to explore scientifically as it is challenging to get funding, some institutions are reluctant to take on potentially polarizing issues, and a lack of theoretical and analytic ingenuity has prevented earlier recognition of the role of discrimination and racism in eliminating health disparities (Drexler 2007; Karlsen and Nazroo 2002).

Health Care Access and Utilization

Socioeconomically disadvantaged individuals are far less likely to utilize the health care system (Henry J. Kaiser Family Health Foundation [KFF] 2007). Specifically, racial and ethnic minority Americans are less likely than whites to have a usual place to receive care or to have regular health care visits. For Hispanics, these differences persist even when accounting for income (KFF

2007). Immigrant status may also play a role. Research reveals a number of barriers to care experienced by immigrant women, for example, that may impede their utilization of health care services. Researchers (Lee-Lin et al. 2007; Remennick 2006) also found that structural barriers to these health care services for immigrants included socioeconomic factors such as poor or lack of health insurance, distance to medical facilities, and the inability to take time off work. Other specific barriers include differences in culture and knowledge, attitudes concerning acculturation and fatalism, and low English proficiency (De Alba et al. 2005).

One study (Deri 2005) found evidence that utilization of health services by immigrants increases with the number of doctors that speak their language in their neighborhood. For many immigrant women, moreover, breast cancer is shrouded in fears, myths, and connotations going beyond the clinical aspect of the disease. Immigrants who are not US citizens may be disproportionately affected by these barriers and may face additional challenges to access and the reception of appropriate health care compared to immigrants who have become US citizens (Carrasquillo et al. 2000). Previous studies have also shown that citizenship independently affects access to health insurance and is therefore an important determinant of health care disparities (Li et al. 2005). These barriers to health care access and utilization may contribute to delays in breast cancer diagnosis, treatment, and eventual higher mortality rates.

Insurance Status

Inadequate health insurance may impede health care utilization and thus underlie certain disparities. The uninsured, for example, are more likely to endure symptoms of disease for longer periods of time before presenting themselves for medical care (Halpern et al. 2008), so their diseases are less likely to be discovered in early stages. The insured, in contrast, are far more likely to seek earlier medical attention and thus to be diagnosed with early stage, and therefore treatable and curable, diseases. Women without insurance, in fact, have been found to increase their use of mammography after receiving Medicare (McWilliams et al. 2003), and most patients coded as having Medicaid actually have no insurance until diagnosis due to symptoms, which then gives them coverage. Despite some regional variations, elderly women in HMOs are generally diagnosed at earlier stages of breast cancer than women in fee-for-service settings, and they are more likely to have BCS and radiation as opposed to mastectomy or modified mastectomy (Riley et al. 1999). Whether these behaviors are influenced most by financial or insurance status per se remains unclear, however. This is because "poor" and "uninsured" are not synonymous terms: all persons who are uninsured are not poor, and all poor persons are not necessarily uninsured.

Additional studies document further disparities in survival by insurance status. The presentation of breast cancer and survival in women with no insurance and with Medicaid is significantly worse than those with private insurance (Ayanian et al.1993; Colburn et al. 2008; McDavid et al. 2003). Breast cancer patients of lower SES in general also tend to have poorer survival (Byers et al. 2008; Kaffashian et al. 2003). Moreover, in a study by Bradley et al. (2002) concluding that black women with breast cancer are more likely to die of their breast cancer disease than white women, the authors associated low SES with later stage breast cancer diagnosis, less adequate treatment, and a poorer prognosis.

Another study found that Hispanic women in an HMO had higher mammography screening rates than Hispanic women in fee-for-service plans, although no such advantage was seen for black or Asian women (Haas et al. 2002). Within node positive disease all treatment disadvantages among younger African American women disappeared with socioeconomic adjustment. The growth of this racial divide implicates social, rather than biological, forces in explaining disparities (Gorey et al. 2008).

Comorbid Disease

The poor tend to have more comorbid disease than their more affluent counterparts, complicating outcomes and making aggressive treatment more difficult to offer. The NCI black-white study of the early 1990s demonstrated that black breast cancer patients had disproportionately more comorbid diseases, such as hypertension, diabetes, and morbid obesity (Muss et al. 1992). Tammemagi (2007) assessed the breast cancer patients treated in one health system. They found that comorbidities (especially hypertension and diabetes) were responsible for nearly half of the overall survival disparities found in 264 black women and 642 white women with breast cancer over the course of a median of 10 years.

Health Communications

At least some of the disparities in treatment, as well as in health outcomes, may be related to variations in factors underlying treatment decisions that depend upon patients' receipt of accurate information and upon clear communication between the patient, doctors, and the family (Fallowfield 2008; Hawley et al. 2007; Roberts et al. 1994). More recent health communications research has begun to focus on drawing attention to inequalities in communication and how these inequalities may contribute to inequalities in health, linking social determinants explicitly with health outcomes (Viswanath et al. 2007).

As defined and explored in detail in Chapter 12 of this book, communication inequality is defined as the differences among social groups in their ability to generate, disseminate, and use information at the macro level and to access, process, and act on information at the individual level (Viswanath et al. 2007). These communication inequalities along with other factors such as cultural and language differences and SES also interact with and contribute to low health literacy, which in turn can hinder communication and adherence to medical advice (Shaw et al. 2008; Viswanath 2006). These factors potentially have important implications for breast cancer outcomes across the cancer continuum.

Communication barriers are particularly likely to affect recent immigrants and ethnic minorities, and may vary by sexual orientation as well. Here lesbians appear to be at particular risk. In one study, for example, Brown and Tracy (2008) found that barriers to adequate screening for breast and cervical cancers include personal factors, poor patient-provider communication, and heath care system factors. This research also revealed the success of tailored risk communication counseling in increasing lesbians' mammography and pap screening and a lack of research regarding this target group for a number of cancers.

Geography

Among the many socioeconomic factors that impact the incidence, mortality, screening, and survival rates of breast cancer, where one lives is key (Grann et al. 2006). The considerable geographic variation among older women, for example, strongly contributes to variation in breast cancer survival and mortality (Goodwin et al. 2002). Travel distance to breast cancer treatment centers and radiotherapy facilities is a challenge, and the time and expense may influence treatment not only for older women, but for black and poor women more so than for white women and middle-class women (Mandelblatt et al. 2002; Prehan et al. 2002; Shea et al. 2008).

The NCI SEER program has compared the cancer incidence, mortality, and 5-year survival data of Americans living in high-poverty ("low resource") areas to the incidence, mortality, and 5-year survival data of those living in non-impoverished areas (Jemal et al. 2008). A low resource area is defined as a county in which more than 20% of residents have family incomes below the US Federal Poverty Level. A high-resource area is defined a county in which less than 10% of residents have family incomes below the FPL. These data show that breast cancer incidence is generally higher among those living in wealthier areas, but mortality is generally 15–20% higher among those living in low resource areas. The 5-year survival rates were better for those in high-resource counties. Furthermore, a higher proportion of advanced-staged cancers were diagnosed among patients living in impoverished areas. These trends occurred irrespective of race: whites from impoverished areas had worse outcomes than whites from non-impoverished areas. These data demonstrate that socioeconomic factors rather than biologic differences significantly influence health status and outcomes. However, it is worth noting that minorities fare worse among the poorest Americans and within the most affluent communities (Ward 2008).

Women in rural settings also have lower mammography screening rates than women in urban settings (66.7% versus 75.4%). Among African American, American Indian, and Alaska Native rural women, women with less formal education and uninsured women have the lowest rates of screening in rural settings (Shea et al. 2008). There are also regional variations in screening among different racial and ethnic groups. Mexican American women have different screening rates depending on the states in which they reside (45% in Texas versus 60% in California) (Ramirez et al. 2000).

Internationally there are large differences in breast cancer occurrence as well. The lowest rates are found in most of Asia and Africa, where the occurrence is less than 25 cases a year for every 100,000 women. The highest rates are seen in North America, Western Europe, Australia, New Zealand, and in the southern part of South America. In these countries, the occurrence rates are more than 75 cases a year for every 100,000 women. The US and the Netherlands are the countries with the highest incidence of breast cancer, with rates as much as 5–8 times those reported for countries in parts of Asia and Africa.

Incidence rates for these other countries may not be directly comparable to those of the US because of large differences in both the tools for diagnosis and tumor reporting amongst different countries. Nonetheless, they can sometimes provide considerable insight into the American situation. For example, Scottish studies of disparities in breast cancer and SES are of interest and may illuminate American observations because the Scots have a rigorous "deprivation index" that distinguishes the poor from the non-poor, middle class, and wealthy. In Scotland, it has been noted that monetary deprivation is associated with a higher stage of cancer at diagnosis, and within-stage deprivation is associated with higher grade disease. This is to say that, even among women with early stage disease, poorer women are more likely to be diagnosed with high grade, ER–, while wealthier women are more likely to be diagnosed with lower grade, ER+ disease. The Scottish studies were done prior to the era of common her 2 neu testing, however, so they cannot be compared to the findings that black and white women in the US have similar her 2 neu despite an excess of ER– disease in black women (Elledge and Allred 1998; Stark et al. 2007).

Summary and Recommendations

While the full effects of SES or deprivation as an extrinsic influence on breast carcinogenesis have yet to be explored, socioeconomic factors in all probability contribute to a great deal of breast cancer disparities and affect breast cancer outcomes across the entire cancer continuum. These factors include many considerations beyond race and ethnicity. Although there are several racial and ethnic differences in incidence, mortality, survival, and treatment protocols, these differences do not explain fully why some groups suffer disproportionately more from breast cancer disparities than others. Regardless of race, poor persons are more likely to have more undesirable breast cancer outcomes, thus again shining the light on poverty, as well as on the devastating toll of a variety of often interrelated factors, including barriers to health care, lack of health insurance, and poor patient–physician communication.

At the same time, racial and ethnic disparities, primarily between blacks and whites, have received significant attention and are better documented than many other disparities, although there are still some gaps about their extent across the cancer continuum. As we go forward, more attention should focus on the interplay of other socioeconomic factors, in addition to race and ethnicity, which would then rightfully give attention to bring other socioeconomically deprived groups into the discussion as well.

Finally, a great deal of the research thus far has focused on screening, treatment, and survival. Much of this research is descriptive and has done very little to offer solutions for eliminating disparities. From this perspective, it is important to remember that SES is also confounded by other factors such as lifestyle, dietary, and cultural factors. To be sure, genetics will complicate the picture further. Considerable attention should be given to genetic ancestry and study designs that better measure SES in investigating breast cancer disparities. Moreover, as we are now in an era of personalized medicine and emerging technologies, understanding better the influence of SES on these new advancements and their relationship to breast cancer disparities will be critical. Finally, and most importantly, the beginning and end goal in reducing and eliminating breast cancer disparities is not to prove the influence of one particular type of factor but rather to achieve equal treatment and, ultimately, equal outcomes for all.

References

American Cancer Society. Breast cancer death rates continue to decline. ACS News Center. 2001. Available from: www.cancer.org/docroot/NWS/content. Accessed June 20, 2008.

Anderson, WF, Chu, KC, Chatterjee, N., Brawley, O., and Brinton, L.A. Tumor variants by hormone receptor expression in white patients with node-negative breast cancer from the surveillance, epidemiology, and end results database. J Clin Oncol. 2001; 19(1):18–17.

Ayanian, J., Kohler, B., Abe, R., and Epstein, A. The relation between health insurance and clinical outcomes among women with breast cancer. New Engl J Med 1993; 329(5):326–331.

Banerjee, M., George, J., Yee, C., Hryniuk, W., and Schwartz, K. Disentangling the effects of race on breast cancer treatment. Cancer. 2007; 110(10):2169–2177.

Baquet, C.R. and Commiskey, P. Socioeconomic factors and breast carcinoma in multicultural women. Cancer. 2000; 88(Suppl 5):1256–64.

Berry, D.A. and Ravdin, P.M. Breast cancer trends: A marriage between clinical trial evidence and epidemiology. J Nat Cancer Inst. 2007; 99(15):1139–1141.

Berstein, L., Teal, C.R., Joslyn, S., and Wilson, J. Ethnicity-related variation in breast cancer risk factors. Cancer. 2003; 97(Suppl 1):222–229.

Bigby, J., Ko, L.K., Johnson, N., David, M.M., and Ferrer, B. REACH Boston 2010 Breast and Cervical Cancer Coalition: a community approach to addressing breast and cervical cancer mortality among women of African descent in Boston. Pub Health Rep. 2003; 118(4):338–347.

Bigby, J. and Holmes, M. Disparities across the breast cancer continuum. Cancer Causes Control. 2005; 16(1):35–44.

Boehmer, U., Linde, R., and Freund, K.M. Sexual minority women's coping and Psychological adjustment after a diagnosis of breast cancer. J Womens Health. 2005; 14(3):214–224.

Bradley, Given, and Roberts. Race, socioeconomic status, and breast cancer treatment and survival. J Nat Cancer Inst. 2002; 94(7):490–496.

Britt, K., Ashworth, A., and Smalley, A. Pregnancy and the risk of breast cancer. Endocrine-Related Cancer. 2007; 14(4):907–933.

Brown, W.M., Consedine, N.S., and Magai, C. Time spent in the United States and breast cancer screening behaviors among ethnically diverse immigrant women: evidence for acculturation? J Immig Minority Health. 2006; 8(4):347–358.

Brown, J.P. and Tracy, J.K. Lesbians and cancer: an overlooked health disparity. Cancer Causes Control. 2008; 19(10):1009–1030.

Byers, T.E., Wolf, H., Bauer, K.R., Bolick-Aldrich, S., Chen, V., Finch, J.L., et al. The impact of socioeconomic status on survival after cancer in the United States: finds from the National Program of Cancer Registries Patterns of Care Study. 2008; 113(3):582–591.

Caban, M.E., Nosek, N.A., Graves, D., Esteva, F.J., and McNeese, M. Breast carcinoma treatment received by women with disabilities compared with women without disabilities. Am Cancer Soc. 2002; 94(5):1391–1396.

Cabeza, E., Esteva, M., Pujol, A., Thomas, V., and Canchez-Contador, C. Social disparities in breast and cervical cancer preventative practices. Eur J Cancer Prev. 2007; 16(4):372–379.

Carey, L., Perou, C.M., Livasy, C.A., Dressler, L.G., Cowan, D., Conway, K., et al. Race, breast cancer subtypes, and survival in the Carolina Breast Cancer Study. JAMA. 2006; 295(21):2492–2502.

Carrasquillo, O., Carrasquillo, A.I., and Shea, S. Health insurance coverage of immigrants living in the United States: Differences by citizenship status and country of origin, Am J Pub Health. 2000; 90(6):917–923.

Centers for Disease Control and Prevention. Use of mammograms among women aged > or = 40 years—United States, 2000–2005. MMWR. 2207; 56(3):49–51.

Chen, V.W., Correa, P., Kurman, R.J., et al. Histologic characteristics of breast cancer in blacks and whites. Cancer Epidem Biomarkers Prev. 1994; 3(2):127–135.

Clark, V.R., and Harrell, J.P. The relationship among Type A behavior, styles utilized in coping with racism and blood pressure. Reprint In: Burlew, K., Banks, C., McAdoo, H., and Azibo, D., eds. African American Psychology. Newbury Park, CA: Sage, 1992.

Clark, R., Anderson, N.B., Clark, V.R., et al. Racism as a stressor for African-Americans. Am Psychol. 1999; 54(10):805–816.

Clegg LX, Li FP, Hankey, B.F., Chu, K., and Edwards, B.K. Cancer survival among U.S. whites and minorities. Arch Int Med. 2002; 162(17):1985–1993.

Colburn, N., Fulton, J., Pearlman, D.N., Law, C., DiPaolo, B., and Cady, B. Treatment variation by insurance status for breast cancer patients. Breast J. 2008; 14(2):128–134.

Colditz, G.A., and Rosner, B. Cumulative risk of breast cancer to age 70 years according to risk factor status: data from the Nurses' Health Study. Am J Epidemiol. 2000; 152(10):950–964.

Colditz, G.A., Egan, K.M., and Stampfer, M.J. Hormone replacement therapy and risk of breast cancer: results from epidemiologic studies. Am J Obstet Gynecol. 1993; 168(5):1473–1480.

Cochran, S.D., Mays, V.M., Bowen, D., Gage, D., Bybee, D., Roberts, S.J., et al. Cancer-related risk indicators and preventive screening behaviors among lesbians and bisexual women. Am J Pub Health. 2001; 91(4):591–597.

Chu, K.C., Lamar, C.A., and Freeman, H.P. Racial disparities in breast cancer survival rates: separating factors that affect diagnosis from factors that affect treatment. Cancer. 2003; 97(11):2853–2860.

Chu, K.C., Miller, B.A., and Springfield, S.A. Measures of racial/ethnic health disparities in cancer mortality rates and the influence of socioeconomic status. J Nat Med Assoc. 2007; 99(10):1092-100-1102-4.

Cui, Y., Whiteman, M.K., Flaws, J.A., et al. Body mass and stage of breast cancer at diagnosis. Int J Cancer. 2002; 98(2):279–283.

Dailey, A.B., Kasi, S.V., Holfrod, T.R., Calvocoressi, L., and Jones, B.A. Neighborhood-level socioeconomic predictors of nonadherence to mammography screening guidelines. Cancer Epidem Biomarkers Prev. 2007; 16(11):2293–2303.

De Alba, I., Hubbel, F.A., McMullin, J.M., Sweningson, J.M., and Saitz, R. Impact of U.S. citizenship status on cancer screening among immigrant women. J Gen Int Med. 2005; 20:290–296.

Deri, C. Social networks and health service utilization. J Health Econom. 2005; 24(6):1076–1107.

Drexler, M. How Racism Hurts—Literally. Boston Globe. July 15, 2007, p. E1.

Eley, J.W., Hill, H.A., Chen, V.W., Austin, D.F., Wesley, M.N., Muss, H.B. et al. Racial differences in survival from breast cancer: results from the National Cancer Institute Black/White Survival Study. JAMA. 1994; 272 (12):947–954.

Emmons KM. Behavioral and social science contributions to the health of adults in the United States. In: Smedley BD, Syme SL, eds. Promoting Health: Intervention Strategies from Social and Behavioral Research. Washington, DC: National Academy Press, 2000, pp. 254–321.

Fallowfield, L.J. Treatment decision-making in breast cancer: The patient-doctor relationship, Breast Cancer Research and Treatment, [Epub ahead of print]. Available at: http://www.springerlink.com.ezp-prod1.hul.harvard.edu/content/ykm6528268w67u87/. Accessed 9-17-2008.

Forshee, R.A., Storey, M.L., and Ritenbaugh, C. Breast cancer risk and lifestyle differences among premenopausal and postmenopausal African-American women and white women. Cancer. 2003; 97(1Suppl):280–288.

Freeman, H.P. and Wasfie, T.J. Cancer of the breast in poor black women. Cancer. 1989; 63 (12): 2562–2569.

Gordon, N.H. Socioeconomic factors and breast cancer in black and white Americans, Cancer Metas Rev. 2003; 22(1):55–65.

Goodwin, P.J., Ennis, M., Pritchard, K.I., et al. Fasting insulin and outcome in early-stage breast cancer: results of a prospective cohort study. J Clin Oncol. 2002; 20(1):42–51.

Gorey, K.M., Luginaah, I.N., Schwartz, K.L., Fung, K.Y., Balagurusamy, M., Bartfay, E., et al. Increased racial differences on breast cancer care and survival in America: historical evidence consistent with a health insurance hypothesis, 1975–2001. Breast Cancer Res Treatment. 2008; 113(3):595–600.

Grann, V., Troxel, A.B., Zojwalla, N., Hershman, D., Glied, S.A., and Jacobson, J.S. Regional and racial disparities in breast cancer-specific mortality. Soc Sci Med. 2006; 62(2):337–347.

Griggs, J.J., Culakova, E., Sorbero, M.E., Poniewierski, M.S., Wolff, D.A., Crawford, J., et al. Social and racial differences in selection of breast cancer adjuvant chemotherapy Regimens. J Clini Oncol. 2007; 25 (18):2522–2527.

Griggs, J.J., Sorbero, M.E., Stark, A.T., et al. Racial disparity in the dose and dose intensity of breast cancer adjuvant chemotherapy. Breast Cancer Res Treat. 2003; 81(1):21–31.

Haas, J.S., Phillips, K.A., Sonneborn, D., McCulloch, C.E., and Liang, S.Y. Effect of managed care insurance on the use of preventive care for specific ethnic groups in the United States. Med Care. 2002; 40(9):743–751.

Halpern, M.T., Bian, J., Ward, E.M., Schrag, N.M., and Chen, A.Y. Insurance status and stage of cancer at diagnosis among women with breast cancer. Cancer. 2007; 110(2):403–411.

Harrell, J.P., Hall, S., and Taliaferro, J. Physiological responses to racism and discrimination: an assessment of the evidence. Am J Public Health. 2003; 93(2):243–248.

Halpern, M.T., Ward, E.M., Pavluck, A.L., Schrag, N.M., and Chen, B.J. Association of insurance status and ethnicity with cancer stage at diagnosis for 12 cancer sites: a retrospective analysis. Lancet Oncol. 2008; 9(3): 222–231.

Hawley, S.T., Lantz, P.M., Janz, N.K., Salem, B., Morrow, M., Schwartz, K., et al. Factors associated with patient involvement in surgical treatment decision making for breast cancer. Patient Educ Couns. 2007; 65(3):387–395.

Hedeen, A.N., and White, E. Breast cancer size and stage in Hispanic American women, by birthplace: 1992–1995. Am J Public Health. 2001; 91(1):122–125.

Hiatt, R.A. and Rimer, B.K. A new strategy for cancer control research, Cancer Epidem Biomarkers Prev. 1999; 8(11):957–964.

House, J.S., Kessler, R.C., Herzog, A.R., Kinney, A.M., Mero, R.P., and Breslow, M.F. Age, socioeconomic status, and health. Milbank Q. 1990; 68:383–411.

Huang, Z., Hankinson, S., Colditz, G., et al. Dual effects of weight and weight gain on breast cancer risk. JAMA. 1997; 278(17):1407–1411.

Institute of Medicine. Care without coverage: Too little, too late. Washington, DC: National Academy Press, 2002.

Israel, B.A., Krieger, J., Vlahov, D., Ciske, S., Foley, M., Fortin, P., et al. Challenges and facilitating factors in sustaining community-based participatory research partnerships: lessons learned from the Detroit, New York City and Seattle Urban Research Centers. J Urban Health. 2006; 83(6):1022–1040.

Jacobellis, J., and Cutter, G. Mammograpy screening and differences in stage of disease by race/ethnicity. Am J Public Health. 2002; 92(7):1144–1150.

James, S.A., Strogatz, D.S., Wing, S.B., and Ramsey, D.L. Socioeconomic status, John Henryism, and hypertension in blacks and whites. Am J Epidemiol. 1987; 126(4):664–673.

Jatoi, I, Becher, H, and Leake, C.R. Widening disparity in survival between white and African-American patients with breast carcinoma treated in the U.S. Department of Defense Healthcare system. Cancer. 2003; 98(5):894–899.

Jemal, A., Ward, E., and Thun, M.J. Recent trends in breast cancer incidence rates by age and tumor characteristics among U.S. women. Breast Cancer Res. 2007; 9(3):R28.

Jemal, A., Ward, E., Anderson, R.N., Murray, T., and Thun, M.J. Widening of socioeconomic inequalities in the U.S. death rates, 1993–2001. PLos ONE. 2008; 3(5):e2181.

Jerant, A.F., Franks, P., Jackson, J.E., and Doescher, M.P. Age-related disparities in cancer screening: analysis of 2001 behavioral risk factor surveillance system data. Ann Fam Med. 2004; 2(5):481–487.

Kaffashian, F., Godward, S., Davies, T., Solomon, L., McCann, J., and Duffy, S.W. Socioeconomic effects on breast cancer survival: proportion attributable to stage and morphology. Br J Cancer. 2003; 89(9):1693–1696.

Karlsen, S., and Nazroo, J.Y. Relation between racial discrimination, social class, and health among ethnic minority groups. Am J Public Health. 2002; 92(4):624–631.

Kaiser Family Foundation. Key Facts: Race, Ethnicity and Medical Care. Update Menlo Park, CA: The Henry J. Kaiser Family Foundation, 2007.

Kerner, J., Rimer, B., and Emmons, K. Introduction to the special section on dissemination. Dissemination research and research dissemination: how we close the gap. Health Psych. 2005; 24(5):443–446.

Kim, J. and Jang, S.N. Socioeconomic disparities in breast cancer screening among U.S. women: trends from 2000 to 2005. J Prev Med Pub Health. 2008; 41(3):186–194.

Krieger, N. Social class and the black/white crossover in the age-specific incidence of breast cancer: a study linking census-derived data to population-based registry records. Am J Epidemiol. 1990; 131(5):804–814.

Krieger, N., van den Eden, S.K., Zava, D., and Okamoto, A. Race/ethnicity, social class, and prevalence of breast cancer prognostic biomarkers: a study of white, black, and Asian women in the San Francisco Bay area. Ethnicity and Disease. 1997; 7(2):137–149.

Krieger, N., Emmons, K., and White, K.B. Cancer disparities: developing a multidisciplinary research agenda – practice. Cancer Causes Control. 2005; 16(1):1–3.

Kawachi, I. and Kennedy, B.P. Health and social cohesion: Why care about income inequality. BMJ. 1997; 314(7086):1037–1040.

Lee-Lin, F., Menon, U., Pett, M., Nail, L., Lee, S., and Mooney, K. Breast cancer beliefs and mammography screening practices among Chinese American immigrants. J Obstet Gynecol Neonatal Nurs. 2007; 36(3):212–221.

Li, A.K., Covinsky, K.E., Sands, L.P., Fortinsky, R.H., Counsell, S.R., and Landefeld, C.S. Reports of financial disability predict functional decline and death in older patients discharged from the hospital. J Gen Med. 2005; 20(2):168–174.

Li, C.L., Malone K.E., and Daling, J.R. Difference in breast cancer stage, treatment, and survival by race and ethnicity. Arch Int Med. 2003; 163(1):49–56.

Linos, E., Holmes, M., and Willett, W.C. Diet and breast cancer. Curr Oncol Rep. 2007; (1):31–41.

Linos, E. and Willett, W.C. Diet and breast cancer risk reduction, J Nat Comp Cancer Network. 2007; 5(8):711–718.

Mandelblatt, J., Kerner, J., Hadley, J., et al. Variations in breast cancer treatment in older, medicare beneficiaries: is it black or white? Cancer 2002; 95(7):1401–1414.

Marmot, M., Bobak, M., Davey Smith, G. Explanations for Social Inequalities in Health in Amick B, et al., eds. Society and Health. New York: Oxford University Press, 1995.

Mayberry, R.M. and Stoddard-Wright, C. Breast cancer risk factors among black women and white women: similarities and differences. Am J Epidem. 1992; 136(12):1445–1456.

Mays, V.M., Cochran, S.D., and Barnes, N.W. Race, race-based discrimination, and health outcomes among African Americans. Annu Rev Psychol. 2007; 58:201–225.

Mays, V.M., Yancey, A.K., Cochran, S.D., Weber, M., and Fielding, J.E. Heterogeneity of health disparities among African American, Hispanic, and Asian American women: unrecognized influences of sexual orientation, Am J Pub Health. 2002; 92(4):639–639.

McCarthy, E.P., Burns, R., Coughlin, S.S., et al. Mammography use helps to explain differences in breast cancer stage at diagnosis between older black and white women. Ann Int Med. 1998; 128(9):729–736.

McCarthy, E.P., Ngo, L.H., Roetzheim, R.G., Chirikos, T.N., Li, D., Drews, R.E., et al. Disparities in breast cancer treatment and survival for women with disabilities. Ann Int Med. 2006; 145(9):637–645.

McDavid, K., Tucker, T.C., Sloggett, A., and Coleman, M.P. Cancer survival in Kentucky and health insurance coverage. Arch Int Med. 2003; 163(18):2135–2144.

McWilliams, J.M,, Zaslavsky, A.M., Meara, E., and Ayanian, J.Z. Impact of medicare coverage on basic clinical services for previously uninsured adults. JAMA. 2003; 290(6):757–764.

Merkin, S.S., Stevenson, L., and Powe, N. Geographic socioeconomic status, race, and advanced stage breast cancer, Am J Pub Health. 2002; 92(1):64–70.

Minkler, M. Using participatory action research to build healthy communities. Pub Health Rep. 2000; 115(2–3):191–197.

Moore, R.J. African American women and breast cancer: notes from a study of narrative. Cancer Nurs. 2001; 24(1):35–42.

Muss, H.B., Hunter, C.P., Wesley, M., Correa, P., Chen, V.W., Greenberg, R.S., et al. Treatment plans for black and white women with stage II node-positive breast cancer. The National Cancer Institute Black/White Cancer Survival Study experience. Cancer. 1992; 70(10):2460–2470.

National Cancer Institute. Eliminating the Suffering and Death Due to Cancer. Bethesda, MD: U.S. Department of Health and Human Services. April 2006. NIH Publication No. 05-5498, Available at: http://www.cancer.gov/ncancerbulletin/NCI_Cancer_Bulletin_041806.pdf. Accessed May 30, 2008.

National Research Council. Preparing for an Aging World: The Case for Cross-National Research. Washington, DC: National Academy Press, 2001.

Newman, L.A., Mason, J., Cote, D., Vin, Y., Carolin, K., Bouwman, D., et al. African-American ethnicity, socioeconomic status and breast cancer survival. Cancer. 2002; 94(11):2844–2854.

Newman, B., Moorman, P.G., Millikan, R., et al. The Carolina Breast Cancer study: integrating population based epidemiology and molecular biology. Breast Cancer Res Treat. 1995; 35:51–60.

Newman, L.A. Breast cancer in African-American women. Oncologist. 2005; 10:1–14.

Newman, L.A. and Martin, I.K. Disparities in breast cancer. Curr Prob Cancer. 2007; 31(3):134–156.

Nosek, M.A. and Howland, C.A. Breast and cervical cancer screening among women with physical disabilities. Arch Phys Med Rehab. 1997; 78(1Suppl 5):S39–S44.

Peek, M.E., and Han, J.H. Disparities in screening mammography. Current status, interventions, and implications. J Gen Intern Med. 2004; 19:184–194.

Petrelli, J.M., Calle, E.E., Rodriguez, C., et al. Body mass index, height, and postmenopausal breast cancer mortality in a prospective cohort of US women. Cancer Causes Control. 2002; 13(4):325–332.

Powles, T.J. Prevention of breast cancer using SERMs. Adv Exp Med Bio. 2008; 620:232–236.

Prehan, A.W., Topol, B., Stewart, S., Glasic, S.L., O'Connor, L., and West, D.W. Differences in treatment patterns for local breast cancer among Asian/Pacific Islander women. Cancer. 2002; 95(11):2268–2275.

Preston, S.H. and Taubman, P. Socioeconomic differences in adult mortality and health status. In: Martin LG, Preston SH, eds. Demography of Aging. Washington, DC: National Academic Press, 1994, pp. 279–318.

Ramirez, A.G., Talavera, G.A., Villarreal, R., et al. Breast cancer screening in regional Hispanic populations. Health Educ Res. 2000; 15(5):559–568.

Randolph, W.M., Goodwin, J.S, Mahnken, J.D, and Freemna, J.L. Regular mammogram use is associated with elimination of age related disparities in size and stage of breast cancer. Ann Int Med. 2002; 137(10):783–790.

Remennick, L. The challenge of early breast cancer detection among immigrant and minority women in multicultural societies. Breast J. 2006; 12(S1):S104.

Riley, G.F., Potosky, A.L., Klabunde, C.N., Warren, J.L., and Ballard-Barbarsh, R. Stage at diagnosis and treatment patterns among older women with breast cancer: an HMO and fee-for-service comparison. JAMA. 1999; 281(8):720–726.

Roberts, C.S., Cox, C.E., Reintgen, D.S., Baile, W.F., and Gibertini, M. Influence of physician communication on newly diagnosed breast patients' psychologic adjustment and decision-making. Cancer. 1994; 74(1 Suppl):336–341.

Roetzheim, R.G., and Chirikos, T.N. Breast cancer detection and outcomes in a disability beneficiary population. J Health Care Poor Underserved. 2002; 13(4):461–476.

Roetzheim, R.G., Pal, N., Tennant, C., Voti, L., Ayanian, J.Z., and Schwabe, A. Effects of health insurance and race on early detection of cancer. J Nat Cancer Inst. 1999; 91(16):1409–1415.

Royak-Schaler, R., Chen, S., Zang, E., Vivacqua, R.J., and Bynoe, M. Does access to screening through health maintenance organization membership translate into improved breast cancer outcomes for African American patients? J Am Med Women's Assoc. 2003; 58(3):154–156.

Rubin, C.H., Burnett, C.A., Halperin, W.E., and Seligman, P.J. Occupation as a risk identifier for breast cancer, Am J Pub Health. 1993; 83(9):1311–1315.

Segman, N. Socioeconomic status and cancer screening. IARC-Sci-Publ. 1997; 138:412.

Shavers, V.L., and Brown, M.L. Racial and ethnic disparities in the receipt of cancer treatment. J Natl Cancer Instit. 2002; 94(5):334–357.

Shaw, S.J., Huebner, C., Armin, J., Orzech, K., and Vivan, J. The role of culture in health literacy and chronic disease screening and management. J Immig Min Health. 2008. [Epub ahead of print]. Available at: http://www.springerlink.com.ezp-prod1.hul.harvard.edu/content/x03720m20857mm86/. Accessed 9-17-2008.

Shea, A.M., Curtis, L.H., Hammill, B.G., DiMartino, L.D., Abernethy, A.P., and Schulman, K.A. Association between the Medicare Modernization Act of 2003 and patient wait times and travel distance for chemotherapy. JAMA. 2008; 300(2):189–196.

Schootman, M. and Jeffe, D.B. Identifying factors associated with disability-related differences in breast cancer screening (United States). Cancer Causes Control. 2003; 14(2):97–107.

Stark, A.M., Anuszkiewicz, B., Mentlein, R., et al. Differential expression of matrix metalloproteinases in brain- and boneseeking clones of metastatic MDA-MB-231 breast cancer cells. J Neurooncol. 2007; 81(1):39–48.

Strzelczyk J.J. and Dignan, M.B. Disparities in adherence to recommended follow-up on screening mammography: interaction of sociodemographic factors. Ethn Dis. 2002; 12(1):77–86.

Swan, J., Breen, N., Coates, R.J., Rimer, B.K., and Lee, N.C. Progress in cancer screening practices in the United States: Results from the 2000 National Health Interview Survey. Cancer. 2003; 97(6):1528–1540.

Tammemagi, C.M. Racial/ethnic disparities in breast and gynecologic cancer treatment and outcomes. Curr Opin Obstet Gynecol. 2007; 19(1):31–36.

Taylor, T.R., Williams, C.D., Makambi, K.H., Mouton, C., Harrell, J.P., Cozier, Y., et al. Racial discrimination and breast cancer incidence in U.S. Black women: The Black Women's Health Study. Am J Epidem. 2007; 166(1):46–54.

United States Government Accountability Office. Mammography: Current National Capacity is Adequate, but Access Problems May Exist in Certain Locations. Government Accountability Office, 2006.

Vainshtein, J. Disparities in breast cancer incidence across racial/ethnic strata and socioeconomic status: a systematic review. J Nat Med Assoc. 2008; 100(7):833–839.

Viswanath, K. Public communication and its role in reducing and eliminating health disparities. In: Thompson, G., Mitchell, F., and Williams, M., eds. Examining the Health Disparities Research Plan of the National Institutes of Health: Unflnished Business. Washington, DC: National Academies Press, 2006.

Viswanath, K., Ramanadhan, S., and Kontos, E.Z. Mass media and population health: a macrosocial view. In: Galea, S.E., ed. Macrosocial Determinants of Population Health. New York: Springer, 2007.

Ward, E., Halpern, M., Schrag, N., Cokkinides, V., DeSantis, C., Bandi, P., and Siegel, R. Association of insurance with cancer care utilization and outcomes. CA Cancer J Clin. January–February 2008; 58(1):9–31.

Williams, D.R., Neighbors, H.W., and Jackson, J.S. Racial/ethnic discrimination and health: findings from community studies. Am J Pub Health. 2003; 93(2):200–2008.

Chapter 7
Disparities and Colorectal Cancer

Eric C. Schneider

Colorectal cancer (CRC) is the third most common cancer of both men and women in the US. In 2007, an estimated 153,760 men and women received a diagnosis of colon or rectal cancer, and 52,180 individuals died of the disease (Cancer of the Colon and Rectum 2007). Substantial literature documents that both the US incidence of CRC and mortality rates from the disease are not evenly distributed throughout the general population but vary by age, gender, race, ethnicity, educational attainment, income, and geography. Other factors, such as lacking health insurance, have also been associated with increased mortality from CRC.

Many explanations potentially underlie these differences. Variations in the incidence and mortality of any disease can be thought of as the product of a complex interplay of numerous factors including biology, environment, social and economic status, personal behavior, and access to health care (Schroeder 2007). Analyses that attempt to apportion the relative contribution of each of these factors to the variation in the incidence and mortality of CRC are complicated by the fact that many of them correlate with, and may also influence, one another. For example, environmental exposures may be determined by economic factors that drive an individual's choice of residence or occupation. Similarly, some environmental exposures, such as smoking, may be determined by both social factors and personal behavior. The impact of these other factors can be modified by the success or failure of the health care system in prevention, diagnosis, and treatment. However, economic factors such as having or lacking health insurance may also play a critical role in defining whether an individual has the opportunity to prevent cancer, detect it early, receive successful treatment, and experience favorable health outcomes.

This chapter aims to describe the factors that are thought to influence the incidence, morbidity, and mortality of CRC in the US. It reviews accumulated evidence on key social and economic factors, placing them within a "cancer continuum" that encompasses all of the relevant phases of CRC, from primary

E.C. Schneider, M.D. (✉)
Harvard School of Public Health, Boston, MA 02115, USA
e-mail: eschneid@hsph.harvard.edu

H.K. Koh (ed.), *Toward the Elimination of Cancer Disparities*,
DOI 10.1007/978-0-387-89443-0_7, © Springer Science+Business Media, LLC 2009

prevention to screening, diagnosis, treatment, survivorship, and mortality. The chapter also offers a framework for understanding the interactions among key social and economic factors that may be useful to those seeking to design effective cancer control strategies.

Disparities in Colorectal Cancer Incidence and Survival

Both incidence and mortality of CRC vary among specific segments of the population (Palmer and Schneider 2005). Chapter 2 of this book addresses some of these trends. Mortality related to CRC has been declining since the 1970s, a change widely attributed to earlier detection and more effective treatment of the disease. Incidence rates have also been falling since the 1980s, presumably also because of early detection and removal of precancerous lesions and perhaps because of changes in lifestyle (Irby et al. 2006). Nevertheless, the favorable trends observed for the population overall appear to mask an increase in disparities among groups defined by characteristics such as age, gender, race/ethnicity, and socioeconomic position (SEP).

Age

Older age is a well-established risk factor for CRC (Fairley et al. 2006). In the US, the median age of death due to CRC is 75 years, and the age-adjusted incidence of CRC is 185.6 per 100,000 (compared to 6.0 per 100,000 individuals under age 50). However, while only 8.5% of CRCs are diagnosed in individuals under 50, the incidence of CRC is increasing among individuals in this age category (Fairley et al. 2006; Pine et al. 2007). Furthermore, the features of CRC appear to differ between those under and those over age 50: individuals under age 50 diagnosed with colon cancer are more likely than those over 50 to have a rectal cancer (37% vs. 26.2%), less likely to have a proximal colon cancer (32.1% vs. 42.6%), more likely to have distant metastases (21.9% vs. 16.0%) and more likely to have poorly differentiated tumors (18.4% vs. 16.3%). Some aspect of these age-related differences may stem from genetic abnormalities such as familial adenomatous polyposis (FAP) or hereditary non-polyposis colorectal cancer (HNPCC) that cause cancer to manifest at an earlier age.

Gender

Colorectal cancer incidence and mortality also vary considerably by gender, with men more likely than women to receive a diagnosis of CRC (Cheng et al. 2001). For example, between 2000 and 2004, the age-adjusted incidence of CRC was 60.8 per 100,000 men, compared to 44.6 per 100,000 women (Cancer of the Colon and Rectum 2007). While the age-adjusted mortality rate is 19.4 per 100,000 overall, the mortality rate is higher among men (23.5 per 100,000) than among women (16.4 per 100,000). These differing rates might be related to differing degrees of disease severity at diagnosis, although the two studies thus far that examined the relationship between stage of diagnosis and gender had conflicting results. One study suggested that after adjustment, women were more likely to have a late-stage diagnosis than men while a later study suggested that a slightly larger percentage of CRCs involved distant metastases in men (18.2%) than in women (17.4%) (Mandelblatt et al. 1996).

Race/Ethnicity

Numerous studies have documented differences in the incidence and mortality of cancer related to race and ethnicity (Polite et al. 2006; Irby et al. 2006; Fairley et al. 2006; Albano et al. 2007; Chien et al. 2005; Chu et al. 2007; Kandula et al. 2006; Polite et al. 2005). Most of the studies, however, are based on census data definitions of race or equivalent classification systems. As such, in classifying individuals, they generally do not distinguish between race and ethnicity (Sequist and Schneider 2006).

Most studies have examined black-white disparities in CRC incidence and mortality. A sizable body of literature indicates that compared to whites, blacks have a higher incidence of CRC, are more likely to be diagnosed with an advanced stage of disease, and have shorter survival even after controlling for health insurance and other sociodemographic characteristics (Krieger et al. 1999; Doubeni et al. 2007). Between 2000 and 2004, for example, white men had a CRC incidence rate of 60.4 per 100,000 compared to 72.6 per 100,000 in black men (see also Chapter 2 of this book). For white women, the incidence was 44.0 per 100,000, while for black women the incidence was 55.0 per 100,000 (Cancer of the Colon and Rectum 2007; Doubeni 2007). In contrast, Hispanic men had an age-adjusted incidence rate of 47.5 per 100,000, and Hispanic women had the lowest age-adjusted incidence rate of all groups at 32.9 per 100,000 (Cancer of the Colon and Rectum 2007). Blacks and whites also have 5-year relative survival rates after CRC diagnosis of 65% and 55%, respectively (Polite et al. 2006). Between 1992 and 2002, moreover, mortality from CRC declined 1.9% per year for whites but only 0.8% per year for blacks.

Stage at diagnosis may be the most important contributor to the black-white disparity in CRC mortality, though it does not seem to explain all of the disparity (Mayberry et al. 1995; Marcella and Miller 2001). Although blacks have a higher incidence of CRC, one study concluded that blacks have a more favorable tumor histology than whites (Chen et al. 1997). However, blacks also present at a younger age, and the younger black cohort seems to have a higher mortality compared to their white counterparts, suggesting both racial and age-related heterogeneity in the biological characteristics of tumors (Polite et al. 2005).

In contrast, a much more limited literature on CRC disparities for other racial/ethnic groups suggest that Asians and Pacific Islanders have better survival rates than their white counterparts, although this finding is controversial. Other racial and ethnic groups are difficult to study because of their relatively small numbers in the US and also because of their sociodemographic and economic heterogeneity. To complicate matters further, many of these populations may contain larger proportions of recent immigrants who may be healthier on average because of the so-called "healthy immigrant" effect—a well-known form of selection bias. A study using Surveillance Epidemiology and End Results (SEER) registry data demonstrated considerable heterogeneity among ethnic subgroups with a higher probability of advanced stage colon cancer at diagnosis among Filipinos, Hawaiians, and Mexicans compared to other ethnic subgroups (Chien et al. 2005). Disentangling the effects of race/ethnicity from other factors in these populations may be especially difficult.

Socioeconomic Position

Socioeconomic position (SEP) is a construct used to encompass educational attainment, occupation, income, and other cultural factors that influence access to resources, including health insurance and health care. Investigators have used varying approaches to define and measure SEP (Braveman 2006). For example, geographic location can be used as a proxy variable for assessing patterns of social deprivation (Subramanian 2006). Despite these variable approaches, a consistent pattern emerges across studies of CRC in which lower SEP (however defined and measured) is associated with a higher incidence of CRC and higher mortality due to the disease (Krieger et al. 1999; Marcella and Miller 2001). More recent studies, using more detailed data and advanced statistical techniques, suggest that SEP is an independent predictor of both stage at diagnosis and survival (Mandelblatt et al. 1996; Albano et al. 2007; Chu et al. 2007; Du et al. 2007; Ward et al. 2004; Schwartz et al. 2003). SEP may be an important mediator of the black-white racial disparities observed by other investigators even though it does not fully explain them (Polite et al. 2006; Mayberry et al. 1995; Marcella and Miller 2001; Du et al. 2007). In the US, health insurance is probably one important mediator of the effects of low SEP. Individuals lacking adequate health insurance are diagnosed with later stages of disease and have an increased mortality risk compared to insured individuals (Mayberry et al. 1995; Kelz et al. 2004; Rogers et al. 2004; McDavid et al. 2003).

Other Factors

Many other factors thought to be related to disparities in health care, including primary language, information literacy, disability, and immigration status may also be associated with the incidence of CRC and mortality from the disease.

However, few studies have evaluated the relationship between CRC and these other factors in detail. Three studies examining the incidence of CRC among Asian and South Asian migrants to the US found that the first-generation immigrant populations have a relatively lower incidence of CRC, though the next acculturated generation experiences a higher incidence rate (Le Marchand et al. 1997; Flood et al. 2000; Blesch et al. 1999). Other immigrant groups have not been well studied. Findings from the few existing studies are an important basis for the assertion that CRC risk is related to environmental or dietary factors rather than ethnic origin.

Geographic location is associated with the incidence of CRC and a higher case-fatality rate (Ries et al. 2000; Cooper et al. 1997). In general, the largest disparity is seen between rural and urban environments, with rural residence conferring a higher risk of death from the disease. The risk appears to vary even among small geographic areas. One study uncovered geographic variation in CRC mortality among counties in Texas with the greatest excess mortality in the urban areas of Houston and Dallas, but with racial/ethnic disparities in excess mortality occurring in a different set of counties (Hsu et al. 2006). Similarly, studies using ZIP codes or census tract data have shown that individuals living in ZIP codes or census tracts with lower income on average experience a greater incidence of CRC (Krieger et al. 1999).

Explaining Observed Disparities in Colorectal Cancer Incidence and Survival

Given the evidence establishing social disparities in the incidence and mortality of CRC, an important next step is to understand the causal contributing factors. Five key categories of contributing factors have to be considered in trying to understand disparities in CRC: (1) disease or tumor biology, (2) environmental exposure, (3) personal behavior, (4) screening and detection, and (5) treatment and follow-up after diagnosis. Factors in the first three categories have a bearing on disparities in the risk of acquiring the disease. All of the categories have a bearing on the subsequent survival experience and mortality outcomes following a diagnosis of CRC.

Disease Biology

A variety of evidence suggests that differences in host and tumor biology could be important contributing factors to disparities. First, the observation that disease incidence and mortality differ among individuals of different ages, between men and women, and across ethnic populations provides suggestive evidence of an underlying biological explanation. Some research studies have suggested that tumor histology varies among populations. Others have noted poorer survival without accompanying differences in tumor histology (Polite et al. 2005).

Some of the genetic risk factors for CRC are also becoming clearer. For example, Jews of Eastern European descent (i.e., Ashkenazi Jews) have the highest CRC risk of any ethnic group in the world. Several genetic mutations may increase the risk of CRC in this group. The most common DNA change, I1307K APC mutation, occurs in about 6% of American Jews and may occur in 10% of CRCs in Jews of Eastern European descent (Syngal et al. 2000). However, the genetic mutations discovered so far do not fully account for the increased number of CRCs in Ashkenazi Jews.

Based on current knowledge, a number of problems arise in trying to ascribe observed sociodemographic variations in the incidence and mortality of CRC to biological mechanisms. First, it can be difficult to isolate genetic predictors of disease activity from the influence of social factors if there is geographic and economic segregation of ethnic subpopulations on the scale that exists within the US and many other countries. To the extent that putative biological factors (such as age and genetic makeup) are correlated with social factors (such as income, education, diet, environmental exposures), epidemiologic studies overestimate the genetic contribution to disparities in disease outcomes, especially in the absence of statistical adjustment or careful stratification. It is conceivable that variation in genetic predisposition may play a minor role relative to the influence of environment, social factors, personal behavior, and treatment patterns as described in the sections that follow.

Environmental Exposures

As noted earlier, immigrants who migrate from areas of low CRC risk experience an increase in CRC risk after moving to a country with a higher rate of the cancer. These recent immigrants do not attain the same rate of CRC as others living in the same area; however, their descendants, second-generation immigrants, appear to have a higher risk, attaining rates of CRC comparable to those of non-immigrant populations living in the same geographic area. Presumably, this change in risk is associated with some sort of dietary change. Evidence about increased CRC risk among individuals living in rural settings (as opposed to more urbanized settings) also supports the notion that environmental exposure can play a role. Nevertheless the evidence for environmental exposure is indirect. Based on epidemiologic evidence, no clear linkages have been established between CRC risk and environmental exposure to specific chemicals or disease pathogens. Rather, the evidence related to migrant populations seems to point to behavioral factors such as dietary practices and tobacco and alcohol use as plausible explanations for geographically based differences in the risk and incidence of CRC.

Personal Behaviors

In addition to biological and environmental factors, a substantial literature indicates a link between the risk of developing CRC and a range of personal behaviors including dietary composition, physical inactivity, and the use of alcohol and tobacco, as well as comorbid clinical conditions such as obesity and diabetes (Gatof and Ahnen 2002). The notion that such factors vary among populations raises the enticing possibility that disparities in CRC incidence might be the result of personal behavioral differences among subpopulations. However, the extent to which differences in personal behaviors and comorbid conditions among populations can explain age, gender, racial/ethnic, and SEP-related disparities in CRC incidence and mortality is not well documented.

Diet seems to play an especially important role in the risk for CRC. Dietary factors that increase risk include foods that are high in fats from animal sources and low in vegetables and fruits. Red meats and processed meats appear to confer a special risk. Heavy alcohol use is an independent risk factor for CRC, perhaps because it depletes protective folate stores. Obesity and physical inactivity appear to contribute independently to the risk of CRC as well. In a related finding, people with diabetes appear to be at greater risk of developing CRC and are more likely than non-diabetic individuals to die if they develop the disease. The current recommendations from the American Cancer Society reflect the emphasis on diet and obesity, advising individuals to eat at least five servings of fruits and vegetables every day and several servings of other foods from plant sources, such as breads, cereals, grain products, rice, pasta, or beans (Can Colorectal Cancer Be Prevented? 2008).

As with other cancers, smoking is also a leading risk factor for CRC. It has been estimated that smokers are 30–40% more likely to die from CRC than non-smokers and that up to 12% of CRC deaths are attributable to smoking. This risk is presumably related to the carcinogens that are ingested by smokers and either transported directly through the gut lumen or absorbed and circulated through the bloodstream (Gatof and Ahnen 2002).

While these behavioral risk factors and related comorbidities are associated with disparities in CRC incidence and mortality, they are also associated with SEP, environment, and the receipt of both screening services and treatment. For example, women who are overweight are less likely to receive CRC screening than men or non-overweight women, and this may increase the likelihood that an obese woman receives a late-stage diagnosis (Rosen and Schneider 2004). Hence, dietary patterns that produce obesity may affect CRC outcomes through pathways other than direct nutritional affects.

Colorectal Cancer Screening

Colorectal cancer (CRC) screening for precancerous polyps and early stage cancer is a highly effective detection and prevention strategy. Because cancer can be detected at an earlier stage or prevented altogether if detected at the precancerous stage, colorectal screening has a favorable cost-effectiveness compared with other preventive services (Frazier et al. 2001; Sonnenberg and Delco 2002; Pignone et al. 2002; Maciosek et al. 2006; Maciosek et al. 2006). Nevertheless, rates of CRC screening have lagged behind rates of prostate screening, for which the evidence of effectiveness is less compelling (Sirovich et al. 2003). Unlike prostate cancer screening, which involves a blood test, CRC screening can involve any of four screening tests: annual fecal occult blood testing (FOBT) with a home test kit, sigmoidoscopy every 5 years, colonoscopy every 10 years, and "air-" or "double"-contrast barium enema (DCBE) every 5 years. In the US, colonoscopy, which allows full visualization of the colon, has become the preferred screening strategy in recent years.

Because of the importance of CRC screening as a prevention strategy, a substantial number of research studies have examined disparities in screening as a potential contributor to overall disparities in incidence and mortality of CRC. These studies have focused on differences in screening based on age, gender, race, ethnicity, and insurance status, Evidence on each is summarized below. However, an important problem with current studies is that CRC screening rates are still low in general, even under ideal circumstances and there are many barriers to population screening (Seeff et al. 2004). Effective CRC screening is a complex and potentially costly undertaking that can require comprehensive organizational systems such as reminders and outreach programs. Insurance is also a potential barrier. Medicare beneficiaries at average risk for colon cancer who lacked supplemental insurance did not gain insurance coverage for invasive and more costly CRC screening procedures until 2003. Thus the special complexity of CRC screening, its costliness, and variability in insurance coverage may all contribute to disparities in the population effectiveness of screening. Screening efficacy, in turn, appears to influence the likelihood of CRC being detected at an early stage or of precursor polyps being removed, both of which prevent CRC (Gross et al. 2006).

Age. A number of studies have examined the relationship between age and CRC screening (Seeff et al. 2004; MMWR 2003, 2007; Cooper and Payes 2005; Koroukian et al. 2006; Meissner et al. 2006; Sewitch et al. 2007; Wee et al. 2005). There are remarkably few studies of CRC screening for individuals over the age of 80 in spite of epidemiological evidence that the risk and incidence of CRC increases markedly with age. At the younger end of the age spectrum, studies have reported underutilization of screening in persons under the age of 64 relative to those who are 65–80 years of age.

Gender. Women are less likely than men to report colorectal screening, but disparities between men and women in colorectal screening rates are small (Rosen and Schneider 2004; Seeff et al. 2004; Meissner et al. 2006; Christie et al. 2005; McMahon et al. 1999; O'Malley et al. 2005). A study based on claims data analysis found little difference in screening rates, but did find that screening was higher among women less than 60 years of age compared to women over 60, suggesting that the gender disparity may be age-specific (Callcut et al. 2006). Questions remain about the reliability of self-reported screening compared to other assessments (Byers et al. 1997).

Race/ethnicity. Early studies based on self-report suggested that rates of CRC screening might be relatively similar between blacks and whites, but lower among Hispanics than whites and relatively low overall (MMWR 2003). However, the finding that black patients present with more advanced disease suggests that screening patterns may differ between races/ethnicities (Mandelblatt et al. 1996). More recent studies suggest the existence of racial/ethnic disparities in screening (Seeff et al. 2004; Swan et al. 2003; Klabunde et al. 2006; Ananthakrishnan et al. 2007; James 2006). A large survey of California residents concluded that many racial/ethnic minority groups have lower rates of screening than whites (Kandula et al. 2006).

Studies are beginning to identify what mediates these disparities, revealing that failure to communicate key health messages and differences in physician counseling and recommendation of screening may account for a large part of racial/ethnic disparities (Kandula et al. 2006; Wee et al. 2005; Fiscella and Holt 2007; Bao et al. 2007; Ponce et al. 2005; Morales et al. 2004; Rao et al. 2004; Goel et al. 2003; Shokar et al. 2007; Wong et al. 2005). Disparities also may be larger in specific geographic locations (such as those in areas with fewer available gastroenterologists or where transportation is not as readily available) suggesting that some delivery systems may face special challenges (Zhao et al. 2006). Finally, race-related differences in the epidemiology of colon cancer have led to a recommendation that screening of black individuals begin at an age earlier than 50 years for this population. Whether this recommendation is routinely followed is not yet clear.

Insurance Status. Research on the role of insurance status has clearly established the relationship between health insurance and CRC screening (Koroukian et al. 2006; Roetzheim et al. 1999, 2000). Increasing the availability of coverage within the Medicare program appears to have had an impact on screening and detection of colon cancer (Gross et al. 2006). However, differences in insurance status or insurance coverage do not appear to explain many of the other sociodemographic disparities in CRC screening, particularly those related to race/ethnicity (Seeff et al. 2004; McMahon et al. 1999; O'Malley et al. 2005; Klabunde et al. 2006; Shih et al. 2006).

Two areas related to screening that have not yet been extensively studied—but that may have relevance to disparities in outcomes—are the quality and effectiveness of the screening tests themselves and the reliability of follow-up of abnormal test results (e.g., positive hemoccult results). As screening becomes more routinely available and uptake increases, both of these issues may become important considerations in evaluating the contribution of screening to overall disparities in the incidence and mortality of CRC. For example, poorly performed colonoscopy and failure to notify patients of abnormal test results may occur more frequently in communities with lower SEP.

Colorectal Cancer Treatment Quality

Observed disparities in survival after diagnosis with colon cancer naturally raise questions about whether disparities in treatment might contribute to disparities in outcomes. In fact, disparities in the quality of colon cancer treatment may take many forms. Physicians may fail to offer potentially beneficial treatments. Patients may refuse offered treatments because of miscommunication or mistrust. Physicians and surgeons may deliver treatments in a substandard manner (e.g., poor quality surgical care or inadequate dosing of chemotherapy and radiation). Finally, patients may fail to receive the full course of sustained treatments like chemotherapy and radiation because of associated toxicities or other issues. On the other hand, while published studies suggest that treatment disparities for colon cancer exist, they are inconclusive about whether these disparities contribute meaningfully to differences in survival and mortality.

Age. Studies of the impact of age on treatment suggest that the rates of adjuvant chemotherapy treatment are relatively lower for the oldest patients (Schrag et al. 2001a, b; Cronin et al. 2006). Because these studies were based on administrative and registry data, however, it is unclear what role patient preference may have appropriately played. Treatment intensity and completion rates among older patients have been less well studied, although the toxicity of traditional colon cancer chemotherapeutic regimens is generally low compared to regimens for other cancers.

Race/ethnicity. There is some controversy about the role of treatment differences among racial/ethnic groups as contributors to survival and mortality. Evidence to date suggests that as much as 20–40% of the survival difference between blacks and whites remains after controlling for known factors such as stage at diagnosis. Furthermore, studies conducted within the Veteran's Administration, where access to care is presumed to be similar, found no observed racial difference in treatment or survival, suggesting that equivalent treatment produces equivalent outcomes (Dominitz and Provenzale 1997).

However, more recent studies suggest that some treatment differences between blacks and whites are not explained by differences in clinical need (Doubeni et al. 2007; Baldwin et al. 2005; Morris et al. 2004, 2006). Blacks with CRC appear less likely than whites to receive surgery, neoadjuvant therapy, and radiation than whites (Roetzheim et al. 2000; Baldwin et al. 2005; Schrag 2002, Clegg et al. 2002; Cooper and Koroukian 2004; Ayanian et al. 2003). Furthermore, some of the treatment disparities seem to be related to provider-specific patterns of care. In one study, the disparities were attenuated when provider specific variables were entered into the regression model (Morris et al. 2006). Disparities in the rate of performing sphincter preserving surgery also seem to exist between Hispanic patients with rectal cancer and other patients (Martinez et al. 2006). Surveillance after treatment may be an important contributor to survival as well. One study found a 25% lower rate of follow-up colonoscopy among blacks compared to whites after non-metastatic CRC, but a second study did not find this disparity (Ellison et al. 2003; Cooper et al. 2000).

Insurance Status/SEP. Few studies have addressed the direct effects of lacking insurance and having a lower SEP on treatment patterns and the quality of treatment. In addition, findings on disparities in the quality of care are somewhat difficult to interpret because of confounding between SEP and the quality of available providers and facilities. For example, patients treated in hospitals that tend to perform lower numbers of operations or treatments (so-called "low volume" hospitals) have lower survival than those treated in higher volume hospitals (Schrag et al. 2000; Hodgson et al. 2001). However, blacks, the uninsured, and those with lower SEP are actually more likely to be treated in high-volume hospitals.

Reducing Social Disparities in Colorectal Cancer

As the above discussion indicates, substantial evidence indicates that age, gender, race/ethnicity, insurance, and SEP have complex and interrelated effects on the incidence, diagnosis, treatment, and outcomes of colon cancer. The variety of studies described in this chapter suggests that no single intervention will reduce disparities. Instead, a series of interventions across the continuum of cancer care will undoubtedly be necessary to address each of the multiple social disparities identified by prior research. How best to prioritize these interventions is an open question. In the context of the US health care delivery system, a number of options may be especially relevant. These can be categorized as public health interventions and delivery system interventions.

Public Health Interventions

In the US, lack of health insurance is a key remediable factor for reducing disparities. Expanding access to health insurance could have an important impact on the incidence, diagnosis, and treatment of CRC because lack of insurance can lead patients to forgo screening, and to delay seeking care for symptoms. Insurance can even prevent the "reverse targeting" of screening whereby the insured individuals, who may ironically be at lower risk than the uninsured, receive frequent screening while the uninsured receive little or no screening (Cairns and Viswanath 2006). Insurance may also enable vulnerable populations to obtain primary care and receive counseling and treatment for major risk factors such as obesity, physical inactivity, diabetes, and alcohol and tobacco use.

Community-based education programs to raise public awareness of a cancer-risk minimizing lifestyle, awareness of the need for screening, and awareness of warning symptoms of colon cancer may also contribute to reducing the incidence of CRC and promoting earlier detection. To date CRC-specific media programs have been somewhat successful (Cram et al. 2003). Targeting these programs to minority communities may enhance their effectiveness.

Delivery System Interventions

A number of improvements to the current health care delivery system may help to reduce disparities in the incidence of CRC. These include shoring up primary care, increasing the availability of high-quality CRC screening services, reducing the barriers that impede population screening, and improving the availability of oncology treatment services and surveillance to patients with a diagnosis of CRC.

Primary care is a critical component of effective cancer control and prevention. This is especially true for CRC because effective screening not only detects cancer, but also provides the means for removing precursor lesions (adenomas) before they transform into cancer. Effective primary-care services can also enhance the detection of early stage disease if symptoms occur and are reported by patients. Finally, effective primary-care collaboration with oncologists may enhance trust during treatment for those with a diagnosis of CRC and may improve adherence to surveillance after cure when an oncologist may no longer be involved as the principle physician. Unfortunately, in the US, a dysfunctional payment system, increased specialization, and disorganized health planning have undermined primary care. To the extent that these trends undermine care in particular for minority patients and those with lower SEP, social disparities in the diagnosis of CRC at an early stage will persist and may even increase.

Colorectal cancer screening is a critical step in the reduction of disparities. Programs to increase screening are needed for all populations because, across the board, rates of screening remain far below what is considered optimal. In the US, "population screening" is a misnomer. CRC screening tied to enrollment in health insurance plans and the delivery system screens only those who have insurance. Other countries with national health systems, such as the United Kingdom, have adopted true population-screening programs based on the use of FOBT administered by mail. They have also been quicker to adopt mass screening with flexible sigmoidoscopy by trained nurse practitioners rather than gastroenterologists. In the US, such an approach could foster the availability of systematic screening at much lower costs than can be achieved by a strategy predicated on primary colonoscopy by gastroenterologists. Training primary-care physicians to carry out colonoscopy could also expand access to screening in rural and underserved communities. These structural changes to the delivery system could reduce disparities related to access to care.

Following a diagnosis of colon cancer, ready access to high quality surgical and medical oncology services may be yet another barrier for patients who are older, members of ethnic minority groups, and/or have lower SEP. In addition to barriers already discussed, such patients may have inordinate difficulty navigating the confusing maze that characterizes many modern oncology centers. Experiments in the use of patient navigators to guide newly diagnosed cancer patients through these confusing settings are only now getting underway (Dohan and Schrag 2005; Fowler et al. 2006; Christie et al. 2008). Enhancing communication between oncologists and patients at risk for disparities is another important objective. Involving the primary-care physician directly may be helpful to establishing trust and improving communication, but co-management approaches have not been formally established in all centers. Training physicians and other staff in techniques that promote cultural competency is yet another new approach to these obstacles that is still being evaluated. Finally, formally clarifying the handoff to primary care once a patient has completed treatment may also serve the needs of the low SEP or minority patients who have to travel greater distances to reach cancer centers. Surveillance reminders may be more effective if they originate from the patient's primary-care physician, but for patients who lack a primary-care physician, the oncologist may also have to take on this role.

Conclusion

Disparities in the incidence of CRC and survival after diagnosis of the disease present an important challenge to current health care delivery systems and public health institutions. While the magnitude of disparities varies greatly, age, gender, race/ethnicity, insurance status, and SEP clearly matter. Racial and ethnic disparities have been studied most extensively, while disparities based on other social factors (such as immigrant status, sexual orientation, or geography) have been less well studied. The points at which these social factors intersect with the continuum of cancer care have been described above. The social factors that create disparities in incidence and survival of CRC interact with one another in a highly complex manner, though it appears that each of the listed factors contributes independently to disparities in at least some populations or settings.

The observed disparities offer numerous targets for intervention. Areas that present fruitful opportunities for reducing disparities include improving public education programs, expanding access to insurance coverage for minority and low SEP patients, tailoring primary care for vulnerable populations, investing in expanded population-based CRC screening programs, increasing access to treatment for patients with a CRC diagnosis, and enhancing the patient's experience through the use of patient navigators or other communication aids. These interventions, taken together, should enhance primary prevention

by reducing risk factors, increasing access to screening and secondary prevention, and assuring equity in treatment and surveillance for those with a cancer
diagnosis. If differences in tumor biology and disease course are due to genetic
or environmental factors, then equity of prevention, screening, treatment, and
surveillance may not eliminate disparities entirely. Nevertheless, establishing
such equity may go a long way toward reducing disparities and augmenting
trust in public health and the health care delivery enterprise.

References

Albano JD, Ward E, Jemal A, et al. Cancer mortality in the United States by education level
    and race. J Natl Cancer Inst 2007;99:1384–1394.
Ananthakrishnan AN, Schellhase KG, Sparapani RA, et al. Disparities in colon cancer
    screening in the Medicare population. Arch Intern Med 2007;167:258–264.
Ayanian JZ, Zaslavsky AM, Fuchs CS, et al. Use of adjuvant chemotherapy and radiation
    therapy for colorectal cancer in a population-based cohort. J Clin Oncol 2003;21:1293–1300.
Baldwin LM, Dobie SA, Billingsley K, et al. Explaining black-white differences in receipt of
    recommended colon cancer treatment. J Natl Cancer Inst 2005;97:1211–1220.
Bao Y, Fox SA, Escarce JJ. Socioeconomic and racial/ethnic differences in the discussion of
    cancer screening: "between-" versus "within-" physician differences. Health Serv Res
    2007;42:950–970.
Blesch KS, Davis F, Kamath SK. A comparison of breast and colon cancer incidence rates
    among Native Asian Indians, US immigrant Asian Indians, and whites. J Am Diet Assoc
    1999;99:1275–1277.
Braveman P. Health disparities and health equity: concepts and measurement. Ann Rev Pub
    Health 2006;27:167–194.
Byers T, Levin B, Rothenberger D, et al. American Cancer Society guidelines for screening
    and surveillance for early detection of colorectal polyps and cancer: update 1997.
    American Cancer Society Detection and Treatment Advisory Group on Colorectal
    Cancer. CA Cancer J Clin 1997;47:154–160.
Cairns CP, Viswanath K. Communication and colorectal cancer screening among the unin-
    sured: data from the Health Information National Trends Survey (United States). Cancer
    Causes Control 2006;17:1115–1125.
Callcut RA, Kaufman S, Stone-Newsom R, et al. Gender disparities in colorectal cancer
    screening: true or false? J Gastrointest Surg 2006;10:1409–1417.
Can Colorectal Cancer Be Prevented? http://www.cancer.org/docroot/CRI/content/CRI_2_4_2X_
    Can_colon_and_rectum_cancer_be_prevented.asp?rnav=cri. Accessed May 18, 2008.
Cancer of the Colon and Rectum. http://seer.cancer.gov/statfacts/html/colorect.html.
    Accessed November 26, 2007.
Chen VW, Fenoglio-Preiser CM, Wu XC, et al. Aggressiveness of colon carcinoma in blacks
    and whites. National Cancer Institute Black/White Cancer Survival Study Group. Cancer
    Epidemiol Biomarkers Prev 1997;6:1087–1093.
Cheng X, Chen VW, Steele B, et al. Subsite-specific incidence rate and stage of disease in colorectal
    cancer by race, gender, and age group in the United States, 1992–1997. Cancer 2001;92:2547–2554.
Chien C, Morimoto LM, Tom J, et al. Differences in colorectal carcinoma stage and survival
    by race and ethnicity. Cancer 2005;104:629–639.
Christie J, Hooper C, Redd WH, et al. Predictors of endoscopy in minority women. J Natl
    Med Assoc 2005;97:1361–1368.

Christie J, Itzkowitz S, Lihau-Nkanza I, et al. A randomized controlled trial using patient navigation to increase colonoscopy screening among low-income minorities. J Natl Med Assoc 2008;100:278–284.

Chu KC, Miller BA, Springfield SA. Measures of racial/ethnic health disparities in cancer mortality rates and the influence of socioeconomic status. J Natl Med Assoc 2007;99:1092–1100, 1102–1094.

Clegg LX, Li FP, Hankey BF, et al. Cancer survival among US whites and minorities: a SEER (Surveillance, Epidemiology, and End Results) Program population-based study. Arch Intern Med 2002;162:1985–1993.

Center for Disease Control and Prevention. Colorectal cancer test use among persons aged > or = 50 years—United States, 2001. MMWR 2003;52:193–196.

Center for Disease Control and Prevention. Colorectal cancer test use—Maryland, 2002–2006. MMWR 2007;56:932–936.

Cooper GS, Koroukian SM. Racial disparities in the use of and indications for colorectal procedures in Medicare beneficiaries. Cancer 2004;100:418–424.

Cooper GS, Payes JD. Receipt of colorectal testing prior to colorectal carcinoma diagnosis. Cancer 2005;103:696–701.

Cooper GS, Yuan Z, Chak A, et al. Patterns of endoscopic follow-up after surgery for nonmetastatic colorectal cancer. Gastrointest Endosc 2000;52:33–38.

Cooper GS, Yuan Z, Rimm AA. Racial disparity in the incidence and case-fatality of colorectal cancer: Analysis of 329 United States counties. Cancer Epidemiol Biomarkers Prev 1997;6:283–285.

Cram P, Fendrick AM, Inadomi J, et al. The impact of a celebrity promotional campaign on the use of colon cancer screening. Arch Intern Med 2003;163:1601–1605.

Cronin DP, Harlan LC, Potosky AL, et al. Patterns of care for adjuvant therapy in a random population-based sample of patients diagnosed with colorectal cancer. Am J Gastroenterol 2006;101:2308–2318.

Dohan D, Schrag D. Using navigators to improve care of underserved patients: current practices and approaches. Cancer 2005;104:848–855.

Dominitz JA, Provenzale D. Patient preferences and quality of life associated with colorectal cancer screening. Am J Gastroenterol 1997;92:2171–2178.

Doubeni CA, Field TS, Buist DS, et al. Racial differences in tumor stage and survival for colorectal cancer in an insured population. Cancer 2007;109:612–620.

Du XL, Meyer TE, Franzini L. Meta-analysis of racial disparities in survival in association with socioeconomic status among men and women with colon cancer. Cancer 2007;109:2161–2170.

Ellison GL, Warren JL, Knopf KB, et al. Racial differences in the receipt of bowel surveillance following potentially curative colorectal cancer surgery. Health Serv Res 2003;38:1885–1903.

Fairley TL, Cardinez CJ, Martin J, et al. Colorectal cancer in U.S. adults younger than 50 years of age, 1998–2001. Cancer 2006;107:1153–1161.

Fiscella K, Holt K. Impact of primary care patient visits on racial and ethnic disparities in preventive care in the United States. J Am Board Fam Med 2007;20:587–597.

Flood DM, Weiss NS, Cook LS, et al. Colorectal cancer incidence in Asian migrants to the United States and their descendants. Cancer Causes Control 2000;11:403–411.

Fowler T, Steakley C, Garcia AR, et al. Reducing disparities in the burden of cancer: the role of patient navigators. PLoS Med 2006;3:e193.

Frazier AL, Colditz GA, Fuchs CS, et al. Cost-effectiveness of screening for colorectal cancer in the general population. JAMA 2001;284:1954–1961.

Gatof D, Ahnen D. Primary prevention of colorectal cancer: diet and drugs. Gastroenterol Clin North Am 2002;31:587–623, xi.

Goel MS, Wee CC, McCarthy EP, et al. Racial and ethnic disparities in cancer screening: the importance of foreign birth as a barrier to care. J Gen Intern Med 2003;18:1028–1035.

Gross CP, Andersen MS, Krumholz HM, et al. Relation between Medicare screening reimbursement and stage at diagnosis for older patients with colon cancer. JAMA 2006;296:2815–2822.

Hodgson DC, Fuchs CS, Ayanian JZ. Impact of patient and provider characteristics on the treatment and outcomes of colorectal cancer. J Natl Cancer Inst 2001;93:501–515.

Hsu CE, Mas FS, Hickey JM, et al. Surveillance of the colorectal cancer disparities among demographic subgroups: a spatial analysis. South Med J 2006;99:949–956.

Irby K, Anderson WF, Henson DE, et al. Emerging and widening colorectal carcinoma disparities between Blacks and Whites in the United States (1975–2002). Cancer Epidemiol Biomarkers Prev 2006;15:792–797.

James TM, Greiner KA, Ellerbeck EF, et al. Disparities in colorectal cancer screening: a guideline-based analysis of adherence. Ethn Dis 2006;16:228–233.

Kandula NR, Wen M, Jacobs EA, et al. Low rates of colorectal, cervical, and breast cancer screening in Asian Americans compared with non-Hispanic whites: Cultural influences or access to care? Cancer 2006;107:184–192.

Kelz RR, Gimotty PA, Polsky D, et al. Morbidity and mortality of colorectal carcinoma surgery differs by insurance status. Cancer 2004;101:2187–2194.

Klabunde CN, Schenck AP, Davis WW. Barriers to colorectal cancer screening among Medicare consumers. Am J Prev Med 2006;30:313–319.

Koroukian SM, Xu F, Dor A, et al. Colorectal cancer screening in the elderly population: disparities by dual Medicare-Medicaid enrollment status. Health Serv Res 2006;41:2136–2154.

Krieger N, Quesenberry C, Jr., Peng T, et al. Social class, race/ethnicity, and incidence of breast, cervix, colon, lung, and prostate cancer among Asian, black, Hispanic, and white residents of the San Francisco Bay Area, 1988–92 (United States). Cancer Causes Control 1999;10:525–537.

Le Marchand L, Wilkens LR, Kolonel LN, et al. Associations of sedentary lifestyle, obesity, smoking, alcohol use, and diabetes with the risk of colorectal cancer. Cancer Res 1997;57:4787–4794.

Maciosek MV, Edwards NM, Coffield AB, et al. Priorities among effective clinical preventive services: methods. Am J Prev Med 2006;31:90–96.

Maciosek MV, Solberg LI, Coffield AB, et al. Colorectal cancer screening: health impact and cost effectiveness. Am J Prev Med 2006;31:80–89.

Mandelblatt J, Andrews H, Kao R, et al. The late-stage diagnosis of colorectal cancer: demographic and socioeconomic factors. Am J Public Health 1996;86:1794–1797.

Marcella S, Miller JE. Racial differences in colorectal cancer mortality: The importance of stage and socioeconomic status. J Clin Epidemiol 2001;54:359–366.

Martinez SR, Chen SL, Bilchik AJ. Treatment disparities in Hispanic rectal cancer patients: a SEER database study. Am Surg 2006;72:906–908.

Mayberry RM, Coates RJ, Hill HA, et al. Determinants of black/white differences in colon cancer survival. J Natl Cancer Inst 1995;87:1686–1693.

McDavid K, Tucker TC, Sloggett A, et al. Cancer survival in Kentucky and health insurance coverage. Arch Intern Med 2003;163:2135–2144.

McMahon LF, Jr., Wolfe RA, Huang S, et al. Racial and gender variation in use of diagnostic colonic procedures in the Michigan Medicare population. Med Care 1999;37:712–717.

Meissner HI, Breen N, Klabunde CN, et al. Patterns of colorectal cancer screening uptake among men and women in the United States. Cancer Epidemiol Biomarkers Prev 2006;15:389–394.

Morales LS, Rogowski J, Freedman VA, et al. Sociodemographic differences in use of preventive services by women enrolled in Medicare + Choice plans. Prev Med 2004;39:738–745.

Morris AM, Billingsley KG, Baxter NN, et al. Racial disparities in rectal cancer treatment: a population-based analysis. Arch Surg 2004;139:151–155; discussion 156.

Morris AM, Wei Y, Birkmeyer NJ, et al. Racial disparities in late survival after rectal cancer surgery. J Am Coll Surg 2006;203:787–794.

O'Malley AS, Forrest CB, Feng S, et al. Disparities despite coverage: gaps in colorectal cancer screening. among Medicare beneficiaries. Arch Intern Med 2005;165:2129–2135.

Palmer RC, Schneider EC. Social disparities across the continuum of colorectal cancer: a systematic review. Cancer Causes Control 2005;16:55–61.

Pignone M, Saha S, Hoerger T, et al. Cost-effectiveness analyses of colorectal cancer screening: a systematic review for the US Preventive Services Task Force. Ann Intern Med 2002;137:96–104.

Pine M, Jordan HS, Elixhauser A, et al. Enhancement of claims data to improve risk adjustment of hospital mortality. JAMA 2007;297:71–76.

Polite BN, Dignam JJ, Olopade OI. Colorectal cancer and race: understanding the differences in outcomes between African Americans and whites. Med Clin North Am 2005;89:771–793.

Polite BN, Dignam JJ, Olopade OI. Colorectal cancer model of health disparities: understanding mortality differences in minority populations. J Clin Oncol 2006;24:2179–2187.

Ponce NA, Huh S, Bastani R. Do HMO market level factors lead to racial/ethnic disparities in colorectal cancer screening? A comparison between high-risk Asian and Pacific Islander Americans and high-risk whites. Med Care 2005;43:1101–1108.

Rao RS, Graubard BI, Breen N, et al. Understanding the factors underlying disparities in cancer screening rates using the Peters-Belson approach: results from the 1998 National Health Interview Survey. Med Care 2004;42:789–800.

Ries LAG, Wingo PA, Miller DS, et al. The annual report to the nation on the status of cancer, 1973–1997, with a special section on colorectal cancer. Cancer 2000;88:2398–2424.

Roetzheim RG, Pal N, Gonzalez EC, et al. Effects of health insurance and race on colorectal cancer treatments and outcomes. Am J Pub Health 2000;90:1746–1754.

Roetzheim RG, Pal N, Tennant C, et al. Effects of health insurance and race on early detection of cancer. J Natl Cancer Inst 1999;91:1409–1415.

Rogers SO, Ray WA, Smalley WE. A population-based study of survival among elderly persons diagnosed with colorectal cancer: does race matter if all are insured? (United States). Cancer Causes Control 2004;15:193–199.

Rosen AB, Schneider EC. Colorectal cancer screening disparities related to obesity and gender. J Gen Intern Med 2004;19:332–338.

Schrag D, Cramer LD, Bach PB, et al. Age and adjuvant chemotherapy use after surgery for stage III colon cancer. J Natl Cancer Inst 2001a;93:850–857.

Schrag D, Cramer LD, Bach PB, et al. Influence of hospital procedure volume on outcomes following surgery for colon cancer. JAMA 2000;284:3028–3035.

Schrag D, Gelfand SE, Bach PB, et al. Who gets adjuvant treatment for stage II and III rectal cancer? Insight from surveillance, epidemiology, and end results – Medicare. J Clin Oncology 2001b;19:3712–3718.

Schrag D. Adjuvant chemotherapy use for Medicare beneficiaries with stage II colon cancer. J Clin Oncology 2002;20:3999–4001.

Schroeder SA. Shattuck Lecture. We can do better—improving the health of the American people. N Engl J Med 2007;357:1221–1228.

Schwartz KL, Crossley-May H, Vigneau FD, et al. Race, socioeconomic status and stage at diagnosis for five common malignancies. Cancer Causes Control 2003;14:761–766.

Seeff LC, Nadel MR, Klabunde CN, et al. Patterns and predictors of colorectal cancer test use in the adult U.S. population. Cancer 2004;100:2093–2103.

Sequist TD, Schneider EC. Addressing racial and ethnic disparities in health care: using federal data to support local programs to eliminate disparities. Health Serv Res 2006;41:1451–1468.

Sewitch MJ, Fournier C, Dawes M, et al. Do physician recommendations for colorectal cancer screening differ by patient age? Can J Gastroenterol 2007;21:435–438.

178   E.C. Schneider

Shih YC, Zhao L, Elting LS. Does Medicare coverage of colonoscopy reduce racial/ethnic disparities in cancer screening among the elderly? Health Aff (Millwood) 2006;25:1153–1162.

Shokar NK, Carlson CA, Weller SC. Prevalence of colorectal cancer testing and screening in a multiethnic primary care population. J Community Health 2007;32:311–323.

Sirovich BE, Schwartz LM, Woloshin S. Screening Men for Prostate and Colorectal Cancer in the United States. JAMA 2003;289:1414–1420.

Sonnenberg A, Delco F. Cost-effectiveness of a single colonoscopy in screening for colorectal cancer. Arch Intern Med 2002;162:163–168.

Subramanian. Comparing individual – and area-based socioeconomic measures for the surveillance of health disparities: a multilevel analysis of Massachusetts births, 1989–1991. Am J Epid 2006;164:12.

Swan J, Breen N, Coates RJ, et al. Progress in cancer screening practices in the United States: results from the 2000 National Health Interview Survey. Cancer 2003;97:1528–1540.

Syngal S, Schrag D, Falchuk M, et al. Phenotypic characteristics associated with the APC gene I1307K mutation in Ashkenazi Jewish patients with colorectal polyps. JAMA 2000;284:857–860.

Ward E, Jemal A, Cokkinides V, et al. Cancer disparities by race/ethnicity and socioeconomic status. CA Cancer J Clin 2004;54:78–93.

Wee CC, McCarthy EP, Phillips RS. Factors associated with colon cancer screening: the role of patient factors and physician counseling. Prev Med 2005;41:23–29.

Wong ST, Gildengorin G, Nguyen T, et al. Disparities in colorectal cancer screening rates among Asian Americans and non-Latino whites. Cancer 2005;104:2940–2947.

Zhao BB, Kilbourne B, Stain SC, et al. Racial disparities and trends in use of colorectal procedures among Tennessee elderly (1996–2000). Ethn Dis 2006;16:412–420.

Chapter 8
Disparities in Prostate Cancer

Otis W. Brawley and Sherrie Flynt Wallington

Introduction

Prostate cancer is the most commonly diagnosed non-skin cancer in the US and the second most common cause of cancer death among American men. In 2008 an estimated 186,320 men will be diagnosed with, and 28,660 will die of, prostate cancer in the US. Incidence rates increased dramatically in the 1990s attributable to prostate cancer screening but then declined after uncovering of prevalent cases. Mortality rates have trended downward in the past 15 years (Fig. 8.1).

Much of the interest in prostate cancer disparities has focused on black versus white men. This is because African Americans have some of the highest incidence and mortality rates of this cancer in the world (Ries et al. 2006). Seventeen percent of Americans diagnosed with prostate cancer (30,870 in 2008) are of African American origin. Compared to white Americans, moreover, African Americans are 1.6 times more likely to be diagnosed with prostate cancer and 2.5 times more likely to die of it. Men of African origin in Jamaica and Brazil also have very high rates of this disease (Glover et al. 1998; Odedina et al. 2006; Phillips et al. 2007). In England, too, the relative risk for prostate cancer is 3.09 (95% CI, 2.85–3.56) for blacks compared to men of Caucasian heritage (Ben-Shlomo et al. 2008). There is also evidence that socioeconomically deprived persons in the US are more likely to die of this disease compared to those who are less deprived (Du et al. 2006; Gilligan et al. 2004; Robbins et al. 2000). In contrast, and for reasons that are not understood, Native Americans, Asian Americans, and Hispanic Americans have even lower rates than whites (Table 8.1).

Disparities in time of diagnosis and death can be seen along racial lines as well. Prostate cancer is largely a disease of the elderly, as indicated in Table 8.2. During the 2000–2005 time period, the median age at diagnosis for white Americans

O.W. Brawley (✉)
Chief Medical Officer, American Cancer Society, Professor of Hematology, Oncology, Medicine and Epidemiology, Emory University, Atlanta, GA 30322, USA
e-mail: otis.brawley@cancer.org

H.K. Koh (ed.), *Toward the Elimination of Cancer Disparities*,
DOI 10.1007/978-0-387-89443-0_8, © Springer Science+Business Media, LLC 2009

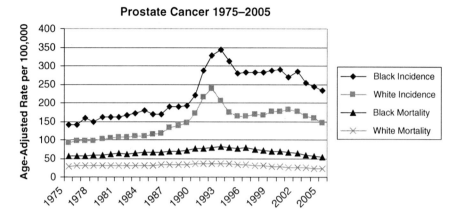

Fig. 8.1 Prostate Cancer 1975–2005
Adapted from Ries et al. 2008.

Table 8.1 Proportion Diagnosed and Dying of Prostate Cancer by Age Range

Age Range	Percent Diagnosed	Percent Dying
35–44	02.5%	0.1%
45–54	8.3%	1.3%
55–64	26.9%	6.5%
65–74	37.0%	21.1%
75–84	22.6%	41.9%
85+	4.7%	29.1%

Adapted from Ries et al. 2006

Table 8.2 Prostate Cancer Incidence in Six Populations of African Origin

Black U.S.	185.4
Martinique	96.3
Zimbabwe	30.7
Uganda	37.1
Mali	7.6
The Gambia	4.7

From Cancer in Five Continents 7th Edition
Age Adjusted to World Standard

was 68 years and median age at death was 80 years. In contrast, the median age at diagnosis for blacks was 70 years and the median age at death was 76 years (Edwards et al. 2005). The number of both blacks and whites diagnosed before the age of 50 is small, with 2.5% of white men diagnosed with prostate cancer under the age of 50, compared to 5.2% of black men. The age-specific diagnosis and death rates of black and white Americans are in Fig. 8.2.

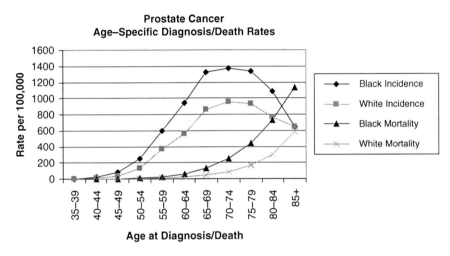

Fig. 8.2 Prostate Cancer Age-Specific Diagnosis/Death Rates
Adapted from Ries et al. 2008

Racial disparities in grade of disease at diagnosis are more subtle, although among men with localized and regional cancers, blacks are twice as likely to have high-grade (Gleason score ≥7) disease (Reed et al. 2007). In clinical studies of those screened for prostate cancer, risk factors for high-grade disease (Gleason score ≥7) are higher PSA level, abnormal digital rectal examination, older age at biopsy, and African American race (Thompson et al. 2006). Despite these disparities, 5-year survival rates from prostate cancer diagnosis have increased dramatically over the past 25 years for all races. US National Cancer Institute Surveillance, Epidemiology and End Results Program (SEER) data show that 92% of whites and 89% of black Americans present with local or regional disease, and 5-year survival rates of both black and white men presenting with local and regional disease are virtually 100%. In addition, approximately 31% of whites and 29% of blacks with distant or metastatic disease are alive 5 years after diagnosis. Nonetheless, many questions continue to focus on the racial and ethnic differences that exist in prostate cancer. These questions present both a challenge and opportunity to better understand the reasons and factors contributing to the differences.

Race and Population Categorization

Persons of African ("black") origin unquestionably have a higher risk of prostate cancer and prostate cancer death than persons of European ("white") origin. However, one must be careful when assessing prostate cancer by racial and ethnic categories. First of all, categorizing a population by race and ethnicity can confound analysis because these categories can overlap with or be influenced by other factors associated with disparities such as socioeconomic status (SES) or education. There is, for example, a correlation between level of education and risk of prostate cancer death, with less education associated with a higher risk. Indeed, black American men who completed 12 or fewer years of education have a prostate cancer death rate that is more than twice that of black men with more schooling (Albano et al. 2007). These kinds of correlations may confound analysis based on a single factor such as race.

Another complication is that American cancer incidence and mortality data are collected by race and ethnicity classifications based not in biology but in sociopolitical categorizations (Brawley 2002, 2003). Race is a construct based in the societal politics and not on anthropologic or biologic principles. In the US, the categories are determined by the US Office of Management and Budget and published 2 years prior to every decennial census. To some extent the scientific literature supports such categorization, with various studies showing small genetic differences among populations when those populations are described by area of geographic origin. For example, persons of African origin have a higher prevalence, but not a monopoly, of the sickle cell mutation than whites of European origin. These genetic differences are often linked to an environmental cause or advantage: a higher resistance to malaria in persons with sickle cell trait.

Placing any given individual into a predetermined racial category, however, is more complicated. Although medical racial profiling is common, collecting data concerning health using sociopolitical categories and drawing scientific conclusions from them can be misleading. This is because race and ethnicity are not true surrogates for genetic variation. Rather, several studies suggest that socially defined race and ethnicity are associated with numerous social determinants of health, including higher levels of poverty, social deprivation, segregation, and discrimination (Fiscella and Williams 2004; Williams 2003, 2005; Williams and Collins 1995; Williams and Jackson 2005). Furthermore, most Americans classified as "black" or "of African origin" are actually some mixture of African, European, and Native American origin.

Prostate Cancer Screening

Prostate cancer incidence rates increased dramatically for both black and white Americans in the 1990s (Fig. 8.1). The rise has been linked both to the increasing use of transurethral resection of the prostate for treatment of benign prostatic hyperplasia and, later, to increased use of serum prostate-specific antigen (PSA) in prostate cancer screening (Potosky et al. 2001). The PSA screening test was introduced in 1986 to monitor patients after diagnosis. It was later adopted for screening, beginning in the late 1980s. By 1998 in the US, almost 40% of white men and 35% of black men over age 65 were being tested each year (Etzioni et al. 2002). In contrast, prostate cancer screening has not been widely adopted in Europe, where the rise in incidence is not nearly as dramatic as in the US (Collin et al. 2008; Shibata et al. 1998; Shibata and Whittemore 2001).

The rapid adoption of the PSA test in the US has occurred amidst tremendous controversy regarding the test's benefits and costs. Most recently, the US Preventative Services Task Force (USPSTF) began recommending no screening at all for prostate cancer in men aged 75 years or older because they found that the incremental benefits of treatment for prostate cancer detected by screening are at best small in this population (US Preventative Task Force 2008). This recommendation further fuels the contentious debate regarding the benefits and harms of screening. Indeed, whether prostate cancer screening truly saves lives remains one of the most important unanswered questions in cancer medicine. At present, prostate cancer screening has not been proven to save lives, but it has been shown to diagnose men who do not need treatment and thus subject them to unnecessary treatment (Etzioni et al. 2002; Miller et al. 2006; Stangelberger et al. 2008; Waldert and Djvan 2008; Telesca et al. 2007). This is true of men of all races.

Some of the increase in 5-year survival specifically is thus probably due to the lead time bias of screening, which suggests that screening per se does not affect the natural history of the disease (Duffy et al. 2008; Kramer et al. 1993; Telesca et al. 2007). At least some of the increase is due to the diagnosis of men who have cancers of no risk to their life as well as those who in earlier times would never have been diagnosed. Many diagnosed men, both black and white, have low-risk disease and might not experience adverse impact to survival or quality of life if treatment were deferred.

The crux of the screening issue is over-detection of prostate cancer by screening leads to over-treatment of an indolent disease process, meaning the treatment of disease that is of no threat and does not need treatment (Cooperberg et al. 2004). This phenomenon is believed to occur in at least 40–60% of men currently diagnosed with localized disease (Yao et al. 2002; Etzioni et al. 2002). Miller et al. (2006) studied the US National Cancer Institute SEER dataset and concluded that of 24,405 American men treated for prostate cancer in the modern PSA era from 2000–2002, an estimated 2,564 men may have been over-treated with surgery and 10,973 may have been over-treated with radiation therapy (Miller et al. 2006).

Evidence that a substantial proportion of American men diagnosed with localized prostate cancer have a disease which is of no threat to their life comes from studies of geographic differences in incidence and mortality. The UK is a country with very little prostate cancer screening and much lower incidence and treatment rates than the US. Even so, the UK has had a prostate cancer mortality rate very similar to that in the US for decades (Shibata et al. 1998; Shibata and Whittemore 2001).

For all these reasons, current screening practices are the subject of considerable controversy. Unfortunately, however, clinical science is hindered by the lack of tests that can accurately predict those cancers that will be of clinical significance during a person's lifetime. There has been much work on development of screening and diagnostic tests and very little on development of tests to determine potentially lethal cancers requiring intervention versus cancers unlikely to cause harm within the patient's natural lifetime and thus requiring only observation (Ingles et al. 1997). The first reports from two long-awaited large, randomized trials designed to provide answers about the effectiveness of prostate cancer screening were released in March 2009 (American Cancer Society (ACS) 2009). Data from the Prostate, Lung, Colorectal, and Ovarian (PLCO) Cancer Screening Trial, a 17-year project of the National Cancer Institute (NCI), finds that six annual screenings for prostate cancer led to more diagnoses of the disease, but no fewer prostate cancer deaths. The second study, the European Randomized Study of Screening for Prostate Cancer (ERSPC), shows a 20 % reduction in the rate of death from prostate cancer, and also found a high risk of over-diagnosis. The ERSPC study concluded that 1,410 men would need to be screened and 48 additional cancers would need to be treated to prevent one death from prostate cancer. The early results from these two major trials suggest that if prostate cancer screening is beneficial, the benefit is small in terms of lives saved. Moreover, the data confirm the following (ACS 2009):

1) As recommended by the American Cancer Society and other organizations, men at average risk should decide whether or not to be screened based on their own concerns and situation and after discussing the benefits and limitations of screening with their doctor.
2) These studies concern men without symptoms. Men who do have urinary symptoms, such as frequent or difficult urination, a weak stream, etc., need to be getting exams, including PSA tests.
3) Men recently diagnosed with prostate cancer should have an open and candid conversation with their physician about these studies to evaluate their plan of care.

Meanwhile, screening is common in the US and is the driving factor behind most diagnosis in all American races and ethnicities. Today, men are rarely diagnosed with metastatic disease. In the 1980s, prior to the PSA screening era, SES appeared not to correlate with stage at diagnosis (Liu et al. 2001). Today fewer than 10% of men are diagnosed with distant disease, and there is evidence linking SES to stage at diagnosis and to survival (Steenland et al. 2004). The cohort with advanced disease at initial diagnosis tends to be disproportionately poorer and less educated (Bennett et al. 1998). Some studies have shown that low literacy is a barrier to diagnosis at early stage, while race itself is not a predictor of presentation with advanced disease (Bennett et al. 1998; Wolf et al. 2006).

The reasons why the poor currently present with more advanced stages are unclear. They may relate to diet and other environmental influences, or they may relate to less attention to health on the part of the poor. Lack of health insurance, a more specific factor than low SES, has also been associated with an increased risk of diagnosis of distant disease (Halpern et al. 2008; Roetzheim et al. (1999). The literature is contradictory concerning this question. Bennett et al. (1998) in a cohort study found that literacy (a marker of SES), but not race, was a predictor of stage at diagnosis. In contrast, Polednak (1997) and Schwartz (2003) found that blacks presented with advanced stage even when SES was considered (Polednak 1997; Schwartz et al. 2003). These findings may be influenced by the time periods in which they were done. The Bennett cohort was diagnosed largely during the PSA screening era, while the Polednak and Schwartz studies were done largely prior to this time.

In the 1990s, there were few good population-based surveys in the US to determine the proportion of men who had had prostate cancer screening. It appears that black men and poor men were relatively less likely to receive screening. Later studies tend to show that the black-white disparity in prostate screening has decreased and perhaps even disappeared (Pan et al. 2003). Additional evidence, such as the leveling out of prostate cancer incidence after the dramatic rise in the early 1990s, suggests that a high proportion of black and white American men at risk for prostate cancer have been screened. This phenomenon has also been seen in breast and colon cancer (Brown and Potosky 1990). Data from the 2000 US National Health Interview Survey (NHIS) shows that 45% of white men and 43% of black men within ages 40–84 had had at least one PSA test by the year 2000 (Mariotto et al. 2007). Data from the 2005 NHIS confirmed the relative equivalence proportions of blacks and whites screened and even suggest a higher proportion of younger black men had been tested compared to whites (Ross et al. 2008). There may be very subtle racial differences in the proportion of men getting routine screening, however, despite a similar proportion of black and white men who have had at least one screening.

Prostate Cancer Risk

The higher prostate cancer incidence and mortality rate of black Americans (and others of African descent) leads to the question: do black Americans or persons of African heritage have a genetic predisposition to develop prostate cancer? In addition, if there is a genetic predisposition to prostate cancer, do blacks or Africans have a predisposition to develop more aggressive forms of prostate cancer or to be diagnosed with prostate cancer at a more advanced stage?

Arguments for a genetic or inherited influence. Many researchers suspect that genetic or familial factors might play a central role in determining prostate cancer predisposition or risk of aggressiveness (Kumar et al. 2004; Ross et al. 1998). Some have suggested that there must be a prostate cancer gene polymorphism, mutation, or series of genetic polymorphisms or mutations that predispose blacks or other men of African heritage to prostate cancer. Chapter 3 of this book explores issues of gene–environment interactions in prostate cancer and other areas.

Many of the genetic polymorphisms or mutations that have been studied increase either the amount of circulating androgen or sensitivity to androgenic stimulation of the prostate. The prostate is an androgen-regulated organ, and prostate cancer is often treated with androgen deprivation. This has led to long-standing interest in the role of androgens in prostate carcinogenesis. Although evidence of a hormonal etiology for prostate cancer is strong, it is almost entirely circumstantial. Ironically, the success of the Prostate Cancer Prevention Trial and its proof that lowering androgen stimulation decreases the incidence of prostate cancer is an important clue in the pathogenesis of the disease (Thompson et al. 2003). While extremely controversial (Litman et al. 2006), some evidence suggests that there may be population-based differences in hormonal levels. Men of African origin are thought to have higher androgenic levels leading to the higher incidence of prostate cancer (Ross et al. 1998). Others have suggested that racial differences in estrogens may contribute to the disparities in prostate cancer (Rohrmann et al. 2007). Much of the problem in proving a relationship is the continued difficulties in reliably measuring human tissue-specific exposure to endogenous steroid hormones.

The enzyme 5-alpha reductase converts testosterone to the more potent androgen dihydrotestosterone (DHT) (Brawley et al. 1994). Inhibition of this enzyme prevents the formation of prostate cancer. When comparing populations, there are varying prevalences of different polymorphisms in the gene (SRD5A2) that codes for 5 alpha reductase (Ross 2001). Certain polymorphisms do appear to increase risk of prostate cancer by promoting more efficient conversion of testosterone to DHT and disproportionately increasing the bioavailability of more potent androgens (Salam et al. 2005). It is unknown, however, as to whether persons originating in sub-Saharan Africa have a higher prevalence of these polymorphisms that portend higher risk of prostate cancer.

UDP-glucuronosyltransferases (UGT) are a family of enzymes that glucuronidate many endogenous chemicals, including androgens. This makes them hydrophilic, alters biologic activity, and facilitates excretion. Certain polymorphisms in UGT reduce the rate of glucuronidation and thus increase available androgen. In a case–control study involving 420 prostate cancer patients (127 black and 293 white) and 487 controls (120 black and 267 white), the UGT217 deletion polymorphism correlated with an increased risk of prostate cancer (Park et al. 2006). Very limited data suggest that a higher proportion of blacks have less active polymorphisms of genes coding for UGT.

CYP3A4 is a protein in the cytochrome p-450 supergene family. It facilitates the oxidative deactivation of testosterone. It has been shown that patients with certain variants of a genetic polymorphism in CYP3A4 are prone to clinically aggressive prostate cancers. These variants may be more prevalent in the black or African population (Bangsi et al. 2006). Similarly, variation in CYP17 and insulin growth factor 1 (IGF1) may be associated with prostate cancer development in the African American population, although all current data remain inconclusive (Hernandez et al. 2007). (See Chapter 3 of this book.)

Polymorphisms in the vitamin D receptor and differences among blacks and whites have also been speculated to cause greater prostate cancer risk in blacks (Kidd et al. 2005; Thompson et al. 2003). Some have also suggested that dietary differences in vitamin D may contribute to differences in prostate cancer rate among populations (Thompson et al. 2003) or that darker complexion of persons of African heritage may portend to lower vitamin D levels and increased risk of prostate cancer. Interestingly, however, the large cohort studies have not shown a correlation between increased vitamin D intake or higher serum levels and lowered prostate cancer risk (Giovannucci 2009).

Irvine et al. (1995) studied the number of repeats in the polymorphic CAG and GGC microsatellites of exon 1 of the androgen receptor gene. A shorter CAG repeat causes tighter androgen binding and greater potency of each androgenic molecule. In normal subjects, the distributions of CAG and GGC micro-satellites differed significantly among the races (two-sided $p = 0.046$ and < 0.0005, respectively). The prevalence of short CAG alleles (< 22 repeats) was highest (75%) in African American males with the highest risk for prostate cancer, intermediate (62%) in intermediate-risk non-Hispanic whites, and lowest (49%) in Asians at very low risk for prostate cancer (Irvine et al. 1995).

Platz et al. (2000) evaluated prospectively the relation between prostate cancer and race among 45,410 American health professionals aged 40–75 years in 1986. They used multivariate, pooled logistic regression to adjust the rate ratio for potential dietary and lifestyle risk factors. They also measured circulating levels of steroid hormones, sex hormone-binding globulin, vitamin D metabolites, and length of the androgen receptor gene CAG repeat in a sample of African American ($n = 43$), Asian ($n = 52$), and white ($n = 55$) participants and used analysis of variance to assess variation by race in these possible prostate epithelial cell growth mediators. The age-adjusted RR for prostate cancer was 1.73 (95% confidence interval [CI], 1.23–2.45) for African American men compared with white men. After multivariate adjustment, the RR increased to 1.81 (95% CI, 1.27–2.58).

The mean number of androgen receptor gene CAG repeats was lower among African Americans (mean $+/-$ standard deviation $= 20.1 +/- 3.5$) than among whites ($22.1 +/- 3.1$; $p = 0.007$) and Asians ($22.1 +/- 3.9$; $p = 0.009$), a group which had a similar rate of prostate cancer to whites. The Platz results confirm the elevated incidence of prostate cancer among African Americans and suggest that this difference cannot be explained by racial differences in dietary and lifestyle risk factors. The study suggested that racial variation in length of the androgen receptor gene CAG repeat may explain a small part of the excess risk of prostate cancer among African American men in this cohort.

Several surveys also demonstrate that men who have a geographic origin from sub-Saharan Africa tend to have shorter CAG repeats than men originating in Europe (Kittles et al. 2001; Sartor et al. 1999). Panz et al. (2001) studied the issue in an 80-men study and, while concluding that the small differences in the number of CAG repeats in both black and white patients do not appear to be a strong indicator of prostate cancer risk, this size polymorphism may be one of many genetic and environmental risk factors involved in prostate cancer.

Some have speculated that CAG repeat length is prognostic, not for risk of prostate cancer, but for aggressiveness and risk of recurrence in men treated for localized disease (Bennett et al. 2002). Powell and colleagues (Powell et al. 2005) studied the association between the number of CAG repeats and extent of disease, Gleason score, and preoperative PSA level at diagnosis in more than 700 prostate cancer patients. Overall, prostate cancer patients who had greater than 18 CAG repeats had a greater risk of recurrence than patients who had less than or equal to 18 CAG repeats (hazard ratio [HR] = 1.52; $p = 0.03$).

Most of the CAG repeat length observations were made more than a decade ago, however, and the contribution of CAG repeat length to prostate cancer risk is still open to debate. Taken together these studies weakly suggest that shorter CAG repeats increase risk of development of prostate cancer; however, among those diagnosed, longer CAG repeats predict for greater likelihood of recurrence and more aggressive disease. These conclusions make some intuitive sense in that they suggest that cancers in those with shorter CAG repeat length are more sensitive to androgen and androgen deprivation.

Two recent studies independently identified polymorphisms strongly associated with prostate cancer risk in the 8q24 region, including a single nucleotide polymorphism (rs1447295). A large, nested, case–control study from the National Cancer Institute Breast and Prostate Cancer Cohort Consortium using 6,637 prostate cancer cases and 7,361 matched controls replicated this finding. The rs1447295 marker was strongly associated with prostate cancer among Caucasians. Among African Americans, the genotype association was statistically significant in men diagnosed with prostate cancer at an early age ($p = 0.011$) and non-significant for those diagnosed at a later age ($p = 0.924$). This difference in risk by age at diagnosis was not present among Caucasians. Although the gene responsible has yet to be identified, the validation of this marker in this large sample of prostate cancer cases leaves little room for the possibility of a false-positive result (Schumacher et al. 2007).

Arguments for an environmental influence. The varying prostate cancer incidence rate in several populations of African origin (Table 8.2) would suggest that some environmental influences underlie prostate cancer as well. It should be noted that the black US population is the only one of the six populations in which screening is common, but that screening has not been shown to affect mortality. The varying international mortality rates even among persons of the same race (Fig. 8.3) would also suggest that that there is an extrinsic environmental influence, even among whites (see Chapter 3 of this book).

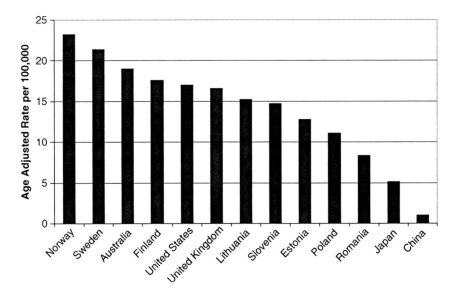

Fig. 8.3 Age-adjusted Prostate Cancer Mortality Rates
Adapted from Greenlee et al. 2000.

Sakr et al. (1994, 2000) studied prostates taken in the autopsy of men dying of trauma in Detroit. They found high proportions of black and white men had small foci of prostate cancer on autopsy. Indeed, several other autopsy studies suggest that the prevalence of small prostate cancers is relatively high among numerous populations (Soos et al. 2005; Sanchez-Chapado et al. 2003). These studies indicate there is little or no racial/ethnic variation in the proportions with small autopsy tumors. There are, however, tremendous international and racial-ethnic variations in clinically diagnosed prostate cancer rates. Promoter factors or environmental influences on genetics might explain the differences in clinical presentation on a background of similar small volume disease. An infectious agent (Klein & Silverman 2008) or an occupational exposure or other causes of oxidative stress (Klein et al. 2006) may be the cause of certain population differences in prostate cancer. The difference in mortality among populations of African origin (Table 8.3), for example, suggests the presence of an environmental component not present in the populations with low mortality rates.

It has also been observed that migration of Asians from areas of low risk (the Far East) to areas of high risk (the US) increases subsequent risk (Haenszel & Kurihara 1968; Haenszel 1985). This strongly suggests that environmental factors (possibly dietary) are important to the development of prostate cancer. Diet has been suggested as playing an important role in the differing pathologies of other cancers, including breast cancer (Harlan et al. 1993), and various aspects of diet have been implicated in prostate cancer as well. These include number of calories consumed, number of calories from carbohydrates, and number of calories from animal fat (Satia-Abouta et al. 2002; Giovannucci et al. 2007). It has been noted that the Asian diet is lacking in cheese and animal fat compared to the western diet. The Asian diet is also high in soy, which has possible prostate cancer preventatives such as the isoflavones and their aglycones (genistein and daidzein) (Akaza et al. 2004; Kumar et al. 2004).

Disparities in body mass index (BMI) and obesity may be the driving force in many black-white cancer disparities as well (Amling et al. 2004; Amling et al. 2001). Black Americans tend to have higher BMIs than white Americans (International data on BMI comparisons are very limited.) Spangler et al. (2007) studied the impact of body mass index on tumor characteristics and treatment failure in prostate cancer. In 924 patients studied (140 black, 784 white), obese men (BMI greater than 30) tended to have worse preoperative and postoperative tumor characteristics and biochemical relapse-free survival than non-obese men (Spangler et al. 2007). A higher proportion of persons of African heritage also have the metabolic syndrome and diabetes. This means that a higher proportion of persons of African heritage have circulating insulin and insulin-like growth factors. The role that these increase circulating growth factors have on prostate cancer risk, while intriguing, is unknown.

The largest study examining each element of dietary influence comes from the Cancer Prevention Study II Nutrition Cohort, where approximately 65,000 men completed an initial questionnaire in 1992–93 and were followed through 2001. Rodriguez et al. reported that, among black men, total red meat intake, including processed and unprocessed meat, was associated with a higher risk of prostate cancer with a two-fold increase in relative risk ($p < 0.05$). The influence of cooked processed meats were especially prominent with a relative risk of 2.7 in the highest quartile versus the lowest (p value for trend = 0.008) (Rodriguez et al. 2006). Other, smaller, studies also have shown that the consumption of cooked processed meats may contribute to prostate cancer in black men in the US.

Selenium, a common dietary element, has been postulated as a prostate cancer preventive agent and is a drug in an ongoing prostate cancer prevention trial (Klein 2004). Vogt and colleagues (2007) analyzed data from the Third National Health and Nutrition Examination Survey (1988–1994) and found that the crude mean serum selenium concentrations for whites were 126.35 ng/ml versus 118.76 ng/ml for blacks. Studies comparing pathologies seem to yield different comparisons by date of study. Studies in the pre-PSA era (pre-circa 1995–1996) seem to suggest more differences among the races, with blacks having a higher prevalence of high-grade tumors. Studies in Americans in the post-PSA era tend to show either no or minimal racial differences.

A post-1995 US Department of Defense (DOD) study of military retirees with prostate cancer found that higher tumor grade (Gleason score ≥ 7) is not correlated with race, but is correlated with rank or SES (Tarman et al. 2000). This finding is quite tantalizing. Enlisted men tend to have a higher risk of high-grade disease than do officers. Officers are generally better educated and have a higher SES. This finding is especially interesting as SES has been correlated with pathologic grade of breast cancer in both American and Scottish studies

(Brewster et al. 2001; Gordon 1995; Harlan et al. 1993). SES is known to correlate with BMI (Chang and Lauderdale 2005; Sarlio-Lähteenkorva and Laheima 1999), and some postulate that SES may correlate with diet as well (Darmon and Drewnowski 2008; Toles 2008).

Patterns of Care

Significant data show disparities by a number of parameters in the amount and type of treatment given. There are clear age, racial, and SES differences in patterns of care received. Specifically, younger, more educated, and wealthier men are far more likely to receive more aggressive treatment (Morris et al. 1999). The wealthier are more likely to receive more expensive and more innovative therapies (Kane et al. 2003). Especially among men aged 75 years and above, the more educated are far more likely to get more aggressive therapy than the less educated. Sadly, efforts to mitigate cancer therapy disparities have been largely unsuccessful, and recent studies of disparities in proportions of the poor and racial minorities going untreated remain largely unchanged from the 1980s up to the present (Gross et al. 2008).

There were and may still be geographic and racial differences in the use of prostatectomy in particular (Harlan et al. 1995). In the early 1990s, black men with local-regional prostate cancer in southeastern registries were less likely to receive aggressive treatment for localized disease, compared to black men with prostate cancer in the northeastern registries. Blacks in northeastern registries were also less likely to receive aggressive prostate cancer treatment than blacks in western US registries. Klabunde et al. (1998) have shown that black men in the SEER-Medicare database were less likely to undergo radical prostatectomy than were white men, while use of radiation therapy did not differ markedly by race. Sociodemographic and clinical characteristics explained approximately half the difference between black men and white men in radical prostatectomy use. Specifically, higher SES and a lack of comorbid conditions were among the factors predictive of use of aggressive therapy (Harlan et al. 2001).

In the mid-1990s, patterns of care studies also demonstrated that blacks were more likely to receive less aggressive therapy for local-regional prostate cancer. Differences in clinical presentation and life expectancy did not explain the disparity in treatment patterns (Shavers et al. 2004). Among men who had localized disease and received observation therapy, there is evidence that black and Hispanic men were more likely to receive less intense monitoring (Shavers et al. 2004). Data on treatment patterns in the late 1990s and beyond are yet to be analyzed. A study of Medicare data linked to population registries shows that 38% of black men and 25% of white men dying of metastatic disease never received hormonal therapy (Lu-Yao et al. 2006). This suggests substantial quality of care issues for both black and white Americans with advanced disease with blacks more likely to get less than optimal care.

Patterns of care differences influence disparities. In a population-based analysis in California, Robbins et al. (2007) found that the large black-white difference in prostate cancer survival was completely explained by known prognostic factors such as comorbid disease.

There is some suggestion that racial differences in the use of prostatectomy may be decreasing over time, at least for men younger than 60. In study of a cohort of men younger than 60 with localized disease treated in the mid-1990s, use of aggressive treatment was similar by race/ethnicity (adjusted percentages are 85.5%, 88.1%, and 85.3% for white, African American, and Hispanic men, respectively). However, among men 60 years old and older, African American men underwent aggressive treatment less often than did white or Hispanic men (adjusted percentages for men aged 60–64 years = 67.1%, 84.7%, and 79.2%, respectively; 65–74 years = 64.8%, 73.4%, and 79.5%, respectively; and 75 years old and older = 25.2%, 45.7%, and 36.6%, respectively) (Harlan et al. 2001).

Treatment Outcomes

Whether black men are at increased risk for biochemical disease recurrence after radical prostatectomy is debatable. Once black men have a recurrence, it is also unknown whether they have more aggressive disease than their white counterparts. Several population studies do show that black American men with localized disease have higher death rates than whites (Oakley-Girvan et al. 2003; Godley et al. 2003). This pattern has been observed in older data, as well as data from the late 1990s.

In a population-based study of California men, Robbins et al. (2000) found that SES differences did not correlate with the higher prostate cancer death rates of blacks, although SES differences did explain racial differences in non-prostate cancer causes of death among prostate cancer patients. In a population-based study of SEER Medicare data, Godley et al. (2003) showed that black men aged 65 years and older treated with radical prostatectomy had a 1.8-year shorter median survival than whites of the same age treated with prostatectomy. The differences were 0.7 years lower for blacks treated with radiation therapy (95% CI, 0.5–1.0 year) and 1.0 year lower for blacks treated with observation therapy (95% CI, 0.7–1.1).

Wood and colleagues analyzed data from a cohort of 2,910 men treated with prostatectomy from 1987 to 2004. They found increases in the rate of organ-confined disease for black and white men diagnosed later in the study. The study found a 11–12% excess in biochemical relapse-free survival for black men compared to whites throughout the study (Wood et al. 2007). The fact that black men continued to show higher rates of biochemical failure after surgery despite an increasing rate of organ-confined disease is an extremely significant finding. It suggests that prostate cancer is more aggressive in blacks and that if screening is beneficial, it may not be as beneficial in black men.

Clinical trials have a selection bias and better guarantee that all patients receive the same quality of care. The predominance of clinical evidence suggests that equal treatment yields equal outcomes and that race need not be a factor in outcomes (Bach et al. 2002). The majority of clinical studies, in fact, conclude that race is not an independent predictor of treatment failure (Shavers and Brown 2002; Peters and Armstrong 2005). Specifically, after considering other prognostic factors such as stage, grade, and comorbid disease, race is not predictive of poor outcomes after treatment with radiation (Young et al. 2000; Hart et al. 1999; Roach et al. 1992; Connell et al. 2001), radical prostatectomy, (Hart et al. 1999; Freedlan et al. 2000; Fowler et al. 1996; Iselin et al. 1998) and hormone therapy (McLeod et al. 1999; Fowler et al. 1997), or chemotherapy (Tannock et al. 2004).

Some studies suggest that race is a dependent variable in outcome (Austin et al. 1990; Austin and Convery 1993; Kim et al. 1995; Moul et al. 1996; Powell et al. 2002; Shekarriz et al. 2000; Tarman et al. 2000). In a select group of black men who were treated in a premier tertiary care center, it was observed that they were more likely to be obese, present with adverse preoperative clinical features at a younger age, and have a higher rate of biochemical progression than whites treated at the same facility. On multivariate analysis black race per se, however, was not an independent predictor of adverse pathological outcome or biochemical recurrence (Nielsen et al. 2006).

It should be noted that the Department of Defense Center for Prostate Disease Research (CPDR) compares the largest cohort of blacks with prostate cancer who have had access to high-quality treatment to a white cohort with the same access to high-quality treatment. In these studies, race did not influence outcome in radical prostatectomy (Amling et al. 2001) or in radiation therapy (Johnstone et al. 2002). These studies did find that obesity was a significant influence in success of therapy for localized disease. The CPDR database noted that the black cohort tended to have higher body mass indexes than the white cohort (Amling et al. 2004).

Conclusion

The cause of the majority of prostate cancers is almost certainly environmental influences upon genetics, the so-called gene–environmental interactions. This is likely true for all races/ethnicities. The environmental influences that cause prostate cancer may be related to diet or perhaps other factors such as infectious agents and occupational exposure as well. Given the current evidence, one cannot rule out the possibility that blacks or persons with a family originating from sub-Saharan Africa may also have a genetic predisposition to prostate cancer. If true, this is likely due to polymorphisms, genetic mutations, or a combination of the two. Such predispositions have been seen in other genetic diseases such as sickle cell anemia or certain BRCA mutations in Askinazi Jewish populations (Brawley 2002). These conditions suggest that if blacks do have a genetic predisposition to prostate cancer, they do not have a monopoly on this predisposition.

The sickle cell trait and its resultant survival advantage (against malaria), for example, is not confined to blacks in sub-Saharan Africa, but to persons in a large contiguous geographic area that includes southern Europe, the Middle East, and sub-Saharan Africa. That is to say, there are also people who are considered white or European with sickle cell trait. It is true that the prevalence of this genetic marker is greater in those with origins in sub-Saharan Africa, but Africans do not monopolize the genetic mutation. The same situation may well pertain to a prostate cancer predisposition.

Some studies also suggest that a higher proportion of blacks presenting with prostate cancer have higher grade disease. A number of clinical trials and DOD data demonstrate that equal treatment yields equal outcome among equal patients (patients with same general health, same stage, and same grade), and race in and of itself need not be a factor in outcome. "What causes high grade disease?" and "How does one distinguish disease destined to cause loss of life from benign cancers?" remain important and as yet unanswered questions, all pertinent to the value of screening.

In contrast, racial differences in the quantity and quality of care received are clear according to population-based patterns of care studies. In the real world of the US, the proportion of black men getting optimal high-quality care is lower than the proportion of whites getting optimal high-quality care. Blacks are less likely to get aggressive therapy for localized disease and less likely to get intense observation while undergoing "watch and wait" therapy. Perhaps as a result, significant disparities remain in treatment outcomes for blacks as well.

Aggressive efforts are needed to close these racial and ethnic prostate cancer disparities along the prostate cancer continuum. Fortunately, more tailored strategies are underway to close the gaps, including targeted efforts to increase communication outreach to provide all men with accurate and balanced prostate cancer information about the advantages and disadvantages of screening, diagnosis, treatment, and diet and lifestyle changes, and to increase the number of racial and ethnic minorities in research studies and clinical trials. These well-documented efforts should be continued as well.

We should also continue to build on the research that has explored how culture and communication with health care providers influence men's knowledge, health beliefs, and practices regarding prostate cancer screening and treatment. This knowledge could contribute to closing some of the known prostate cancer gaps among minority and underserved men as well. Great strides have also already been made, and should continue to be made, in training physicians to familiarize themselves with the health and culture of underserved populations. However, the profession still falls short in increasing the number of physicians from underrepresented populations such as African Americans and Hispanics, and many health facilities and health centers lack an adequate number of bilingual physicians, health professionals, and translators to contend with language barriers that may contribute to poor communication outcomes, lack of understanding of treatment and medicine procedures, and, ultimately, poor health outcomes.

Even more importantly, we must continue to push for greater consensus around screening and equalizing treatment protocols for all men. Further, some emerging research suggests that the type of physician a man sees, the physician's length of time in a particular specialty, and the physician's length of time in performing certain treatment protocol influences the type of balanced information a man receives, which, in turn, may influence prostate treatment decisions and outcomes. This information may be critical in analyzing prostate cancer outcomes and disparities among various populations.

Finally, in this post-"human genome era," researchers and health professionals must continue to ask the hard questions about the biologic influence of race and the social influence of race. Race need not be a factor in outcome. However, discrimination in the health care system by such factors as race, ethnicity, sexual orientation, religion, geography, income, education, and health insurance status are factors that can contribute to the failure of prostate cancer in any other population.

As such, attention should persist regarding the influence of socioeconomic factors and prostate cancer. Researchers such as Tarman and colleagues (2000) and others are right to call for further examination of how social, economic, and racial variables are defined and controlled for. This research is worthy of further study so that accurate conclusions can be drawn regarding the influence of SES and prostate cancer. The reasons for prostate cancer disparities must be determined and must be addressed. This is a moral issue for American society as a whole and not just for American medicine.

References

Akaza, H., Miyanaga, N., Takashima, N., Naito, S., Hirao, Y., Tsukamoto, T. et al. Comparisons of percent equal producers between prostate cancer patients and controls: case-controlled studies of isoflavones in Japanese, Korean, and American residents. Jap J Clin Oncol. 2004; 34(2):86–89.

Albano, J.D., Ward, E., Jemal, A., Anderson, R., Cokkinides, V.E, Murray, T. et al. Cancer mortality in the United States by education level and race. J Natl Cancer Inst. 2007; 99(18):1384–1394.

American Cancer Society (2009). Chief medical officer Otis W. Brawley responds to prostate cancer studies. American Cancer Society. Retrieved March 25, 2008, from http://www.cancer.org/docroot/MED/content/MED_2_1×_Chief_Medical_Officer_Otis_W_Brawley_Responds_to_Prostate_Studies.asp.

Amling, C.L., Kane, C.J., Riffenburgh, R.H., Ward, J.F., Roberts, J.L., Lance, R.S. et al. Relationship between obesity and race in predicting adverse pathologic variables in patients undergoing radical prostatectomy. Urology. 2001; 58(5):723–728.

Amling, C.L., Riffenburg, R.H., Sun, L., Moul, J.W., Lance, R.S., Kusada, L. et al. Pathologic variables and recurrence rates as related to obesity and race in men with prostate cancer undergoing radical prostatectomy. J Clin Oncol. 2004; 22(3):439–445.

Andriole, G.L., Grubb, R.L., III, Buys, S.S., Chia, D., Church, T.R., Fouad, M.N., et al. Mortality results from a radomized prostate-cancer screening trial. New Engl J Med. 2009; 360(13). Retrieved March 26, 2009, from http://content.nejm.org/cgi/content/full/NEJMoa0810696.

Austin, J.P., Convery, K. Age-race interaction in prostatic adenocarcinoma treated with external beam irradiation. Am J Clin Oncol. 1993; 16(2):140–145.

Austin, J.P., Aziz, H., Potters, L., Thelmo, W., Chen, P., Choi, K. et al. Diminished survival of young blacks with adenocarcinoma of the prostate. Am J Clin Oncol. 1990; 13(6):465–469.

Bangsi, D., Zhou, J., Sun, Y., Patel, N.P., Darga, L.L., Heilbrun, L.K. et al. Impact of a genetic variant in CYP3A4 on risk and clinical presentation of prostate cancer among white and African-American men. Urol Oncol. 2006; 24(1):21–27.

Bach, P.B., Schrag, D., Brawley, O.W., Galaznik, A., Yakren, S., Begg, C.B. Survival of black and whites after a cancer diagnosis. J Am Med Assoc. 2002; 287(16):2106–2113.

Barry, M.J. Screening for prostate cancer – The controversy that refuses to die. New Engl J Med. 2009; 360(13). Retrieved March 26, 2009, from http://content. nejm.org/cgi/content/full/NEJMe0901166.

Bennett, C.L., Ferreira, M.R., Davis, T.C., Kaplan, J., Weinberger, M., Kuzel, T. et al. Relation between literacy, race, and stage of presentation among low-income patients with prostate cancer. J Clin Oncol. 1998; 16(9):3101–3104.

Bennett, C.L., Price, D.K., Kim, S., Liu, D., Jovanovic, B.D., Nathan, D. et al. Racial variation in CAG repeat lengths within the androgen receptor gene among prostate cancer patients of lower socioeconomic status. J Clin Oncol. 2002; 20(17):3599–3604.

Ben-Shlomo, Y., Evans, S., Ibrahim, F., Patel, B., Anson, K., Chinegwundoh, F. et al. The risk of prostate cancer amongst black men in the United Kingdom: the PROCESS cohort study. Eur Urology. 2008; 53(1):99–105.

Brawley, O.W. Some perspective on black-white cancer statistics. CA Cancer J Clin. 2002; 52(6):322–325.

Brawley, O.W. Population categorization and cancer statistics. Cancer Metastasis Rev. 2003; 22(1):11–19.

Brawley, O.W., Ford, L.G., Thompson, I., Perlman, J.A., Kramer, B.S. 5-Alpha reductase inhibition and prostate cancer prevention. Cancer Epidemiol Biomarkers Prev. 1994; 3(2):177–182.

Brewster, D.H., Thomson, C.S., Hole, D.J., Black, R.J., Stroner, P.L., Gillis, C.R. Relation between socioeconomic status and tumor stage in patients with breast, colorectal, ovarian, and lung cancer: results from four national, population based studies. BMJ. 2001; 322(7290):830–831.

Boyle, P. Screening for prostate cancer: have you had your cholesterol measured? BJU Int. 2003; 92(3):191–199.

Brown, M.L., Potosky, A.L. The presidential effect: the public health response to media coverage about Ronald Reagan's colon cancer episode. Pub Op Quarterly. 1990; 54(3):317–329.

Collin, S.M., Martin, R.M., Metcalfe, C., Gunnell, D., Albertsen, P.C., Neal, D. et al. Prostate-cancer mortality in the USA and UK in 1975–2004: an ecological study. Lancet Oncol. 2008; 9(5):445–452.

Connell, P.P., Ignacio, L., Haraf, D., Awan, A.M., Halpern, H., Abdalla, I. et al. Equivalent racial outcome after conformal radiotherapy for prostate cancer: a single departmental experience. J Clin Oncol. 2001; 19(1):54–61.

Cooperberg, M.R., Lubeck, D.P., Meng, M.V., Mehta, S.S., Carroll, P.R. The changing face of low-risk prostate cancer: trends in clinical presentation and primary management. J Clin Oncol. 2006; 22(11):2141–2149.

de Koning, H.J., Auvinen, A., Berenguer-Sanchez, A., Calais da Silva, F, Ciatto, S., Denis, L. et al. Large-scale randomized prostate cancer screening trials: program performances in the European Randomized Screening for Prostate Cancer trial and the Prostate, Lung, Colorectal and Ovary Cancer trial. Int J Cancer. 2002; 97(2):237–244.

Du, X.L., Fang, S., Coker, A.L., Sanderson, M., Aragaki, C., Cormier, J.N. Racial disparity and socioeconomic status in association with survival in older men with local/regional stage prostate carcinoma: findings from a large community-based cohort. Cancer. 2006; 106(6):1276–1285.

Duffy, S.W., Nagtegaal, I.D., Wallis, M., Cafferty, F.H., Houssami, Warwick, J. et al. Correcting for lead time and length bias in estimating the effect of screen detection on cancer survival. Am J Epid. 2008; 168(1):98–104.

Edwards, B.K., Brown, M.L., Wingo, P.A., Howe, H.L., Ward, E., Ries, L.A. et al. Annual report to the nation on the status of cancer, 1975–2002, featuring population-based trends in cancer treatment. J Natl Cancer Inst. 2005; 97(19):1407–1427.

Etzioni, R., Penson, D.F., Legler, J.M., di Tommaso, D., Boer, R., Gann, P.H. et al. Over-diagnosis due to prostate-specific antigen screening: lessons from U.S. prostate cancer incidence trends. J Natl Cancer Inst. 2002; 94(13):981–990.

Fiscella, K., Williams, D.R. Health disparities based on socioeconomic inequities: implications for urban health care. Acad Med. 2004; 79(12):1139–1147.

Fowler, J.E., Bigler, S.A. Renfroe, D.L., Dabagia, M.D. Prostate specific antigen in black and white men after hormonal therapies for prostate cancer. J Urol. 1997; 158(1): 150–154.

Fowler, J.E., Jr., Terrell, F.L., Renfroe, D.L. Co-morbidities and survival of men with localized prostate cancer treated with surgery or radiation therapy. J Urol. 1996; 156(5):1714–1718.

Freedland, S.J., Jalkut, M., Dorey, F., Sutter, M.E., Aronson, W.J. Race is not an independent predictor of biochemical recurrence after radical prostatectomy in an equal access medical center. Urology. 2000; 56(1):87–91.

Gilligan, T., Wang, P.S., Levin, R., Kantoff, P.W., Avorn, J. Racial differences in screening for prostate cancer in the elderly. Arch Int Med. 2004; 164:1858–1864.

Giovannucci, E. Vitamin D and cancer incidence in the Harvard cohorts. Ann Epid. 2009; 19(2):87–88.

Giovannucci, E., Liu, Y., Platz, E.A., Stampfer, M.J., Willet, W.C. Risk factors for prostate cancer incidence and progression in the health professionals follow-up study. Int J Cancer. 2007; 121(7):1571–1578.

Glover, F.E., Jr., Coffey, D.S., Douglas, L.L., Cadogan, M., Russell, H., Tulloch, T. et al. The epidemiology of prostate cancer in Jamaica. J Urol. 1998; 159(6):1984–1986.

Godley, P.A., Schenck, A.P., Amamoo, M.A., Schoenbach, V.J., Peacock, S., Manning, M. et al. Racial differences in mortality among Medicare recipients after treatment for localized prostate cancer. J Natl Cancer Inst. 2003; 95(22):1702–1710.

Gordon, N.H. Association of education and income with estrogen receptor status in primary breast cancer. Am J Epid. 1995; 142(8):796–803.

Greenlee, R.T., Murray, T., Bolden, S., Wing, P.A., Cancer Statistics, 50: 7–33, 2000.

Gross, C.P., Smith, B.D., Wolf, E., Andersen, M. Racial disparities in cancer therapy: did the gap narrow between 1992 and 2002? Cancer. 2008; 112(4):900–908.

Haenszel, W. Studies of migrant populations. Am J Pub Health. 1985; 75(3):225–226.

Haenszel, W., Kurihara, M. Studies of Japanese migrants: mortality from cancer and other diseases among Japanese in the United States. J Natl Cancer Inst. 1968; 40(1):43–68.

Halpern, M.T., Ward, E.M., Pavluck, A.L., Schrag, N.M., Bian, J., Chen, A.Y. Association of insurance status and ethnicity with cancer stage at diagnosis for 12 cancer sites: a retrospective analysis. Lancet Oncol. 2008; 9(3):222–231.

Harlan, L., Brawley, O., Pommerenke, F., Wali, P., Kramer, B. Geographic, age, and racial variation in the treatment of local/regional carcinoma of the prostate. J Clin Oncol. 1995; 13(1):93–100.

Harlan, L.C., Coates, R.J., Block, G., Greenberg, R.S., Ershow, A., Forman, M. et al. Estrogen receptor status and dietary intakes in breast cancer patients. Epid. 1993; 4(1):25–31.

Harlan, L.C., Potosky, A., Gilliland, F.D., Hoffman, R., Albertsen, P.C., Hamilton, A.S. et al. Factors associated with initial therapy for clinically localized prostate cancer: prostate cancer outcomes study. J Natl Cancer Inst. 2001; 93(24):1864–1871.

Hart, K.B., Wood, D.P., Jr., Tekyi-Mensah, S., Porter, A.T., Pontes, J.E., Forman, J.D. The impact of race on biochemical disease-free survival in early-stage prostate cancer patients treated with surgery or radiation therapy. Int J Rad Oncol Biol Phys. 1999; 45(5):1235–1238.

Hernandez, W., Grenade, C., Santos, E.R., Bonilla, C., Ahaghotu, C., Kittles, R.A. IGF-1 and IGFBP-3 gene variants influence on serum levels and prostate cancer risk in African-Americans. Carcinogenesis. 2007; 28(10):2154–2159.

Ingles, S.A., Ross, R.K., Yu, M.C., Irvine, R.A., La, P.G., Haile, R.W. et al. Association of prostate cancer risk with genetic polymorphisms in vitamin D receptor and androgen receptor. J Natl Cancer Inst. 1997; 89(2):166–170.

Irvine, R.A., Yu, M.C., Ross, R.K., Coetzee, G.A. The CAG and GGC microsatellites of the androgen receptor gene are in linkage disequilibrium in men with prostate cancer. Cancer Res. 1995; 55(9):1937–1940.

Iselin, C.E., Box, J.W., Vollmer, R.T., Layfield, L.J., Robertson, J.E., Paulson, D.F. Surgical control of clinically localized prostate carcinoma equivalent in African-American and white males. Cancer. 1998; 83(11):2353–2360.

Johnstone, P.A., Kane, C.J., Sun, L., Wu, H., Moul, J.W., McLeod, D.G. et al. Effect of race on biochemical disease-free outcome in patients with prostate cancer treated with definitive radiation therapy in an equal-access health care system: radiation oncology report of the Department of Defense Center for Prostate Disease Research. Radiology. 2002; 225(2):420–426.

Kane, C.J., Lubeck, D.P., Knight, S.J., Spitalny, M., Downs, T.M., Grossfeld, G.D. et al. Impact of patient educational level on treatment for patients with prostate cancer: data from CaPSURE. Urology. 2003; 62(6):1035–1039.

Kidd, L.C., Paltoo, D.N., Wang, S., Chen, W., Akereyeni, F., Issacs, W. et al. Sequence variation within the 5' regulatory regions of the vitamin D binding protein and receptor genes and prostate cancer risk. Prostate. 2005;64(3):272–282.

Kim, J.A., Kuban, D.A, el-Mahdi, A.M., Schellhammer, P.F. Carcinoma of the prostate: race as a prognostic indicator in definitive radiation therapy. Radiology. 1995; 194(2):545–549.

Kittles, R.A., Young, D., Weinrich, S., Hudson, J., Argyropoulos, G., Ukoli, F. et al. Extent of linkage disequilibrium between the androgen receptor gene CAG and GGC repeats in human populations: implications for prostate cancer risk. Hum Genet. 2001; 109(3):253–261.

Klabunde, C.N., Potosky, A.L., Harlan, L.C., Kramer, B.S. Trends and black/white differences in treatment for nonmetastatic prostate cancer. Med Care. 1998; 36(9):1337–1348.

Klein, E.A. Selenium and vitamin E cancer prevention trial. Ann NY Acad Sci. 2004; 1031:234–241.

Klein, E.A., Silverman, R. Inflammation, infection, and prostate cancer. Curr Op Urol. 2008; 18(3):315–319.

Klein, E.A., Casey, G., Silverman, R. Genetic susceptibility and oxidative stress in prostate cancer: integrated model with implications for prevention. Urology 2006; 68(6):1145–1151.

Kramer, B.S., Brown, M.L., Prorok, P.C., Potosky, A.L., Gohagen, J.K. Prostate cancer screening: what we know and what we need to know. Ann Int Med. 1993; 119(9):914–923.

Kripalani, S., Sharma, J., Justice, E., Justice, J., Spiker, C., Laufman, L.E. et al. Low-literacy interventions to promote discussion of prostate cancer: a randomized controlled trial. Am J Prev Med. 2007; 33(2):83–90.

Kumar, R.J., Baha Barqawi, A.B., Crawford, E.D. Epidemiology of prostate cancer. Business Briefing: US Oncology Review 2004: 42–45.

Liu, L., Cozen, W., Bernstein, L., Ross, R.K., Deapen, D. Changing relationship between socioeconomic status and prostate cancer incidence. J Natl Cancer Inst. 2001; 93(9):705–709.

Litman, H.J., Bhasin, S., Link, C.L., Araujo, A.B., McKinlay, J.B. Serum androgen levels in black, Hispanic, and white men. J Clin Endocrin Metab. 2006; 91(11):4326–4334.

Lu-Yao, G., Albertsen, P.C., Stanford, J.L., Stukel, T.A., Walker-Corkery, E.S., Barry, M.J. Natural experiment examining impact of aggressive screening and treatment on prostate cancer mortality in two fixed cohorts from Seattle area and Connecticut. BMJ. 2002; 325(7367):740.

Lu-Yao, G., Moore, D.F., Oleynick, J., DiPaola, R.S., Yao, S.L. Use of hormonal therapy in men with metastatic prostate cancer. J Urol. 2006; 176(2):526–531.

Mariotto, A.B., Etzioni, R., Krapcho, M., Feuer, E.J. Reconstructing PSA testing patterns between black and white men in the US from Medicare claims and the National Health Interview Survey. Cancer. 2007; 109(9):1877–1886.

McLeod, D.G., Schellhammer, P.F., Vogelzang, N.J., Soloway, M.S., Sharifi, R., Black, N.L. et al. Exploratory analysis on the effect of race on clinical outcome in patients with advanced prostate cancer receiving bicalutamide or flutamide, each in combination with LHRH analogues. The Casodex Combination Study Group. Prostate. 1999; 40(4):218–224.

Miller, D.C., Gruber, S.B., Hollenbeck, B.K., Montie, J.E., Wei, J.T. Incidence of initial local therapy among men with lower-risk prostate cancer in the United States. J Natl Cancer Inst. 2006; 98(16):1134–1141.

Morris, C.R., Snipes, K.P., Schlag, R., Wright, W.E. Sociodemographic factors associated with prostatectomy utilization and concordance with the physician data query for prostate cancer (United States). Cancer Causes Control. 1999; 10(6):503–511.

Moul, J., Douglas, T., McCarthy, W., McLeod, D. Black race is an adverse prognostic factor for prostate cancer recurrence following radical prostatectomy in an equal access health care setting. J Urol. 1996; 155(5):1667–1672.

Nielsen, M.E., Han, M., Mangold, L., Humphreys, E., Walsh, P.C., Partin, A.W. et al. Black race does not independently predict adverse outcome following radical retropubic prostatectomy at a tertiary referral center. J Urol. 2006; 176(2): 515–519.

Oakley-Girvan, I., Kolonel, L.N., Gallagher, R.P., Wu, A.H., Felberg, A., Whittemore, A.S. Stage at diagnosis and survival in a multiethnic cohort of prostate cancer patients. Am J Pub Health. 2003; 93(10):1753–1759.

Odedina, F.T., Ogunbiyi, J.O., Ukoli, F.A. Roots of prostate cancer in African-American men. J Natl Med Assn. 2006; 98(4):539–543.

Pan, C.C., Lee, J.S., Chan, J.L., Sandler, H.M., Underwood, W., McLaughlin, P.W. The association between presentation PSA and race in two sequential time periods in prostate cancer patients seen at a university hospital and its community affiliates. Int J Rad Oncology, Biology, Physics. 2003; 57(5):1292–1296.

Panz, V.R., Joffe, B.I., Spitz, I., Lindenberg, T., Farkas, A., Haffejee, M. Tandem CAG repeats of the androgen receptor gene and prostate cancer risk in black and white men. Endocrine. 2001; 15(2):213–216.

Park, J., Chen, L., Ratnashinge, L., Sellers, T.A., Tanner, J.P., Lee, J.H. et al. Deletion polymorphism of UDP-glucuronosyltransferase 2B17 and risk of prostate cancer in African American and Caucasian men. Cancer, Epidemiology, Biomarkers, and Prevention. 2006; 15(8):1473–1478.

Parkin, D.M., Whelan, S.L., Ferlay, J., Raymond, L., Young, J., eds. Cancer Incidence in Five Continents, Vol 7. Lyon (France), IARC Scientific Publication No. 143, IARC Press; 1997.

Peters, N., Armstrong, K. Racial differences in prostate cancer treatment outcomes. Cancer Nurs. 2005; 28(2):108–116.

Phillips, A.A., Jacobson, J.S., Magai, C., Consedine, N., Horowicz-Mehler, N.C., Neugut, A.I. Cancer incidence and mortality in the Caribbean. Cancer Invest. 2007; 25(6):476–483.

Platz, E.A., Rimm, E.B., Willett, W.C., Kantoff, P.W., Giovannucci, E. Racial variation in prostate cancer incidence and in hormonal system markers among male health professionals. J Natl Cancer Inst. 2000; 92(24):2009–2017.

Polednak, A.P. Stage at diagnosis of prostate cancer in Connecticut by poverty and race. Ethnicity and Disease. 1997; 7(3):215–220.

Potosky, A.L., Feuer, E.J., Levin, D.L. Impact of screening on incidence and mortality in the United States. Epidem Rev. 2001; 23(1):181–186.

Powell, I.J., Dey, J., Dudley, A., Pontes, J.E., Cher, M.L., Sakr, W. et al. Disease-free survival difference between African Americans and whites after radical prostatectomy for local prostate cancer: a multivariable analysis. Urol. 2002; 59: 907–912.

Powell, I.J., Land, S.J., Dey, J., Heilbrun, L.K., Hughes, M.R., Sakr, W. et al. The impact of CAG repeats in exon 1 of the androgen receptor on disease progression after prostatectomy. Cancer. 2005; 103(3):528–537.

Reed, A., Ankerst, D.P., Pollack, B.H., Thompson, I.M., Parekh, D.J. Current age and race adjusted prostate specific antigen threshold values delay diagnosis of high grade prostate cancer. J Urol. 2007; 178(5):1929–1932.

Ries L.A.G., Melbert, D., Krapcho, M., Stinchcomb, D.G., Howlader, N., Horner, M.J., Mariotto, A., Miller, B.A., Feuer, E.J., Altekruse, S.F., Lewis, D.R., Clegg, L., Eisner, M.P., Reichman, M., Edwards, B.K., (Eds). SEER Cancer Statistics Review, 1975–2005, National Cancer Institute. Bethesda, MD, http://seer.cancer.gov/csr/1975_2005, based on November 2007 SEER data submission, posted to the SEER web site, 2008.

Ries, L.A.G., Harkins, D., Krapcho, M., Mariotto, A., Miller, B.A., Feuer, E.J. et al. SEER cancer statistic review, 1975–2003. Bethesda: National Cancer Institute, 2006 http://www.seercancer.gov/csr/1975–2002. Accessed August 4, 2008.

Roach, M., III. Krall, J., Keller, J.W., Perez, C.A., Sause, W.T., Doggett, R.L. et al. The prognostic significance of race and survival from prostate cancer based on patients irradiated on Radiation Therapy Oncology Group protocols (1976–1985). Int J Rad Oncol Biol Phys. 1992; 24(3):441–449.

Robbins, A.S., Whittemore, A.S., Thom, D.H. Differences in socioeconomic status and survival among white and black men with prostate cancer. Am J Epidem. 2000; 151(4):409–416.

Robbins, A.S., Yin, D., Parikh-Patel, A. Differences in prognostic factors and survival among white men and black men with prostate cancer, California, 1995–2004. Am J Epidem. 2007; 166(1):71–78.

Rodriguez, C., McCullough, M.L., Mondul, A.M., Jacobs, E.J., Chao, A., Patel, A.V. et al. Meat consumption among blacks and white men and risk of prostate cancer in the Cancer Prevention Study II Nutrition Cohort. Cancer Epidem Biomarkers Prev. 2006; 15(2):211–216.

Roetzheim, R.G., Pal, N., Tennant, C., Voti, L., Ayanian, J.Z., Schwabe, A. et al. Effects of health insurance and race on early detection of cancer. J Natl Cancer Inst. 1999; 91(16):1409–1415.

Rohrmann, S., Nelson, W.G., Rifai, N., Brown, T.R., Dobs, A., Kanarek, N. et al. Serum estrogen, but not testosterone, levels differ between black and white men in a nationally representative sample of Americans. J Clin Endo Met. 2007; 92(7):2519–2525.

Ross, R.K. The role of molecular genetics in chemoprevention studies of prostate cancer. IARC Scientific Publications. 2001; 154:207–213.

Ross, L.E., Berkowitz, Z., Ekwueme, D.U. Use of the prostate-specific antigen test among U.S. men: findings from the 2005 National Health Interview Survey. Cancer, Epidemiology, Biomarkers, and Prevention. 2008; 17(3):636–644.

Ross, R.K., Pike, M.C., Coetzee, G.A., Reichardt, J.K., Yu, M.C., Feigelson, H. et al. Androgen metabolism and prostate cancer: establishing a model of genetic susceptibility. Cancer Res. 1998; 58(20):4497–4504.

Sakr, W.A., Billis, A., Ekman, P., Wilt, T., Bostwick, D.G. Epidemiology of high-grade prostatic intraepithelial neoplasia. Scand J Urol Nephr. Supp, 2000; 205:11–18.

Sakr, W.A., Grignon, D.J., Crissman, J.D., Heilbrun, L.K., Cassin, B.J., Pontes, J.J. et al. High grade prostatic intraepithelial neoplasia (HGPIN) and prostatic adenocarcinoma between the ages of 20–69: an autopsy study of 249 cases. In Vivo. 1994; 8(3):439–443.

Salam, M.T., Ursin, G., Skinner, E.C., Dessissa, T., Reichardt, J.K. Associations between polymorphisms in the steroid 5-alpha reductase type II (SRD5A2) gene and benign prostatic hyperplasia and prostate cancer. Urol Oncol. 2005; 23(4):246–253.

Sanchez-Chapado, M., Olmedilla, G., Cabeza, M., Donat, E., Ruiz, A. Prevalence of prostate cancer and prostatic intraepithelial neoplasia in Caucasian Mediterranean males: an autopsy study. Prostate. 2003; 54(3):238–247.

Sarter, O., Zheng, Q., Eastham, J.A. Androgen receptor gene CAG repeat length varies in a race-specific fashion in men without prostate cancer. Urol. 1999; 53(2):378–380.

Satia-Abouta, J., Patterson, R.E., Schiller, R.N., Kristal, A.R. Energy from fat is associated with obesity in U.S. men: results from the Prostate Cancer Prevention Trial. Prev Med. 2002; 34(5):493–501.

Schröder, F.H., Hugosson, J., Roobol, M.J., Tammela, T.L.J., Ciatto, S., Nelen, V., et al. Screening and prostate-cancer mortality in a randomized European study. New Engl J Med. 2009; 360(13). Retrieved March 26, 2009, from http://content.nejm.org/cgi/ content/ full/NEJMoa0810084.

Schumacher, F.R., Feigelson, H.S., Cox, D.G., Haiman, C.A., Albanes, D., Buring, J. et al. A common 8q24 variant in prostate and breast cancer from a large nested case-control study. Cancer Res. 2007; 67(7):2951–2956.

Schwartz, K.L., Crossley-May, H., Vigneau, F.D., Brown, K., Banerjee, M. Race, socio-economic status and stage at diagnosis for five common malignancies. Cancer Causes Control. 2003; 14(8):761–766.

Shavers, V.L., Brown, M.L. Racial and ethnic disparities in the receipt of cancer treatment. J Natl Cancer Inst. 94(5):334–357.

Shavers, V.L., Brown, M.L., Potosky, A.L., Klabunde, C.N., Davis, W.W., Moul, J.W. et al. Race/ethnicity and the receipt of watchful waiting for the initial management of prostate cancer. J General Int Med. 2004; 19(2): 146–155.

Shekarriz, B., Tiguert, R., Upadhyay, J., Gheiler, E., Powell, I.J., Pontes, J.E. et al. Impact of location and multifocality of positive surgical margins on disease-free survival following radical prostatectomy: a comparison between African-American and white men. Urol. 2000; 55(6):899–903.

Shibata, A., Ma, J., Whittemore, A.S. Prostate cancer incidence and mortality in the United States and the United Kingdom. J Natl Cancer Inst. 1998; 90(16):1230–1231.

Shibata, A., Whittemore, A.S. Re: Prostate cancer incidence and mortality in the United States and the United Kingdom. (Letter). J Natl Cancer Inst. 2001; 93(14):1109–1110.

Soos, G., Tsakiris, I., Szanto, J., Turzo, C., Haas, P.G., Dezso, B. The prevalence of prostate carcinoma and its precursor in Hungary: an autopsy study. Eur Urol. 2005; 48(5):739–744.

Spangler, E., Zeigler-Johnson, C.M., Coomes, M., Malkowicz, S.B., Wein, A., Rebbeck, T.R. Association of obesity with tumor characteristics and treatment failure of prostate cancer in African-American and European American men. J Urol. 2007; 178(5):1939–1944.

Stangelberger, A., Waldert, M., Djavan, B. Prostate cancer in elderly men. Rev Urol. 2008; 10(2):111–119.

Steenland, K., Rodriguez, C., Mondul, A., Calle, E.E., Thun, M. Prostate cancer incidence and survival in relation to education (United States). Cancer Causes Control. 2004; 15(9):939–945.

Tannock, I.F., de Wit, R., Horti, J., Pluzanska, A., Chi, K.N. et al. Docetaxel plus prednisone or mitoxantrone plus prednisone for advanced prostate cancer, NEJM. 2004; 351(15):1502–1512.

Tarman, G.J., Kane, C.J., Moul, J.W., Thrasher, J.B., Foley, J.P., Wilhite, D. et al. Impact of socioeconomic status and race on clinical parameters of patients undergoing radical prostatectomy in an equal access health care system. Urol. 2000; 56(6):1016–1020.

Taylor, K.L., Davis, J.L., III., Turner, R.O., Johnson, L., Schwartz, M.D., Kerner, J.F. et al. Educating African American men about the prostate cancer screening dilemma: A randomized intervention. Cancer Epidem Biomarkers Prev. 2006; 15:2179–2188.

Telesca, D., Etzioni, R., Gulati, R. Estimating lead time and overdiagnosis associated with PSA screening from prostate cancer incidence trends. Biometrics. 2007; 64(1):10–19.

Thompson, I.M., Ankerst, D.P., Chi, C., Goodman, P.J., Tangen, C.M., Lucia, M.S. et al. Assessing prostate cancer risk: results form the Prostate Cancer Prevention Trial. J Natl Cancer Inst. 2006; 98(8):529–534.

Thompson, I.M., Basler, J.A., Leach, R., Troyer, D., Klein, E., Brawley, O. Challenges and opportunities to the design and implementation of chemoprevention trials for prostate cancer. Urol Oncol. 2003; 21(1):73–78.

Thompson, I.M., Goodman, P.J., Tangen, C.M., Lucia, M.S., Miller, G.J., Ford, L.G. et al. The influence of finasteride on the development of prostate cancer, NEJM. 2003; 349(3):215–224.

U.S. Preventive Services Task Force. Screening for prostate cancer: U.S. Preventive Task Force Recommendation Statement. Ann Int Med. 2008; 149 (3):185–191.

Vogt, T.M., Ziegler, R.G., Patterson, B.H., Graubard, B.I. Racial differences in serum selenium concentration: analysis of US population data from the Third National Health and Nutrition Examination Survey. Am J Epidem. 2007; 166(3):280–288.

Williams, D.R. Race, health, and health care. St. Louis Univ Law J. 2003; 48(1):13–35.

Williams, D.R. The health of men: Structured inequalities and opportunities. Am J Pub Health. 2003; 93(5):724–731.

Williams, D.R. The health of U.S. racial and ethnic populations. Journal of Gerontology. Series B. Psych Sci Soc Scie. 2005; 60(2):53–62.

Williams, D.R., Collins, C. U.S. socioeconomic and racial differences in health. Annual Review of Sociology. 1995; 21:349–386.

Williams, D.R., Jackson, P.B. Social sources of racial disparities in health. Health Affairs (Millwood). 2005; 24(2):325–334.

Wolf, M.S., Knight, S.J., Lyons, E.A., Durazo-Arvizu, R., Pickard, S.A., Arseven, A. et al. Literacy, race, and PSA level among low-income men newly diagnosed with prostate cancer. Urol. 2006; 68(1):89–93.

Wood, H.M., Reuther, A.M., Gilligan, T.D., Kupelian, P.A., Modlin, C.S., Jr., Klein, E.A. Rates of biochemical remission remain higher in black men compared to white men after radical prostatectomy despite similar trends in prostate specific antigen induced stage migration. Journal of Urology. 2007; 178(4 Pt 1):1271–1276.

Yao, S.L., Lu-Yao, G. Understanding and appreciating overdiagnosis in the PSA era. J Nat Cancer Inst. 2002; 94(13):958–960.

Young, C.D., Lewis, P., Weinberg, V., Lee, T.T., Coleman, C.W., Roach, M, III. The impact of race on freedom from prostate-specific antigen failure in prostate cancer patients treated with definite radiation therapy. Semin Urol Oncol. 2000; 18(2):121–126.

Chapter 9
Disparities and Cervical Cancer

Marcela del Carmen and Teresa Diaz-Montez

Introduction

Cervical cancer became a preventable disease with the introduction of the Papanicolaou smear (Pap smear) in the 1940s. Trend data show that incidence rates have decreased steadily over the past several decades in both white and African American women living in the United States (American Cancer Society 2007). Mortality rates have declined steadily over the past several decades as well due to screening-related prevention and early detection (American Cancer Society 2007). Despite these trends, however, striking social and racial/ethnic inequities affect the entire cervical cancer continuum in different domains, including prevention, vaccination, diagnosis, follow-up, treatment, and survival (del Carmen et al. 2007; Newmann et al. 2005).

The factors underlying these inequities affect each domain in a variety of ways. As one moves along the cervical cancer continuum, moreover, some barriers dissipate while others emerge (del Carmen et al. 2007). Potential sources of racial/ethnic disparities in health care, for example, may include discrimination, stereotyping, and bias (del Carmen et al. 2007). These sources may be encountered at different levels: the individual level (patient or health care provider), the institutional level, and the health system level (del Carmen et al. 2007). At the patient level, factors such as patient preferences, refusal of treatment, difficulty participating in health care plans, and biological differences may play a role. At the health system level, financing, the structure of care, and cultural and linguistic differences may influence the degree of disparity (del Carmen et al. 2007). Developing target cancer control and prevention strategies requires recognizing and addressing these and other disparities at all points of the cervical cancer continuum.

M. del Carmen (✉)
Division of Gynecologic Oncology, Massachusetts General Hospital, Harvard Medical School, Boston, MA
e-mail: mdelcarmen@partners.org

H.K. Koh (ed.), *Toward the Elimination of Cancer Disparities*,
DOI 10.1007/978-0-387-89443-0_9, © Springer Science+Business Media, LLC 2009

Epidemiology

Worldwide

Amongst all malignancies, cervical cancer is the second most common cancer affecting women (Sankaranarayanan et al. 2006). It is also the number one killer of women in developing countries. Worldwide, in fact, cervical cancer is the most common gynecologic malignancy (Sankaranarayanan et al. 2006), accounting for 492,800 new cases and 273,200 deaths during the year 2002 alone (Sankaranarayanan et al. 2006). In developing countries, cervical cancer is the most common female malignancy as well, accounting for 83% (409,400) of new cases diagnosed and 85% (233,700) of cancer-related deaths (Sankaranarayanan et al. 2006). In developed countries, cervical cancer is the third most common cause of female malignancy, accounting for 17% (83,400) of the new cases diagnosed and 15% (39,500) of cancer-related deaths (Sankaranarayanan et al. 2006). The highest incidence rates worldwide are observed in sub-Saharan Africa, Melanesia, Latin America and the Caribbean, South-Central Asia, and Southeast Asia (Sankaranarayanan et al. 2006). One-third of the cervical cancer burden in the world is experienced in South-Central Asia.

Age-specific incidence rates reveal unique patterns. In developed countries, cervical cancer rates are higher among young individuals but plateau after age 40. In developing countries, cervical cancer rates are low among young individuals but subsequently increase and, after age 40, exceed those in developed countries (Kamangar et al. 2006). The low risk in developed countries is attributed to availability of effective screening programs. Prior to the introduction of cervical cancer screening, the incidence rates of developed countries were similar to those found in developing countries today. Estimates note that only about 5% of women in developing countries have been screened for cervical dysplasia in the past 5 years compared with some 40–50% of women in developed countries (Denny et al. 2006). The highest mortality rates are observed in Eastern Africa (Sankaranarayanan et al. 2006). The high mortality rates in developing countries are due to advanced clinical stage at presentation, as well as deficiencies in treatment availability, accessibility, and affordability that impede ability to receive or complete prescribed treatment.

United States of America

During the year 2007 in the United States, an estimated 11,150 new cervical cancer cases will be diagnosed and 3,670 cervical cancer related deaths are expected (Jemal et al. 2007). Accounting for 1.6% of new cancer diagnoses and 1.4% of cancer-related deaths in the United States, it is the third most common cause of gynecological malignancy and the 14th most common cause of new cancer diagnosis and cancer-related cause of death (Jemal et al. 2007; American Cancer Society 2007).

Disparity in Incidence and Mortality

Cervical cancer incidence and death rates vary considerably among racial and ethnic groups despite the steady decrease in incidence and mortality rates over the past several decades in both white and African Americans (American Cancer Society 2007). While overall cervical cancer incidence in the United States (1999–2003) was estimated at 9.1/100,000, for example, Hispanic Latino and African American groups had significantly higher incidence rates (14.7/ 100,000 and 13.0/100,000, respectively) than white (8.6/100,000), Asian American/Pacific Islander (9.3/100,000), and American Indian/Alaska Native (7.2/ 100,000) groups (Howe et al. 2006; Ries et al. 2006). Similarly, while the overall cervical cancer death rate in the United States (1999–2003) was estimated as 2.7/ 100,000, African Americans (5.1/100,000) and Hispanic Latinos (3.4/100,000) groups had significantly higher death rates than whites (2.4/100,000), Asian American/Pacific Islanders (2.5/100,000), and American Indian/Alaska Natives (2.6/100,000) (Howe et al 2006; Ries et al. 2006).

Saraiya and colleagues, while evaluating the incidence of cervical cancer by geography, race/ethnicity, and histology, reported that cervical cancer rates were especially high among Hispanic Latinos aged 40 years or older ($\geq$26.5/ 100,000) and African Americans older than 50 years ($\geq$23.5/100,000) (Saraiya et al. 2007). The rates of squamous cell carcinoma (75% of all cases) were significantly higher among African Americans and Hispanic Latinos than among their white counterparts. In contrast, rates of adenocarcinoma (18% of all cases) were significantly lower among African Americans than in whites (rate ratio = 0.88, $P<0.05$). Rates of adenocarcinoma were significantly higher among Hispanic Latino women than among non-Hispanic Latino groups (rate ratio = 1.71, $P<0.05$). Although no regional differences were noted for adenocarcinoma, rates of squamous cell carcinoma were higher in the South than in other regions (Saraiya et al. 2007).

African Americans diagnosed with cervical cancer are also less likely than whites to be diagnosed with cancer at a localized stage (45% versus 53%), when the disease may be more easily and successfully treated, and more likely to be diagnosed with cancer at a regional stage of disease (38% versus 33%) (Reis et al. 2006). The 5-year relative survival is lower in African Americans than in whites within each stratum of diagnosis (localized: 86% versus 93%; regional: 48% versus 56%; distant: 7% versus 16%; all stages: 63% versus 73%) (Reis et al. 2006). Patel et al., while evaluating the racial/ethnic differences in survival after diagnosis with invasive cervical cancer in a population-based sample of patients (while adjusting for patient, tumor characteristics, and treatment types), reported that Hispanic Latino subjects were at 26% decreased risk of death from any cause (OR = 0.74, 95% CI: 0.66–0.83) and African American subjects were at 19% increased risk of death (OR = 1.19, 95% CI: 1.06–1.33) compared to white women (Patel et al. 2005).

Table 9.1 summarizes the average annual incidence and mortality rates by racial or ethnic group, as reported by the Surveillance Epidemiology and End Results (SEER) database from 2000 to 2004 (Reis et al. 2006). This table also depicts lifetime risks of being diagnosed with or dying from cervical cancer.

Table 9.1 Average annual rates and lifetime risks associated with cervical cancer in the United States, by racial and ethnic group (Reis et al. 2006)

	SEER average annual incident rates[a]	Average annual mortality rates[b]	% lifetime risk of diagnosis[c]	% lifetime risk of dying[c]
Non-Hispanic white	7.2	2.2	0.67	0.21
Black	11.4	4.9	0.92	0.43
Hispanic	13.8	3.3	1.19	0.35
Asian American/ Pacific Islander	8.0	2.4	0.76	0.32

[a]per 100,000 persons, 2000–2004, age-adjusted; calculated from 17 SEER areas
[b]per 100,000 persons, 2000–2004, age-adjusted; calculated from data provided by the National Center for Health Statistics
[c]2002–2004

Disparity in Prevention/HPV Vaccination

The incidence of cervical cancer in the United States has declined substantially since the widespread introduction of Pap smear screening in the 1940s. Pap smear screening can detect preclinical lesions and is recognized as an effective means of reducing cervical cancer incidence, morbidity, and mortality. However, these declines have not eliminated racial/ethnic disparities in incidence rates. These disparities are primarily due to differences in the utilization of cervical cancer screening and follow-up of abnormal results by race/ethnicity. The conventional method of cervical cancer screening involves sequential testing and is difficult to implement ubiquitously in developing countries and in certain pockets of the US population, where access to services may be limited and disparities more prominent. The difficulties in implementing successful screening programs may be due to requirements for compliance with repeated testing, expertise in specimen preparation, diagnostic interpretation, and cost.

A Healthy People 2010 goal is to increase the percentage of US women ever receiving a Pap test to 97%. In 2000, the following groups of women reported ever receiving a Pap test (age-adjusted, aged 18 years and over): 95% of American Indian/Alaska Native, 95% of African American, 95% of white, 87% of Hispanic Latino, and 77% of Asian American/Pacific Islander (Healthy

People 2010). A related Healthy People 2010 goal is to increase the percentage of women having received a Pap test within the past three years to 90%. In 2000, the following groups of women reported receiving a Pap test within the past three years (age-adjusted, aged 18 years and over): 84% of African Americans, 83% of whites, 77% of Hispanic Latinos, 76% of American Indian/Alaska Natives, and 66% of Asian American/Pacific Islanders (Healthy People 2010).

Human papilloma virus (HPV) has been implicated in the development of virtually all cervical cancers. Notably, HPV DNA is detected in approximately 100% of invasive squamous cervical cancers (Nuovo et al. 1990; Lorincz et al. 1992; Lorincz et al. 1989). HPV is classified into high-, intermediate-, and low-risk types based on its association with invasive cancer. Types 16 and 18, considered high-risk (oncogenic) types, are associated with aggressive forms of cervical cancers (Stone 1995; Bosch et al. 1995). Conversely, infection with low-risk HPV subtypes is unlikely to progress to invasive cancer (Lorincz et al 1992). HPV infection is the most common sexually transmitted disease, with reported prevalence rates of 19–46% in the United States (Cuzick et al. 1995; Hildeshien et al. 1993; Ho et al. 1998). The major risk factor is sexual behavior, including early age at onset of sexual activity, multiple sexual partners, failure to use barrier methods of contraception, and co-infection with other sexually transmitted diseases, particularly HIV (Peyton et al. 2001). The prevalence of HPV declines with increasing age, and persistent infection after age 30 is usually associated with oncogenic types of HPV (Ley et al. 1991; Burk et al. 1996; Sherman et al. 1992). Two recent vaccines—a quadrivalent vaccine containing HPV 16, 18, 6, and 11, and a bivalent formula of 16 and 18—have the potential to prevent about 70% of cervical cancers when available and administered correctly (Clifford et al. 2003).

Disparity in Screening

Cultural/Personal Barriers

Cervical cancer risks and rates may be influenced by cultural and genetic factors. In approximately half of the new US cervical cancer cases, women report sub-optimal screening. Behbakht and colleagues studied the behaviors, attitudes, and beliefs that pose barriers to optimal screening for cervical cancer (Behbakht et al. 2004). Using an advisory panel, inventories from national cancer organizations, and a literature review, they developed a questionnaire that addressed lifestyle issues, fatalistic attitudes, and patient relationships with health care professionals. The responses of women who have never had a Pap smear were compared with those who reported receiving at least one Pap smear before being diagnosed with cancer. Nearly a quarter (36/146) patients recently diagnosed with cervical cancer reported never being screened for cervical cancer. Women in this group were more likely to be Hispanic Latino, recent immigrants, and to have limited education, little family support, and no health insurance. They also were much more likely to believe that cancer occurred because of bad luck, and to report not wanting to know their diagnosis. The two groups did not differ in age, influence of religion on health care choices, access to physicians, trust for physicians, or aspects of knowledge about cancer causation, detection, prevention, and treatment. Only 16% stated that they would rather do a home test for cancer than have a physician perform a conventional Pap smear. The authors concluded that fatalistic attitudes, lack of family support, and low levels of information about cervical cancer are associated significantly with lack of Pap screening in women with cervical cancer, as are the previously identified risk factors of recent immigration and low levels of education.

Bazargan et al., while evaluating cervical cancer screening practices among the underserved Hispanic Latino and African American women, reported that only 51% of the former and 22% of the latter population interviewed had received a screening for cervical cancer within the past year (Bazargan et al. 2004). Twenty-nine percent of the women claimed that no health care provider ever told them that they needed a screening test for cervical cancer. Hispanic Latino and older women were also far less likely to adhere to screening guidelines. Multivariate analysis shows that affordability, continuity of care, and receiving advice from health care providers regarding a Pap smear were significant predictors of up-to-date cervical cancer screening. The continuity of obtaining medical services and receiving recommendations from a physician remain the core factors significantly associated with obtaining cervical cancer screening.

Racial/ethnic groups comprised largely of foreign-born individuals also have lower rates of cancer screening than whites (Goel et al. 2003). In analyses adjusted for sociodemographic characteristics and illness burden, African American respondents were more likely to report cancer screening than white respondents. However, Hispanic Latino and Asian American/Pacific Islander respondents were significantly less likely to report screening for most cancers. When race/ethnicity and birthplace were considered together, US-born Hispanic Latino and Asian American/Pacific Islander respondents were as likely to report cancer screening as US-born whites. However, foreign-born white (adjusted OR = 0.58, 95% CI: 0.41–0.82), Hispanic Latino (adjusted OR = 0.65, 95% CI: 0.53–0.79), and Asian American/Pacific Islander respondents (adjusted OR = 0.28, 95% CI: 0.19–0.39) were less likely than US-born whites to report having had Pap smears. After adjusting for access to care, the disparities among foreign-born respondents were partially attenuated.

Language and acculturation could also be significant barriers in terms of cervical cancer screening for some of these groups. Hispanic Latino women, particularly those speaking only or mostly Spanish, are the least likely group to have received a Pap smear within the last three years (Harlan et al. 1991). Aside from the language barrier, other reasons cited for not having had a recent Pap smear were procrastination and not believing this test was necessary

(Harlan et al. 1991). On the other hand, acculturation levels tended to be inversely correlated with no Pap smear. Women who were highly acculturated were less likely to never have had a Pap smear than their less-acculturated counterparts (OR $= 0.86$, 95% CI: $0.58-1.27$ for moderately acculturated women and OR $= 0.51$, 95% CI: $0.29-0.89$ for highly acculturated women) (Shah et al. 2006). Similar results were found for having had no Pap smear within the past three years (OR $= 0.83$, 95% CI: $0.61-1.13$ for moderately acculturated women and OR $= 0.73$, 95% CI: $0.49-1.08$ for highly acculturated women) (Shah et al. 2006).

Thus, while developing a cervical cancer screening program, targeting Hispanic Latino women, particularly Spanish speakers, appears critical. In addition, educational programs should target unscreened women who forego the test due to ignorance (e.g., underestimating its importance), procrastination, or lack of awareness (e.g., because a medical care provider did not suggest the procedure). Women in these underserved groups must be intensively educated that Pap smears should be scheduled routinely to detect precancerous lesions or asymptomatic cervical cancer.

It is also critical to target personal beliefs that have the potential to become a barrier to screening. Byrd and colleagues, for example, evaluated the beliefs, attitudes, and personal characteristics that correlated with self-reported cervical cancer screening history among Hispanic women aged 18–25 years old (Byrd et al. 2004). Sixty-nine percent reported ever having had a Pap test and 56% reported having had a test in the past year. Eighty percent reported that they were sexually active and, of these, 63% reported using birth control. Respondents understood the seriousness of cervical cancer, their susceptibility to cervical cancer, and the benefits of Pap testing; however, only 61% agreed that most young women whom they know have Pap tests. Greater acculturation and the belief that most young unmarried women have Pap tests were positively associated with ever having screening. The perception that the test would be painful and not knowing where to go for the test were negatively associated with ever having a Pap test.

Socioeconomic Barriers

Socioeconomic deprivation has also been found to be a strong predictor of screening, diagnosis, treatment, and survival differentials. Part of the explanation may lie in lower Pap smear screening rates, which—since socioeconomic status is related to health care access and coverage—can translate into later stage at diagnosis and poorer outcomes. Among women on Medicare, for example, 51% were diagnosed with late-stage disease at the time of initial diagnosis (O'Malley et al. 2006). Relative to women without Medicaid coverage adjusted odds ratios for late-stage diagnosis were 2.8 times higher and 1.3 times higher among women enrolled or intermittently enrolled in Medicaid at the time of their diagnosis, respectively. Women of low socioeconomic status and older women were at particularly high risk of not being screened.

Both income and educational levels appear to be good predictors of screening. Only 75.4% (95% CI: 73.8−77.1) of 3947 women (18 years of age and older) who had a reported household income of less than $15,000 dollars per year had received a Pap test in the previous three years. This compared with 92.2% (95% CI: 91.2−93.1) of 18,698 women with a household income of $50,000+ per year. Overall, 77.5% (95% CI: 75.7−79.3) of women without a high-school education had received a Pap test compared with 91.7% (95% CI: 91.0−92.3) of college graduates. Multivariate analysis showed that educational level was positively associated with Pap smear testing rates, especially among women residing in areas where relatively few residents had a low education level ($P<0.0001$) (Coughlin et al. 2006).

Low socioeconomic status also influences the prevalence of underlying risk factors for cancer (such as smoking) as well as access to services (American Cancer Society 2007). Compared with 11% of whites, 24% of African Americans and 23% of Hispanic Latinos live below the poverty line (American Cancer Society 2007). Moreover, 18% of African Americans and 35% of Hispanic Latinos are uninsured compared to 12% of white Americans (American Cancer Society 2007). Low-income and uninsured people in particular are more likely to be diagnosed with cancer at late stages of disease, to receive substandard clinical care and services, and to die from the disease. It is therefore not surprising that incidence rates of cervical cancer increase with higher levels of socioeconomic deprivation among all four racial/ethnic groups: white, African American, Asian American/Pacific Islander, and Hispanic Latino (Krieger et al. 1999). Poverty, in fact, has been found to be the biggest predictor of invasive cervical cancer. Poor and working-class white women had an invasive cervical cancer incidence that was four times higher than in professional women of the same race (Krieger et al. 1999).

Finally, comorbid diseases may contribute to sub-optimal cervical cancer treatment in these populations as well. This is because minority women of low socioeconomic status tend to have comorbid diseases that contribute to poorer treatment outcomes for cervical cancer. Cervical cancer screening has been shown to be inversely proportional to the number of comorbid conditions (Kiefe et al. 1998).

Structural Barriers

Large gaps exist between urban and rural populations in terms of cervical cancer screening. Baker and colleagues, for example, reported that the highest cervical cancer rates occurred among rural African American women over age 45 (Baker et al. 2000). One explanation for this gap may be that preventive care in primary care practices is often more difficult to deliver in rural medical practices, contributing to lower screening rates. Rural women tend, on average, to be older, poorer, less educated, and, therefore, less frequently screened than their urban counterparts. These patients tend to spend less time with their physicians and more time traveling to health care providers (Harris et al. 1993).

Inadequate health insurance creates yet another structural barrier to care. Several studies have reported that medically uninsured women have lower cancer screening rates and often present at later stages of disease. Compared with health maintenance organization-insured women too, uninsured women tend to have later stages of cervical cancer diagnosis (Ferrante et al. 2000). Among Medicare patients with cervical cancer, those enrolled in health maintenance organizations are less likely than fee-for-service enrollees to be diagnosed with late-stage disease (Riley et al. 1994). In addition, Hiatt et al. found that the strongest predictors of cancer screening were having private health insurance and frequent use of medical services (Hiatt et al. 2001).

Lack of Knowledge Regarding HPV, Cervical Cancer, and Screening

To make appropriate, evidence-based choices among existing prevention strategies (Pap smear, HPV DNA test, and HPV vaccination), women first need to understand the link between HPV and cervical cancer. An analysis of cross-sectional data from women (18−75 years old) responding to the 2005 Health Information National Trends Survey (n = 3,076) revealed that among the 40% of women who had ever heard about HPV, less than half knew it caused cervical cancer. Also, of those who had previously heard of HPV, 64% acknowledged that HPV is sexually transmitted and 79% that HPV infection can increase the incidence of abnormal Pap tests (Tiro et al. 2001). Factors associated with having heard about HPV included younger age, non-Hispanic white race/ ethnicity, higher educational attainment, exposure to multiple health information sources, trusting health information, regular Pap tests, awareness of changes in cervical cancer screening guidelines, and having tested positive for HPV. Accurate knowledge of the HPV-cervical cancer link leads to screening and then is associated with abnormal Pap and positive HPV test results (Tiro et al. 2001).

Lack of knowledge of cervical cancer screening and HPV is associated with lower socioeconomic status and educational level. In one study of women with abnormal screening cervical cytology attending university colposcopy clinics (n = 178), for example, only 74% (131) of the 176 responding women understood that Pap tests evaluate the cervix, whereas 78% (138/ 176) understood that Pap tests should be repeated at intervals of 1−3 years. The cancer screening function of a Pap test was identified by 69% (122/177), but only 56% (99/177) knew HPV is sexually transmitted and causes warts and premalignant changes. Rural residence was not associated with level of knowledge, but older (≥40 years of age) women were more likely to know the nature of the Pap test ($P=0.005$) and the meaning of an abnormal Pap test

($P=0.04$). Women in higher income strata were more likely to understand the meaning of an abnormal Pap test ($P=0.03$), the nature of HPV ($P=0.005$), and risk factors for cervical cancer ($P=0.03$). College graduates were better able ($P=0.0005$), and women of greater parity (parity greater than 3) were less ($P=0.02$) able than others to identify the nature of HPV, although neither differed from others in ability to answer other questions correctly ($P>0.1$) (Massad et al. 2006).

Disparity in Treatment

Disparities in cancer survival and mortality also exist across racial/ethnic minority groups. Several investigators have documented this disparity even after adjusting for stage of disease at diagnosis (Shavers et al. 2002; Dignamm et al. 2000; del Carmen et al. 1999), with racial differences in treatment efficacy and failure to provide adequate care proposed as additional contributing factors (Dignamm et al. 2000). Racial disparities occur in the receipt of definitive primary therapy, conservative surgery, and adjuvant therapy, as well as in follow-up after treatment with curative intent (Shavers et al. 2002; Dignamm et al. 2000).

Several studies have demonstrated disparities among racial/ethnic minorities in cervical cancer treatment. Some of these disparities affect the assignment of a stage to the cancer, and the receipt of surgical treatment, intracavitary radiation, and definitive treatment for the cancer (del Carmen et al. 1999; Russell et al. 1998; Howell et al. 1999; Merrill et al. 2000; Thoms et al. 1998; Mundt et al. 1998). Based on SEER data, African Americans, compared to whites, were less likely to be treated with surgery alone and more likely to receive no treatment or to have radiation therapy alone for their cervical cancer (Howell et al. 1999). This difference was seen after adjusting for age and stage of disease (Howell et al. 1999). A different SEER data study noted that African American women with cervical cancer were less likely to have clinical staging and those with unstaged tumors were more likely to be untreated (Merrill et al. 2000).

Although the studies exploring these disparities in cervical cancer are rather limited, several additional studies suggest that African Americans are less frequently treated, or treated appropriately, for cervical cancer than white women (Howell et al. 1999; Merrill et al. 2000). Microscopically invasive cervical cancer is sub-categorized into Stage IA, IA_1, and Stage IA_2 lesions. Stage IA_1 lesions have a depth of invasion less than or equal to 3 mm and a horizontal spread of less than or equal to 7 mm. This sub-category of microscopically invasive cervical cancer can be treated with either a cervical conization or loop electrocautery excision procedure (LEEP) or with an extrafascial hysterectomy. Stage IA_2 lesions are 3.1−5 mm in depth and less than or equal to 7 mm in horizontal spread and require surgical treatment with a modified radical hysterectomy and bilateral pelvic lymph node dissection. In a 1999 study, del Carmen et al. found that African Americans were more likely than their white counterparts to receive inappropriate fertility-sparing therapies for Stage IA_2 lesions in place of radical curative surgery (del Carmen et al. 1999). This study also found that African American women with early stage, surgically resectable cervical cancer (Stage IA_1 and Stage IA_2) and Hispanic women with Stage IA_2 disease were more often treated with less adequate, fertility-sparing treatments than the recommended hysterectomy (del Carmen et al. 1999). In another study of women with operable Stage IB (clinically visible cervical tumor) cervical cancer, African American women were more likely to be offered radiation therapy and less likely to be treated surgically or with combined therapy than were their white counterparts (Thoms et al. 1998). When compared to white women, African American patients have also been reported to receive intracavitary brachytherapy less often than external beam radiation (Mundt et al. 1998). Among patients who had cervical-cancer-directed surgery as part of their primary treatment, significantly more African Americans had local surgery compared to other racial/ethnic groups, whereas Hispanics underwent a relatively greater proportion of radical hysterectomies (Patel et al. 2005). This finding was noted despite the fact that African Americans had a greater proportion of later stage tumors (stages II, III, and IV) than Hispanics or non-Hispanic whites (Patel et al. 2005).

Proposed explanations for these disparities in treatment include structural barriers, comorbidities, patient's choice to decline recommended treatment, and physician's bias in making treatment recommendations (Shavers et al. 2002; Merrill et al. 2000; Mundt et al. 1998). Shavers, in fact, has proposed three categories of factors that may contribute to optimal cancer treatment: (1) structural factors, (2) factors related to provider recommendations, and (3) factors related to freedom of choice (Shavers et al. 2002). Some of the suggested structural barriers include health insurance status and geographic location (accessibility) of the treatment facility (Shavers et al. 2002). In making their treatment recommendations, physicians may be influenced by prognostic indicators, stage, perception of the patient's desire and ability to participate in her treatment plan, and personal preferences and biases (Shavers et al. 2002). Patients, in turn, may be influenced as a result of their attitudes/beliefs about treatment options and their ability and resources to overcome structural barriers, as well as their own personal biases and preferences (Shavers et al. 2000). A critical component in the reduction of cervical cancer disparities may be identifying and correcting both clinical and non-clinical factors at the level of cancer treatment that contribute to those disparities—in part by conducting better studies and developing strategies to facilitate appropriate cancer treatments (Shavers et al. 2000).

Disparity in Survival

As noted earlier, while there have been declines in both the incidence and mortality rates for cervical cancer across all racial and ethnic groups in the United States, marked disparities in survival rates persist (Ries et al. 2005). The following have been reported in 2004 as the cervical cancer mortality rates per 100,000 based on racial/ethnic categories (DATA 2010):

- Non-Hispanic whites: 2.1
- Asian/Pacific Islander: 2.1
- Hispanics: 3.1
- African Americans: 4.5

The reported 5-year cervical cancer survival rates for Hispanics and non-Hispanics are similar—71% and 68%, respectively (Patel et al. 2005). However, the 5-year survival rate for African Americans is much lower, estimated to be 56% (Patel et al. 2005). African Americans have been reported to have a significantly increased risk of death compared to non-Hispanic whites among women with stage I tumors, but not higher stages (Patel et al. 2005). Geographic disparities, often correlating with the geographical distribution of minority groups, have also been reported. For example, states in the Deep South have 11–38% higher cervical cancer death rates than the total US rates (Ries et al. 2005). The incidence and mortality rates for Hispanic women are even higher than reported, as speculation exists that these women return to their countries of origin to receive "traditional" treatments or to die. Furthermore, studies may not accurately capture the death rate of Hispanic women. Until recently, Hispanic ethnicity was often excluded as a specific ethnic category in many studies and surveys capturing death rates from different causes.

The differences in cervical cancer survival may be a result of differences in screening, as detailed above, follow-up, or treatment. Non-adherence to screening and follow-up plans may lead to later stages of diagnosis, which, in turn, can result in increased morbidity and mortality. Similar potential barriers affecting the receipt of optimal cancer treatment—structural barriers, as well as physician and patient barriers—may also play a role.

Disparities, Demographics, and Potential Societal Impact

Understanding the changing demographics in the United States is critical to framing these disparities, as well as to understanding their potential impact on the health care system. Over the next few decades, minority groups will increase in size and make up a larger percentage of the US population. As of 2006, Hispanics constitute 20% of the total US population under the age of 18, making them second only to non-Hispanic whites (57.4%) in this age category (US Census Bureau 2007). When each population is analyzed individually, non-Hispanic whites have the lowest proportion of females under the age of 18 (20.14%) when compared to Hispanics (34%), African Americans (28%), and Asian Americans (21.7%) (US Census Bureau 2007).

The US Census Bureau projects that by the year 2050, the Hispanic population will have increased by 187.9% of the 2000 estimates, and will then constitute 24.4% of the US population, up from 12% in 2000 (US Census Bureau 2004). Similar increases are projected for African Americans (12.7% in 2000 versus 14.6% in 2050) and Asian Americans (3.8% in 2000 versus 8.0% in 2050) (US Census Bureau 2004), Fig. 9.1. If today's health disparities continue, these changes will have a significant impact on the societal infrastructure of the growing populations and, due to increased morbidity and mortality, will result in ever-increasing burdens on the US health care system.

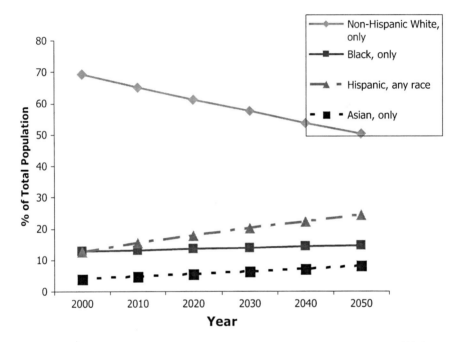

Fig. 9.1 Projected percentage population changes, 2000–2050 (US Census Bureau 2004)

Proposed Approaches to Reducing Disparities in Cervical Cancer Prevention

Given that disparities in cervical cancer screening and follow-up rates among minority populations have been shown to contribute to higher incidence and mortality rates, many projects have been launched at the federal, state, and local levels to determine effective methods to reduce these disparities. Such methods include federally funded initiatives to promote screening, increase awareness in target communities, aid minority access to health care, and create community partnerships to educate health care providers and community leaders and support outreach programs. Other initiatives include providing culturally appropriate educational materials to at-risk populations; utilizing lay health care workers representative of target populations to educate and guide women, and telephoning women to remind them to participate in screening or in follow-up of an abnormal Pap smear.

National and State Initiatives

National initiatives such as the National Breast and Cervical Cancer Early Detection Program and the National Institute's Patient Navigator Academy have tried to overcome barriers to screening and cervical cancer care. Chapters 11 and 14 of this book review many of these initiatives. The National Breast and Cervical Cancer Early Detection Program (NBCCEDP) was established in 1991 to provide screening to low-income, uninsured women (The Centers for Disease Control and Prevention. National Breast and Cervical Cancer Early Detection Program 2007; Ryerson et al 2005). An estimated 11–18% of US women are eligible, based on their status as uninsured, or underinsured at or below 250% of the federal poverty level (The Centers for Disease Control and Prevention. National Breast and Cervical Cancer Early Detection Program 2007; Ryerson et al 2005). The program provides cervical cancer screening services for women aged 18–64 and breast cancer screening for women aged 40–64 (The Centers for Disease Control and Prevention. National Breast and Cervical Cancer Early Detection Program 2007; Ryerson et al 2005). In 2005, 14.7% of all women eligible had a mammogram, and 6.7% had a Pap smear (The Centers for Disease Control and Prevention. National Breast and Cervical Cancer Early Detection Program 2007; Ryerson et al 2005).

From 1991 to 2005, there was a 81.2% increase in the total number of women who were provided Pap smears through NBCCEDP as a result of partnerships and outreach programs established by this initiative (The Centers for Disease Control and Prevention. National Breast and Cervical Cancer Early Detection Program 2007; Ryerson et al 2005). In 2001–2002, 49% of women who received Pap smear services were white, 14% were African American, 23% were Hispanics, and 5% were Asian/Pacific Islander (Ryerson et al. 2005). The Breast and Cervical Cancer Prevention and Treatment Act of 2000, signed into law on October 24, 2000, gives states the option to provide medical assistance through Medicaid to eligible women who are screened through NBCCEDP and found to have breast or cervical cancer, including pre-cancerous lesions (Department of Health and Human Services 2007).

Under current funding levels, however, the NBCCEDP program can only provide screening to one out of every five eligible women. This is not uniform for all states; some have enough money for only 1 in 20 eligible women (Finkelstein et al. 2007). Many states have developed successful outreach programs, but due to lack of funding, they have to turn away women (Finkelstein et al. 2007). On the other hand, data collected from the Behavioral Risk Factor Surveillance System (BRFSS) revealed that the NBCCEDP program did have a positive influence on increasing screening among low-income women. From 1996 to 2000, Pap screening increased from 63.9% to 68.0% among white women, 59.0% to 66.9% among Hispanic women, and 66.5%–69.9% among African American women (Adams et al. 2007). The increase among African American women was not considered significant, but their rates were similar to those observed among low-income white women. Even so, disparities in screening behaviors persisted after five years of the program (Adams et al. 2007). Although the program was successful in increasing the screening rate among minority women, Hispanics and African American women were still less likely to be screened appropriately even after this program's intervention.

Another national initiative is the National Cancer Institute's (NCI) Patient Navigator Academy (Fowler et al. 2006). This initiative, funded through The Patient Navigator Outreach and Chronic Disease Act of 2005, provides patient navigator services with the goal of reducing barriers through the recruitment, training, and employment of patient navigators (Winstead et al. 2005). Patient navigators assist patients to overcome barriers to care, helping them "navigate" the health care system to receive timely diagnosis and treatment. Navigators represent a wide range of racial and ethnic populations from different geographical locations and are involved in scheduling appointments, coordinating insurance, community outreach, forming community partnerships, and encouraging clinical trial participation (Fowler et al. 2006). Chapter 13 of this book adds more information on these important topics.

Community-Based Initiatives

A series of community partnerships have also been organized with the purpose of addressing and disseminating cervical cancer screening and care disparities (see also Chapters 11, 13, and 14 of this book). The Asian American Network for Cancer Awareness, Research, and Training (AANCART), for example, is a cooperative effort between the NCI and the University of California, Davis, and comprises six NCI cancer centers and associated universities (Asian American Network for Cancer Awareness, Research, and Training 2007). An important component of this organization is its commitment to improving the quality of research in cancer care disparities (Asian American Network for Cancer Awareness, Research, and Training 2007). Another program, Racial and Ethnic Approaches to Health (REACH 2010), is designed to help eliminate racial and ethnic disparities in health and targets disparities in cardiovascular disease, immunizations, breast and cervical cancer screening and management, diabetes, HIV/AIDS, and infant mortality among African Americans, Native Americans, Alaska natives, Asian Americans, Hispanics, and Pacific Islanders

(Mensah et al. 2006). REACH 2010 supports community coalitions in designing, implementing, and evaluating community-driven strategies to eliminate disparities (Mensah et al. 2006).

Yet another initiative, the Special Populations Networks (SPNs), was established by the NCI in 2000, to reduce cancer disparities (see also Chapters 11 and 14). While this initiative ended in 2005, its lessons learned and best practices were rolled into the current Community Networks Program (CNP) (Freeman et al. 2006). The SPN program included 5 national, 2 regional, and 11 local programs, with the major goal of promoting cancer awareness research in minority and underserved communities, targeting most ethnic and racial populations (Jackson et al. 2006). The SPN's goals were reached by training minority researchers, developing culturally appropriate educational materials, and training lay workers in the target communities (Jackson et al. 2006).

One particularly effective SPN program was in Maryland, where a community and academic partnership that combined community-based outreach with evidence-based education interventions such as print and broadcast media, health fairs, tribal and community centers, and sporting events. Baseline screening services and health evaluations were available when appropriate (Baquet et al. 2006). Data from the BRFSS indicate that Maryland's SPN was successful in improving positive health behaviors in the program's target areas (2000 to 2002 versus 1995 to 1999) (Baquet et al. 2006). Women aged 18 and older in the program's target areas showed a 2.89% increase in having Pap smears within 3 years, as opposed to only a 1.31% increase in other areas (Baquet et al. 2006).

Another promising community initiative is Colorado's Special Population Network-Greater Denver Latino Cancer Prevention/Control Network, a special project of the Latino/a Research & Policy Center (LRPC) (Flores et al. 2006). Part of this program is *Día de la Mujer Latina* in Denver. This cultural, family-centered health fair offers breast and cervical cancer screening, provides counseling and education, ethnic music, food, entertainment, and giveaways (Flores et al. 2006). The Cancer Monologues, another program under LRCP, comprises a set of skits that use culturally proficient methods (e.g., parody and humor in dealing with death) to educate and raise awareness at community fairs, on public television, and at SPN sites. The goal is to reach underserved, uninsured Latinos with low literacy levels who may be less likely to read brochures or talk to health care providers. Educational materials in English and Spanish are always provided at each performance (Flores et al. 2006).

Finally, The Cancer Awareness Network for Immigrant Minority Populations (CANIMP), part of SPN was based out of the Center for Immigrant Health at New York University School of Medicine and ended in 2005. This program was a network of community- and faith-based organizations, local and federal government institutions, as well as health care providers, researchers, immigrant services, and advocacy groups (Gany et al. 2006). This initiative addresseed specific needs of immigrant populations, especially vulnerable to disparities, concentrating on programs that help them access and navigate the health care system (Gany et al. 2006).

Telephone-Based Intervention

Telephone-based intervention can also help to reduce certain disparities, specifically by improving compliance with follow-up. For example, telephone confirmation of initial colposcopy visits has been shown to increase likelihood of compliance (68%) compared to standard care (no phone call, 50%), and telephone counseling has been shown to result in even higher adherence rates than telephone confirmation (76% versus 68%, OR 1.50; 95% CI 1.04–2.17) (Miller et al. 1997). Another successful program is the Screening Adherence Follow-Up (SAFe) intervention model, another telephone-based intervention, which combines health education, counseling, and systems navigation (improving communication and access to resources) to improve follow-up among low-income Hispanic women (Ell et al. 2002). In this program, a bilingual, bicultural Hispanic peer counselor targets intervention patients deemed at risk for loss of follow-up after an abnormal Pap smear. The intervention involves contact by telephone to alert these at-risk patients to SAFe services and to invite them to participate in the program. Women enrolled in the program have been shown to have significantly higher follow-up rates than unenrolled women: adherence to at least one follow-up appointment for low-grade dysplasia smears was 83% for the program versus 58% for the control (no telephone contact) cohort (Ell et el. 2002). For patients with high-grade dysplasia on their Pap smears, adherence to follow-up appointments for program patients was 93% compared to 67% for controls (Ell et al. 2002).

Lay Health Care Workers

Lay health care workers can also play a role in diminishing disparities in the cervical cancer spectrum. *Promotoras* are Hispanic female cancer survivors who are trained to be health educators in their communities (Hansen et al. 2005). They usually speak with women they already know, and often in their homes, successfully encouraging other women to participate in screening programs by sharing information, personal contact, and frequent follow-up reminders (Hansen et al. 2005). Meta-analysis of intervention programs reported in the literature shows that clinic-based, *promotora*-based, and combined approaches can all increase use of key preventive health services by Hispanic women (Wasserman et al. 2007). Other studies have shown that reminder/recall interventions that utilize lay health care workers (in person, by telephone, or by letter) increase use of prenatal care, Pap smear screening, and immunizations by Hispanic women (Wasserman et al 2007). One investigation demonstrated that programs using lay health advisors resulted in increased compliance rates for cancer screening by 10–15%, with a remarkable 20–25% increase seen for Southeast-Asian women (Margolis et al. 1998).

In a randomized, controlled trial among Chinese women in Seattle and Vancouver, furthermore, interventions via direct mail or contact by multi-lingual outreach workers significantly improved screening behavior (Taylor et al. 2002). Among Vietnamese women in Santa Clara, California, for example, Pap smear testing increased significantly when the intervention involved a combination of both media-based education and outreach by lay health care workers. This combination program was also more effective than media-based intervention alone: in the combination intervention group, the percentage of women who became up-to-date in screening after one year of intervention rose from 45.7% to 67.3%, while in the media-only group, compliance rose from 50.9% to 55.7% (Mock et al. 2007).

Other Approaches

Other interventions that may help eradicate disparities include introducing cross-cultural curriculum for residents and medical students to increase "cultural competence" and thus faciliate greater communication and understanding between physicians and their minority patients (Carillo et al. 1999). Other programs have proposed strengthening the relationship between low-income, African American women and their physicians to enhance quality of care and health outcomes, including cervical cancer screening. This goal could be accomplished by making primary care sites more accessible, linking patients to the same physician for each visit, and organizing primary health care centers to provide for all of a woman's health care needs and coordinated specialty services, since these factors have been associated with improved patient–physician relationships (O'Malley et al. 2002). Community pharmacies, particularly in rural areas, may prove to be effective venues for disseminating information about breast and cervical cancer screening as well (McGuire et al. 2007). Yet another promising intervention explored the role of a culturally appropriate 1-hour curriculum about cervical cancer for high-school students, mainly Hispanic, in rural Eastern Washington State. The study showed a significantly increased knowledge regarding Pap smear testing and improved attitudes about screening and cervical cancer among the students exposed to the curriculum (Tejada et al. 2006).

Conclusion

While disparities in health care along the entire spectrum for cervical cancer are well recognized, their elimination will require further investigation and effort so that barriers to equitable care can be better understood and addressed (del Carmen et al. 2007). These disparities affect each component of the spectrum from screening to follow-up to diagnosis to treatment. Research efforts, focused on individual parts of the spectrum, such as screening and treatment, have attempted to identify and alleviate barriers that lead to these disparities.

Eradication of disparities, however, will require turning this knowledge into action, and, indeed, a variety of promising educational and outreach efforts are already underway. Culturally appropriate education regarding cervical cancer, its link to oncogenic HPV types, and the importance of cervical cancer screening, for example, have the potential to significantly reduce both the incidence and mortality rate from cervical cancer for all populations. To be effective, these education efforts should not only target members of high-risk populations, but also the physicians who care for them. Developing culturally competent physicians will also make a significant impact in reducing many barriers to care and resulting health disparities.

As discussed earlier too, community-based outreach, such as follow-up reminders and lay health care workers (e.g., *promotoras*), can enhance communication between health care providers and underscreened women as well. Most of the programs discussed above that are designed to reduce cervical cancer disparities could incorporate cervical cancer vaccination education into their programs. Furthermore, cervical cancer vaccination programs can be incorporated into the other standard immunizations that adolescents receive, as has been recommended by the ACIP (Committee on Infectious Diseases 2007). Although the broad-based implementation of such vaccination programs would not eliminate the need for screening, they would undoubtedly reduce the impact of screening disparities on minority populations.

Given that minority populations in the United States are younger, and are increasing in proportion at a faster rate than the white population, cervical cancer will undoubtedly become a growing burden on the health care system should these disparities persist. We must therefore immediately take action to understand and address these barriers.

References

Adams EK, Breen N, Joski PJ. 2007. Impact of the National Breast and Cervical Cancer Early Detection Program on mammography and pap test utilization among white, Hispanic, and African American women: 1996–2000. Cancer. (Nov 29) 109(S2):348–358.

American Cancer Society. Cancer Facts & Figures, 2007. Atlanta, Georgia. http://www.cancer.org/downloads/STT/CAFF2007PWSecured.pdf

Asian American Network for Cancer Awareness, Research and Training. http://www.aancart.org. Accessed October 18, 2007.

Baker P, Hoel D, Mohr L, Lipsitz S, Lackland D. 2000. Racial, age, and rural/urban disparity in cervical cancer incidence. Ann Epidemiol 10(7):466–467.

Baquet CR, Mack KM, Mishra SI, et al. 2006. Maryland's Special Populations Network. A model for cancer disparities research, education, and training. Cancer. 107(8 Suppl):2061–2070.

Bazargan M, Bazargan SH, Farooq M, Baker RS. 2004. Correlates of cervical cancer screening among underserved Hispanic and African-American women. Prev Med 39(3):465–473.

Behbakht K, Lynch A, Teal S, Degeest K, Massad S. 2004. Social and cultural barriers to Papanicolaou test screening in an urban population. Obstet Gynecol 1046:1355–1361.

Bosch FX, Manos MM, Munoz N, Sherman M, Jansen AM, Peto J, Schiffman MH, Moreno V, Kurman R, Shah KV. 1995. Prevalence of human papillomarivus in cervical cancer: a worldwide perspective. International biological study on cervical cancer (IBSCC) study group. J Natl Cancer Inst 87(11):796–802.

Burk RD, Kelly P, Feldman J, Bromberg J, Vermund SH, DeHovitz JA, Landesman SH. 1996. Declining prevalence of cervicovaginal human papillomavirus infection with age is independent of other risk factors. Sex Transm Dis 23(4):333–341.

Byrd TL, Peterson SK, Chavez R, Heckert A. 2004. Cervical cancer screening beliefs among young Hispanic women. Prev Med 38(2):192–197.

Carrillo JE, Green AR, Betancourt JR. 1999. Cross-cultural primary care: a patient-based approach. Ann Intern Med. 130(10):829–834.

Clifford GM, Smith JS, Plummer M, Munoz N, Franceschi S. 2003. Human papillomavirus types in invasive cervical cancer worldwide: a meta-analysis. Br J Cancer 88(1):63–73.

Committee on Infectious Diseases. Recommended Immunization Schedules for Children and Adolescents – United States, 2007. Pediatrics. 119(1):207–208.

Coughlin SS, King J, Richards TB, Ekwueme DU. 2006. Cervical cancer screening among women in metropolitan areas of the United States by individual-level and area-based measures of socioeconomic status, 2000 to 2002. Cancer Epidemiol Biomarkers Prev 15(11):2154–2159.

Cuzick J, Szarewski A, Terry G, Ho L, Hanby A, Maddox P, Anderson M, Kocjan G, Steele ST, Guillebaud J. 1995. Human papillomavirus testing in primary cervical screening. Lancet 345(8964):1533–1536.

DATA 2010. The Healthy People 2010 database. The Centers for Disease Control and Prevention. http://wonder.cdc.gov/scripts/broker.exe. Accessed May 15, 2007.

del Carmen MG, Fidnley M, Muzikansky A, Roche M, Verrill CL, Horowtiz NE, Seiden M. 2007. Demographic, risk factor, and knowledge differences between Latinas and non-Latinas referred to colposcopy. Gynecol Oncol. (Jan) 104(1):70–76.

del Carmen MG, Montz FJ, Bristow RE, Bovicelli A, Cornelieson T, Trimble E. 1999. Ethnic differences in patterns of care of stage IA1 and stage IA2 cervical cancer: A SEER database study. Gyn Oncol 75:113–117.

Denny L, Quinn M, Sankaranarayanan R. 2006. Screening for cervical cancer in developing countries. Vaccine 24(3):S71–S77.

Department of Health and Human Services. Medicaid Special Coverage Conditions. Breast and Cervical Cancer: Prevention and Treatment. http://www.cms.hhs.gov/MedicaidSpecialCovCond/02_BreastandCervicalCancer_PreventionandTreatment.asp. Accessed November 01, 2007.

Dignamm JJ. Differences in breast cancer prognosis among African American and Caucasian women. 2000. CA Cancer J Clin. 50:50–64.

Ell K, Vourlekis B, Muderspach L, et al. 2002. Abnormal cervical screen follow-up among low-income Latinas: Project SAFe. J Womens Health Gend Based 11(7):639–651.

Ferrante JM, Gonzalez EC, Roetzheim RG, Pal N, Woodard L. 2000. Clinical and demographic predictors of late-stage cervical cancer. Arch Fain Med 9(5):439–445.

Finkelstein JB. 2007. Screening program serves fraction of those eligible. J Natl Cancer Inst. (Feb 21) 99(4):270–271.

Fowler T, Steakley C, Garcia AR, Kwok J, Bennett LM. 2006. Reducing disparities in the burden of cancer: the role of patient navigators. PLoS Med. (Jul) 3(7):e193.

Flores E, Espinoza P, Jacobellis J, Bakemeier R, Press N. 2006. The greater Denver Latino Cancer Prevention/Control Network: prevention and research through a community-based approach. Cancer. 107(8 Suppl):2034–2042.

Freeman HP, Vydelingum NA. 2006. The role of the special populations networks program in eliminating cancer health disparities. Cancer. (Oct 15) 107(8 Suppl):1933–1935.

Gany FM, Shah SM, Changrani J. 2006. New York City's immigrant minorities. Reducing cancer health disparities. Cancer. 107(8 Suppl):2071–2081.

Goel MS, Wee CC, McCarthy EP, Davis RB, Ngo-Metzger Q, Phillips RS. 2003. Racial and ethnic disparities in cancer screening: the importance of foreign birth as a barrier to care. J Gen Intern Med 18(12):1028–1035.

Hansen LK, Feigl P, Modiano MR, et al. 2005. An educational program to increase cervical and breast cancer screening in Hispanic women: a Southwest Oncology Group study. Cancer Nurs. 28(1):47–53.

Harlan LC, Bernstein AB, Kessler LG. 1991. Cervical cancer screening: who is not screened and why? Am J Public Health 81(7):885–890.

Harris R, Leininger L. 1993. Preventive care in rural primary care practice. Cancer 72(3 Suppl):1113–1118.

Healthy People 2010. The Centers for Disease Control and Prevention. http://wonder.cdc. gov/DATA2010.

Healthy People 2010. US Department of Health and Human Services. http://www.healthy-people.gov/default.htm. Accessed May 16, 2007.

Hiatt RA, Pasick RJ, Stewart S, Bloom J, Davis P, Gardiner P, Johnston M, Luce J, Schorr K, Brunner W, Stroud F. 2001. Community-based cancer screening for underserved women: design and baseline findings from the Breast and Cervical Cancer Intervention Study. Prev Med. 33(3):190–203.

Hildesheim A, Gravitt P, Schiffman MH, Kurman RJ, Barnes W, Jones S, Tchabo JG, Brinton LA, Copeland C, Epp J, et al. 1993. Determinants of genital human papillomavirus infection in low-income women in Washington, D. C. Sex Transm Dis 20(5):279–285.

Ho GY, Bierman R, Beardsley L, Chang CJ, Burk RD. 1998. Natural history of cervicovaginal papillomavirus infection in young women. N Engl J Med 338(7):423–428.

Howe HL, Wu X, Ries LA, Cokkinides V, Ahmed F, Jemal A, Miller B, Williams M, Ward E, Wingo PA, Ramirez A, Edwards BK. 2006. Annual report to the nation on the status of cancer, 1975–2003, featuring cancer among U.S. Hispanic/Latino populations. Cancer 107(8):1711–1742.

Howell EA, Chen YT, Concato J. 1999. Differences in cervical cancer mortality among black and white women. Obstet Gynecol. 94:509–15.

Jackson FE, Chu KC, Garcia R. 2006. Special Populations Networks – how this innovative community-based initiative affected minority and underserved research programs. Cancer. 107(8 Suppl):1939–1944.

Jemal A, Siegel R, Ward E, Murray T, Xu J, Thun MJ. Cancer statistics, 2007. CA Cancer J Clin 57(1):42–66.

Kamangar F, Dores GM, Anderson WF. 2006. Patterns of cancer incidence, mortality, and prevalence across five continents: defining priorities to reduce cancer disparities in different geographic regions of the world. J Clin Oncol 224(14):2137–2150.

Kiefe CI, Funkhouser E, Fouad MN, May DS. 1998. Chronic disease as a barrier to breast and cervical cancer screening. J Gen Intern Med 13(6):357–365.

Krieger N, Quesenberry C Jr, Peng T, Horn-Ross P, Stewart S, Brown S, Swallen K, Guillermo T, Suh D, Alvarez-Martinez L, Ward F. 1999. Social class, race/ethnicity, and incidence of breast, cervix, colon, lung, and prostate cancer among Asian, Black, Hispanic, and White residents of the San Francisco Bay Area, 1988–92 (United States). Cancer Causes Control 10(6):525–537.

Ley C, Bauer HM, Reingold A, Schiffman MH, Chambers JC, Tashiro CJ, Manos MM. 1991. Determinants of genital human papillomavirus infection in young women. J Natl Cancer Inst 83(14):997–1003.

Lorincz AT, Reid R, Jenson AB, Greenberg MD, Lancaster W, Kurman R J. 1992. Human papillomavirus infection of the cervix: relative risk associations of 15 common anogenital types. Obstet Gynecol 79(30):328–337.

Lorincz AT, Reid R. 1989. Association of human papillomavirus with gynecologic cancer. Curr Opin Oncol 1(1):123–132.

Margolis KL, Lurie N, McGovern PG, Tyrrell M, Slater JS. 1998. Increasing breast and cervical cancer screening in low-income women. J Gen Intern Med. 13(8):515–521.

Massad LS, Verhulst SJ, Hagemeyer M, Brady P. 2006. Knowledge of the cervical cancer screening process among rural and urban Illinois women undergoing colposcopy. J Low Genit Tract Dis. 10(4):252–255.

McDougall JA, Madeleine MM, Dailing JR, Li CI. 2007. Racial and ethnic disparities in cervical cancer incidence rates in the United States, 1992–2003. Cancer Causes Control 18(10):1175–1186.

McGuire TR, Leypoldt M, Narducci WA, Ward K. 2007. Accessing rural populations: role of the community pharmacist in a breast and cervical cancer screening programme. J Eval Clin Pract. 13(1):146–149.

Mensah G. 2006. Racial and Ethnic Approaches to Community Health (REACH) 2010. The Centers for Disease Control and Prevention. Atlanta, GA: U.S. Department of Health and Human Services.

Merrill RM, Merrill AV, Mayer LS. 2000. Factors associated with no surgery or radiation therapy for invasive cervical cancer in Black and White women. Ethn Dis. 10:248–56.

Miller SM, Siejak KK, Schroeder CM, Lerman C, Hernandez E, Helm CW. 1997. Enhancing adherence following abnormal Pap smears among low-income minority women: a preventive telephone counseling strategy. J Natl Cancer Inst. 89(10):703–708.

Mock J, McPhee SJ, Nguyen T, et al. 2007. Effective Lay Health Worker Outreach and Media-Based Education for Promoting Cervical Cancer Screening Among Vietnamese American Women. Am J Public Health 97:1693–1700.

Mundt AJ, Connell PP, Campbell T, Hwang JH, Rotmensch J, Waggoner S. 1998. Race and clinical outcome in patients with carcinoma of the uterine cervix treated with radiation therapy. Gynecol Oncol. 71:151–8.

Newmann SJ, Garner EO. 2005. Social inequities along the cervical cancer continuum: a structured review. Cancer Causes Control. 16: 63–70.

Nuovo GJ, Pedemonte B. M. 1990. Human papillomavirus types and recurrent cervical warts. JAMA 263(9):1223–1226.

O'Malley AS, Forrest CB, Mandelblatt J. 2002. Adherence of low-income women to cancer screening recommendations. J Gen Intern Med. 17(2):144–154.

O'Malley AS, Forrest CB. 2002. Beyond the examination room: primary care performance and the patient-physician relationship for low-income women. J Gen Intern Med. 17(1):66–74.

O'Malley CD, Shema SJ, Clarke LS, Clarke CA, Perkins CI. 2006. Medicaid status and stage at diagnosis of cervical cancer. Am J Public Health 96(12):2179–2185.

Patel DA, Barnholtz-Sloan JS, Patel MK, Malone JM Jr, Chuba PJ, Schwartz K. 2005. A population-based study of racial and ethnic differences in survival among women with invasive cervical cancer: analysis of Surveillance, Epidemiology, and End Results data. Gynecol Oncol 97(2):550–558.

Peyton CL, Gravitt PE, Hunt WC, Hundley RS, Zhao M, Apple RJ, Wheeler CM. 2001. Determinants of genital human papillomavirus detection in a U. S. population. J Infect Dis 183(11):1554–1564.

Population Estimates. The US Census Bureau. 2007. http://www.census.gov/popest/estimates.php. Accessed November 1, 2007.

Ries L, Harkins D, Krapcho M, Mariotto A, Miller BA, Feuer EJ, Clegg L, Eisner MP, Horner MJ, Howlader N, Hayat M, Hankey BF, Edwards BK (eds). 2005. SEER Cancer Statistics Review, 1975–2004, National Cancer Institute. Bethesda, MD, based on November 2005 SEER data submission, posted to the SEER web site. http://seer.cancer.gov/csr/1975_2004/.

Ries LAG, Harkins D, Krapcho M, Mariotto A, Miller BA, Feuer EJ, Clegg L, Eisner MP, Horner MJ, Howlader N, Hayat M, Hankey BF, Edwards BK (eds). 2006. SEER Cancer Statistics Review, 1975–2003, National Cancer Institute. Bethesda, MD, http://seer.cancer.gov/csr/1975_2003/, based on November 2005 SEER data submission, posted to the SEER web site, 2006.

Riley GF, Potosky AL, Lubitz JD, Brown ML. 1994. Stage of cancer at diagnosis for Medicare HMO and fee-for-service enrollees. Am J Public Health 84(10):1598–1604.

Russell AH, Shingleton HM, Jones WB, Stewart AK, Fremgen A, Winchester DP, et al. 1998. Trends in the use of radiation and chemotherapy in the initial management of patients with carcinoma of the uterine cervix. Int J Radiat Oncol Biol Phys. 40:605–13.

Sankaranarayanan R, Ferlay J. 2006. Worldwide burden of gynaecological cancer: the size of the problem. Best Pract Res Clin Obstet Gynaecol 20(2):207–225.

Ryerson AB, Benard, V. B., and Major, A.C. 2005. The National Breast and Cervical Cancer Early Detection Program: 1991–2002 National Report. Atlanta, GA: The Centers for Disease Control and Prevention.

Saraiya M, Ahmed F, Krishnan S, Richards TB, Unger ER, Lawson HW. 2007. Cervical cancer incidence in a prevaccine era in the United States, 1998–2002. Obstet Gynecol 109(2 Pt 1):360–370.

Shah M, Zhu K, Wu H, Potter J. 2006. Hispanic acculturation and utilization of cervical cancer screening in the US. Prev Med 42(2):146–149.

Shavers VL, Brown ML. 2002. Racial and ethnic disparities in the receipt of cancer treatment. J Natl Cancer Inst. Mar 94(5):334–357.

Stone KM. 1995. Human papillomavirus infection and genital warts: update on epidemiology and treatment. Clin Infect Dis 20(Suppl 1):S91–S97.

Taylor VM, Hislop TG, Jackson JC, et al. 2002. A randomized controlled trial of interventions to promote cervical cancer screening among Chinese women in North America. J Natl Cancer Inst. 94(9):670–677.

Tejeda S, Thompson B, Coronado GD, Rees JM. 2006. A cervical cancer curriculum for Hispanic adolescents in rural high schools: a pilot study. J Health Care Poor Underserved. 17(4):734–744.

The Centers for Disease Control and Prevention. National Breast and Cervical Cancer Early Detection Program. http://www.cdc.gov/cancer/nbccedp/. Accessed March 29, 2007.

Thoms WW, Unger ER, Carisio R, Nisenbaum R, Spann CO, Horowitz IR, et al. 1998. Clinical determinants of survival from stage Ib cervical cancer in an inner-city hospital. J Natl Med Assoc. 90:303–8.

Tiro JA, Meissner HI, Kobrin S, Chollette V. 2007. What do women in the U.S. know about human papillomavirus and cervical cancer? Cancer Epidemiol Biomarkers Prev 16(2):288–94.

U.S. Census Bureau, 2004, "U.S. Interim Projections by Age, Sex, Race, and Hispanic Origin". http://www.census.gov/ipc/www/usinterimproj/.

Wasserman M, Bender D, Lee S-Y D. 2007. Use of Preventive Maternal and Child Health Services by Latina Women. Med Care Res Rev. 64(1):4–45.

Winstead E. 2005. tHelping Patients Navigate the Health Care System. NCI Cancer Bulletin. NCI Cancer Bulleting. Vol 2.

Chapter 10
Melanoma and Primary Hepatocellular Carcinoma

Christopher A. Aoki, Alan Geller, and Moon S. Chen

Melanoma and primary hepatocellular carcinoma (HCC) are two cancers with distinct disparity profiles. In the case of melanoma, while fair-skinned individuals with high education and income are more likely to be diagnosed, those of low socioeconomic status (SES) have a higher case-fatality rate. Greater awareness of warning signs of melanoma and access to primary care/dermatologists likely account for disparities between persons of moderate-high SES and those of lower SES. In the case of HCC, however, the highest incidence and mortality rates in the United States occur among Asian and Pacific Islanders (APIs); all other people of color have higher rates compared to non-Hispanic whites (Miller et al. 1996). Worldwide, APIs are approximately four times more frequently affected, and blacks and Hispanics approximately two times more frequently affected, than non-Hispanic whites. Even so, in the United States, the largest absolute number of HCC cases still occur among whites (El-Serag 2007).

This chapter presents the clinical and public health significance of both melanoma and primary HCC, including the magnitude, etiology, and risk factors for each. It then discusses disparities in access to screening by social class, race and ethnicity, age and gender and then reviews the rising disparity in survival between developed and less-developed regions of the world. The chapter concludes by suggesting a series of solutions to address disparities at both the individual and policy levels.

Melanoma

Clinical and Public Health Significance of Melanoma

Melanoma—a potentially lethal melanocytic neoplasm with a propensity for distant metastasis (Koh 1991)—is the sixth most common cancer in the United

C.A. Aoki (✉)
Division of Gastroenterology and Hepatology, Department of Internal Medicine, School of Medicine, University of California, Davis, CA
e-mail: christopher.aoki@ucdmc.ucdavis.edu

H.K. Koh (ed.), *Toward the Elimination of Cancer Disparities*,
DOI 10.1007/978-0-387-89443-0_10, © Springer Science+Business Media, LLC 2009

States with more than 60,000 new cases diagnosed annually (Jemal et al. 2007). In the past five years, there have been notable strides toward earlier recognition and discovery of this cancer, including new technologies to complement and augment the clinical examination and new insights to help clinicians recognize early stages of the disease (Geller et al. 2007). Nonetheless, in the past 25 years, incidence and mortality rates throughout most of the developed world have risen, while education, early detection, and screening, the potentially best means for reducing the disease, continue to be severely underutilized (Geller et al. 2007). The most recent data indicate that only 14–21% of Americans report having ever received a skin cancer examination (Saraiya et al. 2004, Santmyire et al. 2001).

Current Language Regarding Melanoma Screening

It should be noted that no randomized trial or definitive data about mortality reduction from screening exist; therefore, there are no current positive or negative recommendations for skin cancer screening. Ideally, evaluating melanoma screening would involve a randomized trial demonstrating sustained reductions in the melanoma mortality in a defined population (compared with a control population). Without this evidence, esteemed Federal bodies have not recommended screening across a whole population.

For example, The 1996 US Preventive Services Task Force (USPSTF) (US Preventive Services Task Force 1996) found insufficient evidence to recommend either for or against routine screening for skin cancer by primary care providers. The Third United States Preventive Services Task Force (2001) concluded "evidence is lacking that the skin examination by clinicians is effective in reducing mortality or morbidity from skin cancer," and The Institute of Medicine (Institute of Medicine 2000) stated:

> In summary, the committee concluded that evidence for the effectiveness of skin cancer screening is insufficient to support positive or negative conclusions about the adoption of a new program of clinical screening of asymptomatic Medicare beneficiaries.

In the same Institute of Medicine report (2000), they indicated the benefits of early detection and treatment by stating:

> Because evidence does support benefits of early detection and treatment as part of usual medical care, clinicians and patients should continue to be alert to the common signs of skin cancer-with a particular emphasis on older white males and on melanoma—and should investigate suspicious signs further (Institute of Medicine 2000).

Magnitude of Melanoma

Both in the United States and throughout most of the world, the incidence of melanoma has been increasing steadily over the past few decades (Crocetti et al. 2004, Ries et al. 1975–2002). In fact, in the United States, the age-adjusted incidence among non-Hispanic whites has increased from 7.5 cases per 100,000 (1973) to 21.9 cases per 100,000 (2002) (Ries et al. 1975–2002). Although the overall mortality rate has only recently stabilized, this rate has increased 28% since 1975 (Ries et al. 1975–2002).

Etiology and Risk Factors for Melanoma

Risk factors for melanoma have been well documented and are generally categorized as constitutional predispositions (e.g., increasing age, fair skin and hair color, total number of moles, tendency for freckling, presence or absence of three or more atypical moles, propensity to burn in the sun rather than tan, and family history of melanoma), risk behaviors (e.g., history of three or more episodes of sunburn, ultraviolet (UV) exposures at tanning salons), and environmental factors (e.g., residing in latitudes closer to the equator) (Rhodes et al. 1987, Kirkpatrick et al. 1990).

Disparities in Access and by Geography

Limited access to care is likely to be associated with poor outcomes, including diagnosis at late-stage and decreased survival. Inequalities between patients of low and moderate/higher SES include underinsurance, lack of access to dermatologists and/or primary care physicians, and physical barriers to care, such as travel.

In an ecological analysis, Roetzheim et al., for example, strongly suggested that physician workforce issues could impact health outcomes in melanoma. They found that with each additional dermatologist per a population of 10,000, there was a 39% increased odds of earlier diagnosis (Roetzheim et al. 2000). Recent studies using Medicare data, moreover, suggest that diagnosis by a dermatologist (as opposed to non-dermatologist physicians) significantly improves the chances of melanoma survival at 2 years (Pennie et al. 2007), indicating the potential significance of an expert, thorough examination. Notably, nearly all of the ten states with highest melanoma mortality rates are among the least populous and often have the fewest number of dermatologists per capita. These states show striking state-by-state disparities for mortality rates—which exceed 3.5 per 100,000 in states with the fewest dermatologists (such as New Hampshire, Oklahoma, Maine, Utah, and Idaho), compared with rates as low as 1.5–2 per 100,000 in other states (Ries et al. 1975–2002, Geller et al. 2007).

While determining exactly how specialty and physician workforce issues are associated with earlier diagnosis requires further investigation, more physicians and more dermatologists could plausibly facilitate and expedite referrals from primary care physicians. Other benefits of more dermatologists in a community might include prompt removal of atypical moles and one-to-one expert education regarding self-screening and family screening. Also, more dermatologists in a particular area might generate shorter wait times for scheduling appointments, although recent studies indicate that patient reports of changing moles to dermatology offices paradoxically often generate longer waiting times (Resneck et al. 2006). While higher density of specialists is a possible indicator for access to care, it does not guarantee increased access even in urban/suburban areas, particularly in situations in which medical dermatologists may refuse to accept Medicare and Medicaid patients. In fact, the very availability of specialists such as dermatologists in a particular community may reflect underlying economic inequalities.

Yet another factor that may limit access to care is the patient's insurance status. In a separate study by Roetzheim et al., Medicaid patients had nearly a fivefold risk of receiving a late-stage diagnosis and uninsured patients had a 2.6-fold risk compared with patients with commercial indemnity insurance (Roetzheim et al. 1999). An earlier stage of diagnosis was found for HMO patients compared with those receiving fee-for-service (FFS) (Kirsner et al. 2005). For all patients, HMO enrollees were less than half as likely as FFS enrollees to receive a diagnosis at a distant stage (OR, 0.46; 95% CI, 0.24–0.80).

Geography is clearly a factor as well. In a study of 42 counties in North Carolina (including many rural counties), Stitzenberg et al. found that greater distance from home to a dermatologist predicted melanoma Breslow thickness (an important prognostic indicator for melanoma survival) (Stitzenberg et al. 2007, Di Quinzio et al. 2005, Reyes-Ortiz et al. 2006). They speculated that proximity to dermatologic care was an indicator of local health resources and noted that patients who lived in counties with at least one dermatologist traveled approximately eight fewer miles to care than those in counties without a dermatologist (Stitzenberg et al. 2007). Similarly, researchers in Nova Scotia who used a billing system within their province to examine access to family practitioners and its association with melanoma thickness found that patients with multiple visits to the same physician (rather than to many different providers) had lower risk for having a melanoma thicker than 0.75 mm at time of diagnosis (Di Quinzio et al. 2005). In fact, patients having 2–5 visits to the same provider were 66% less likely to have a thicker melanoma than those patients who were not seen by a family physician in the two-year period before diagnosis. Men, older persons, and patients living in rural areas were also more likely to have thicker melanomas at time of diagnosis. The authors speculated that geographic barriers to care may have had a role in delayed diagnosis and thus, thicker melanoma (Kirkpatrick et al. 1990, Di Quinzio et al. 2005).

Disparities by social class. While melanoma is more commonly diagnosed in fair-skinned individuals with higher education and income, lower SES individuals experience higher case-fatality rates, later stage disease at diagnosis, and decreased survival. This is true whether SES is measured at the individual level (e.g., occupation) or aggregate levels (e.g., median household income, education, socioeconomic deprivation, or poverty percentage) (Reyes-Ortiz et al. 2006). Many US studies support the inverse relationship between low SES or lack of insurance and poorer stage of diagnosis. In addition, not only is lower SES associated with less knowledge of melanoma, but patients with lower SES or without health insurance are also less likely to undergo either self-examination or physician screening (Miller et al. 1996). Greater awareness of warning signs of melanoma and lack of access to primary care/dermatologists (see section above) likely account for disparities between persons of moderate-high SES and lower SES (Miller et al. 1996, Koh et al. 1991, Girgis et al. 1991, Geller et al. 1992).

Recently, for example, Reyes-Ortiz linked the tumor registry records from the US SEER program and Medicare claims from the Centers for Medicare and Medicaid Services. After adjustment for sociodemographic variables, stage at diagnosis, comorbidities, and tumor thickness, residence in low-income areas was found to be an independently poor prognostic factor in melanoma survival (Reyes-Ortiz et al. 2006). Similarly, a US population-based study found that men and women with invasive melanoma residing in poor areas had lower survival rates (83%) than those living in wealthier areas (91%). A population-based study in Massachusetts too found that advanced stage and higher case-fatality of melanoma was associated with lower income census tract or ZIP code (Geller et al. 1996). Finally, a case study of patients in California and Michigan found that men with the least amount of education, i.e., less than high school, had greater melanoma thickness at diagnosis and thus a worse prognosis than persons from all other educational strata (Swetter et al. 2009).

Reyes-Ortiz et al. speculated that low SES influenced melanoma survival through at least two mechanisms: biological features of the tumor or stage or thickness at diagnosis, and host factors (Reyes-Ortiz et al. 2006). For example, at the biological level, nodular tumors, which comprise only 10% of all melanoma, are responsible for nearly 50% of all melanoma diagnosed at greater than 2 mm (Demierre et al. 2005). Nodular tumors have been found to be relatively more frequent in patients with the least education (Geller et al. 2009).

Disparities by race and ethnicity. Although diagnoses are rare in persons of color, the latest examination of the US Surveillance Epidemiology and End Results (SEER) registry found that the overall 5-year survival was demonstrably less for minorities (72%–81%) than for whites (89.6%) (Ries et al. 1975–2002). While melanoma is very uncommon in African Americans (1.0 per 100,000,or less than 1/20th the rate of Caucasians (Ries et al. 1975–2002)), the anatomic location and the severity of disease in low SES populations— particularly the high rates of acral melanoma in African Americans (Cress and Holly 1997, Byrd et al. 2004, Hemmings et al. 2004), and recently found among Hispanics in California (Cockburn et al. 2006)—may make these lesions harder to discover at an earlier, curable stage. In a recent analysis of more than 1,600 cases of melanoma in Miami Dade County, Florida (1997–2002), for example, regional and distant disease was more common in non-Hispanic blacks (52%) than in Hispanics (27%) or whites (16%), although there were only 29 diagnoses of melanoma among non-Hispanic blacks (Hu et al. 2006). Similarly, although rates of invasive melanoma for Hispanic California men are far less than those for non-Hispanic California men (2.8 per 100,000 vs. 17.2 per 100,000), estimated annual percent change rates increased 1.8 per year for the Hispanic men between 1988 and 2001. Thicker lesions (greater than 1.5 mm) were more common in the Hispanic (35%) than the non-Hispanic men (24%) as well. Both Hispanic men and women in this study, moreover, experienced sharper increases in the incidence of thick tumors than in thin (<0.75 mm) or moderate (0.75–1.49 mm) tumors (Cockburn et al. 2006).

Although some degree of disparity in incidence between races is linked to UV exposure, evidence elucidating specific linkages is currently contradictory. Eide et al. found that melanoma incidence was associated with increased UV Index and lower latitude only in non-Hispanic whites, with no evidence to support the association of UV exposure and melanoma incidence in black or Hispanic populations (Eide and Weinstock 2005). In contrast, Hu et al. found significant correlations of UV Index and melanoma incidence in white men, white women, and black men but not in black women, Hispanic men, or Hispanic women (Hu et al. 2004).

Disparities by age and gender. In the United States, incidence rates from 1973 to 2002 have risen in all age groups and in men and women. Even more strikingly, over these same 30 years, men aged 55 through 64 years have experienced more than a fourfold increase (12.4–56.1 per 100,000), and rates have risen more than fivefold in men aged 65 years and older (18.8–104.4 per 100,000) (Ries et al. 1975–2002, Geller et al. 2002).

With regard to mortality, from 1973 to 2002, rates decreased by 23% in women aged 20 through 54 years and by 11% in men of the same age. In contrast, mortality rates rose 15% in women aged 55 through 64 years and 64% in men of the same age. Mortality rates increased 130% (8.6–19.8 per 100 000) in men aged 65 years or older and 73% in women of the same age. In all, nearly 50% of US melanoma deaths today are in white men aged 50 and above (Ries et al. 1975–2002, Geller et al. 2002).

Worldwide, mortality rates are highest in the following five countries: New Zealand, Australia, Norway, Denmark, and South Africa (Crocetti et al. 2004, Ferlay et al. 2004, de Vries et al. 2003, Diepgen and Mahler 2002, Severi et al. 2000). Mortality rates are uniformly higher in men than women. Rates are rising worldwide, most precipitously in older men (ages 65+), with older women experiencing smaller increases. In contrast, mortality rates are decreasing or stabilizing for younger women, while rates among younger men vary by country. For example, since the mid-1980s mortality has leveled off in Sweden, with a statistically significant downward trend observed for women (Cohn-Cedermark et al. 2000).

Some of these disparities may be related to behavioral differences between the sexes. Men are also less likely than women to examine their skin for melanoma (Diepgen and Mahler 2002), and less commonly seek physician examinations (Miller et al. 1996). In a recent multi-institutional study of men diagnosed with thin ($n = 170$) and thick ($n = 57$) melanoma, thinner tumors correlated with men who had heard of melanoma ($p = 0.007$), paid attention to their health ($p = 0.002$), regularly taken interest in reading or watching stories about health topics ($p = 0.003$), believed it was important to have a doctor examine their skin for signs of melanoma ($p = 0.05$), and carefully paid attention to information about skin cancer detection ($p = 0.02$) (Swetter et al. 2009).

Finally, data from the SEER registry-Medicare linked database suggest that older widowed persons were more likely to be diagnosed at later stage and to die from melanoma than were older married persons (odds ratio = 1.31, 95% CI 1.13–1.51) (Reyes Ortiz et al. 2007). Hence, health knowledge and action of one partner can improve the health of the other. It has been long speculated that female spouses play an important role in the discovery of lesions and encouraging their husbands to seek prompt referrals for a suspect lesion.

Disparities by nation. While 5-year survival rates in many countries such as the United States, Scotland, Australia, and Sweden exceed 90%, many nations have not benefited from early detection and educational programs (Globocan http://www-dep.iarc.fr/globocan/downloads.html). Low rates of 5-year survival have been found among men in Northern Ireland (53.5), Poland (Cracow) (55.8), the Czech Republic (60.3), and Slovenia (60.6), equivalent to survival rates in the United States and Australia from over 40 years ago (Globocan http://www-dep.iarc.fr/globocan/downloads.html) (Fig. 10.1). Survival rates for women—who had surprisingly high rates of trunk melanoma (over 30% of all melanoma in women)—generally fared no better in these four countries (World Health Organization and Globocan http://www-dep.iarc.fr/globocan/downloads.html).

Four Eastern European countries (Croatia, Slovenia, Macedonia, and the Slovak Republic) are on the list of ten nations in the world with the highest

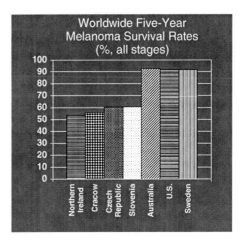

Fig. 10.1 Disparities in 5-year melanoma survival rates (worldwide)

Table 10.1 Variables associated with heightened disparities in melanoma survival

Social Class	Low SES > middle/High SES
Gender	Men > women
Race and ethnicity	African Americans and Hispanics > Caucasians
Age	Age 65+ > age≤55
Nation	Eastern European > North America, Australia, and Western Europe
Geography	Rural, small states > populous states
Access to care	Uninsured, persons without private dermatologists > insured, open access to dermatologists

melanoma mortality rates in men, while five Eastern Europeans nations (Latvia, Estonia, Lithuania, Slovak Republic, and Macedonia) are on the comparable list for women (World Health Organization). Disparities are particularly striking when contrasting developed to undeveloped nations. For women, mortality/incidence ratios (MIR) are 0.460 for less-developed regions and 0.179 for more developed regions. In fact, for three countries with more than 200 cases per year among women (Ethiopia, Zaire, and Indonesia), the MIR exceeds 60%. In contrast, the US MIR is less than 15% (World Health Organization).

There is some evidence that these high mortality rates may be attributable, at least in part, to late detection. Notably, in Croatia, one of the countries with the lowest 5-year survival rates in the world, a 20-year epidemiological study of one of the more populous districts there uncovered large disparities in late-stage melanoma detection. For example, nodular melanoma comprised 35% of all diagnoses, more than threefold the percentage found in countries with higher melanoma survival. Most lesions had a thickness of 1.50–2.49 mm. The authors called for more effective community information and a commitment to mass education (Zamolo et al. 2000).

Suggested Next Steps for Addressing Disparities

In general, melanoma control requires increasing public education and widening access to care for disadvantaged populations. The sections below identify some future research tasks and political, professional, and public education strategies to address the disproportionate burden of late-stage melanoma among individuals with low SES, minority groups, and middle-aged and older men.

Research agenda. First, new qualitative studies are needed to understand barriers that low-SES individuals face when seeking skilled dermatologic exams for skin cancer. Extensive interviewing of low-SES and high-SES individuals should explore and contrast psychosocial factors complicating melanoma diagnosis, such as comorbidities, inadequate perception and awareness of risk factors, and other reasons for delay in diagnosis.

Second, interventions that jointly target high-risk residents, their physicians, and health care systems should be funded for communities with high melanoma MIRs. New attention should also be given to developing specific information on factors that may be associated with state-by-state rates of mortality such as incidence, social class, rural vs. urban residence, and surgical care, information that is currently unavailable (Ries et al. 1975–2002, Geller et al. 2007).

There is also no current information documenting the proportion of at-risk Americans who have yet to receive a full skin cancer examination. Therefore, cancer control planners should be asking regular questions on the receipt of screening and on barriers to screening as part of the US and state population-based surveillance studies (e.g., the National Health Interview Survey or the Behavioral Risk Factor Surveillance Survey [BRFSS]).

Fourth, serious consideration must be given to the development and design of a randomized screening trial to decrease melanoma mortality. Physicians and insurers alike look for evidence that screening saves lives before recommendations are made available to the public. Proof that melanoma screening saves lives could lead to new training programs for physicians and nurses, inclusion of the skin exam in medical schools and nursing schools, and universal reimbursement for the complete skin examination. If a screening trial proves to be beneficial, and positive recommendations are forthcoming, there are ample opportunities to receive a skilled exam as high-risk persons make 3–4 visits per year to their primary care physicians—in fact, two-thirds of all melanoma patients report having seen a primary care doctor in the year before their diagnosis (Geller et al. 1992).

Over the past year, the Melanoma Screening Group, led by dermatologists, cancer educators, screening experts, and epidemiologists, have met to design a rigorous, scientific screening trial. For such a trial, persons would be randomized to one of two study conditions and the severity of their cancers and reduction in deaths from melanoma would be compared. In one group, an estimated 350,000 persons would receive an expert skin cancer examination coupled with instruction in the skin self-examination. For the other condition, nearly 700,000 patients would receive the routine practice of skin cancer screening in primary care. The study would require four years to screen the entire group and eight more years to follow all individuals to determine differences in melanoma severity and reduction of deaths caused by melanoma. While it may be intuitive that screening saves lives, scientific recommendations must be based on carefully constructed studies with a large enough sample size to make these crucial determinations.

Educational efforts. Educational efforts to overcome disparities must strive to expand public outreach and education, educate health care providers and the public, and recruit new screeners in light of the shortage of medical dermatologists in high-risk areas. Increasing the availability of free screenings for individuals previously unscreened should be a cornerstone of national campaigns led by the American Academy of Dermatology and rapidly proliferating US melanoma foundations. Professional education programs with physicians and physicians-in-training must alert them not only to well-established risks such as adverse sun exposure and atypical moles but also to the disproportionate burden of late-stage disease related to social class and gender. The lack of medical dermatologists and long waiting times for mole checks must be ameliorated through the use of mid-level providers or physician extenders, such as physician assistants or nurse practitioners.

Patient navigation systems that have drawn increased attention for other "early detectable" cancers (Freeman 2006) should be used to assist patients with significant risk factors for melanoma as well. Such patients could be easily identified and provided personal instruction in skin self-examination and in finding prompt referrals to physicians or physician extenders. In more impoverished areas, novel patient navigation systems may enhance high-risk patients' opportunities to access skilled and expert evaluations.

Policy arena. Improved screening and outreach for underserved individuals will be best accomplished through a concerted combination of the following: (a) policy changes to provide melanoma screening as a benefit of health care, (b) embedding melanoma screening in health plans, and (c) advocacy for legislation to support melanoma screening and education. To overcome suboptimal access to specialty care, for example, federally funded melanoma screening and education programs, with Medicare coverage and Medicaid options for follow-up and treatment services, should be increased or piloted as part of demonstration projects in high-risk states. Furthermore, other states should follow the Florida legislature that adopted legislation to allow residents speedy access to a dermatologist (A Journey through the Dream (1930–2005): A History of Florida Dermatology and Dermatologic Surgery, (fsdds.org/commemorative)). Cost-benefit studies should also be done to determine the effectiveness of expedited referrals leading to earlier diagnoses, as well as ways to increase initiatives to provide reimbursed screening as part of overall health promotion packages (Geller et al. 2006). One promising development along these lines is the US House and Senate Appropriations Committee's recent endorsement of the Strategic Plan for Melanoma and their request to the National Cancer Institute to consider a national screening study for early melanoma detection.

Conclusion

Disturbingly low screening rates in the presence of persistent and avoidable mortality prompts a call for new and far-reaching approaches, including ways to make screening more available to underserved individuals, education targeted to the high-risk public, and early education to health professional students in all disciplines. In many parts of the developed world, early detection efforts have stabilized previously increasing melanoma mortality rates. However, education and screening, potentially the best means for reducing the disease, continue to be severely underutilized. In particular, much progress still needs to be made to reach middle-aged and older men and persons of lower SES—groups that suffer a disproportionate burden of death from melanoma.

In Australia, for example, where early detection (or screening) campaigns were initiated earlier than in Europe, a shift toward thinner lesions (without an appreciable reduction in thick melanoma) has been observed over time, accompanied by improvements in melanoma survival. In most industrialized nations, considerable progress has been made as well in detecting lesions earlier, reducing case-fatality, and improving survival. However, building on these improvements and extending them to developing nations requires a deeper understanding of some of the following questions:

1) Can new technologies and advances in vigilant surveillance of persons with key risk factors for melanoma, such as dermoscopy, be extended more broadly to individuals, communities, and nations with less access to expert dermatologic care?
2) Can we deepen our understanding of the biological, clinical, and behavioral features of nodular melanoma that all underlie disproportionately late melanoma diagnosis?
3) Can the worldwide and widespread proliferation of Internet information for physicians and the public alike now be harnessed and then tailored to help identify and improve screening for persons of disproportionately high mortality, particularly those of lower SES and men (Harris et al. 2001, Gerbert et al. 2002, Geller et al. 2007) who suffer a disproportionate burden of melanoma deaths and are often seeing primary care physicians for other health reasons?

We also need to generate more convincing evidence that widespread screening effectively reduces melanoma mortality. With the abrupt cessation of the population-based, randomized screening trial in Queensland (Mark Elwood personal communication), randomized studies of large cohorts in the United States and other nations with high melanoma rates—required to rigorously demonstrate that early detection of melanoma is desirable—may never be funded anywhere. The lack of scientific evidence has important implications for individuals yet to be screened as positive findings from large screening studies such as those for breast and cervical cancer often result in new population-wide screening.

Primary Hepatocellular Carcinoma (HCC)

Clinical and Public Health Significance of HCC

Clinical significance. While the US SEER definition of primary liver cancer includes both intrahepatic bile duct cancer and fibrolamellar liver cancer, this chapter focuses solely on primary HCC, which originates from intraparenchymal cells of the liver and makes up between 85% and 90% of all primary liver cancers (Parkin 2001). HCC, the fifth most common cancer in the world, has the third highest mortality rate. Approximately 560,000 cases are diagnosed annually, resulting in 550,000 deaths per year (Parkin 2001). While the incidence and mortality rates for the majority of cancer sites between 1995 and 2004 have been declining, the incidence of liver cancer in the United States increased by 22% and the mortality rate for liver cancer increased by 17% (National Cancer Institute Fact Book 2006, 2007, Jemal et al. 2008). Liver cancer affects men more than four times greater than women (McGlynn et al. 2001).

Hepatocellular carcinoma is often asymptomatic until it has metastasized to other structures or has grown to the point at which therapy cannot be offered. Useful laboratory tests in identifying HCC include a high alkaline phosphatase and a high alpha-fetoprotein (AFP), measures which have a high specificity but low sensitivity. Most lesions can be diagnosed with specific characteristics on a four phase-CT of the abdomen and a blood AFP greater than 200 mg, if the patient has cirrhosis or chronic hepatitis B (Bruix and Sherman 2005). If there is a question of diagnosis, biopsy is preferably done with radio-frequency ablation to prevent tumor seeding. Staging methods that take into account the degree of liver injury include the Cancer of the Liver Italian Program (CLIP) (Investigators 1998) and the Barcelona-Clinic-Liver Cancer (BCLC) staging system (Llovet et al. 1999).

Currently the only curative treatments for HCC include liver resection and liver transplantation. Unfortunately most patients are diagnosed at an advanced stage or are too ill from their underlying chronic liver disease for these therapies to be offered; without them, survival rate is less than 10% after 5 years (Bruix and Sherman 2005). Thus, prevention and control remain the cornerstones for stemming the spread and devastating effects of HCC.

Public Health Significance

The etiology of HCC has been principally attributed to infection with the hepatitis B virus (HBV) and the hepatitis C virus (HCV), the first two viruses classified as human carcinogens by the US Department of Health and Human Services (US Department of Health and Human Services 2004). Worldwide, about one out of three people are infected with HBV, which is responsible for 60–80% of all HCC cases. HBV-induced HCC is the third most common cause of cancer death. The World Health Organization considers HBV infection the second most important cause of cancer after tobacco (www.who.int/csr/disease/hepatitis/whocdscsrlyo20022/en/index1.html).

More than 400 million people are infected with HBV, making it one of the most common and serious infections in the world. More than ten times as many people are infected with HBV compared to those living with HIV (approximately 33 million people) (El-Serag 2002) In endemic countries, HBV is typically transmitted from mother to infant during childbirth or from child to child through close living conditions, and can also be sexually transmitted or by contact with infected blood. Hence, HBV and HIV are transmitted in similar ways; however, HBV is up to 100 times more infectious [www.cdc.gov/ncidod/diseases/hepatitis/b/aqb.htm]. Without appropriate treatment, 25% of those chronically infected with HBV will die of liver diseases such as cirrhosis and liver cancer.

Exposure to these viruses varies based on geography and human behavior. HCC has the highest incidence rates in countries where hepatitis B is endemic, which include sub-Saharan Africa, Amazon River, most of Eastern Asia and a number of Pacific Islands, parts of the Middle East, and some countries in eastern Europe and Central Asia. China, which in some provinces has some of the highest incidence rates of chronic hepatitis B, accounts for over 50% of all liver cancer deaths in the world (Parkin et al. 2001). Western Europe, Australia, New Zealand, and North America are low-endemicity areas.

In the United States, approximately two million people are thought to be chronically infected with HBV, up from 1.25 million used in previous estimates (Cohen et al. 2007, Lin et al. 2007). Those born in endemic counties who have immigrated to the United States carry with them a 10–15% risk of being infected with hepatitis B. The risks of HCC vary with duration of disease and mode of infection. In patients who obtained the virus in endemic areas (e.g., Asia and Africa) during infancy or early childhood, the risk of HCC in carriers of HBV is 100 times greater than in the general population and can occur independent of developing cirrhosis (Lin et al. 2007). In contrast, patients who acquire hepatitis B as an adult, which is the primary method of transmission in the Western world, develop HCC only if they have cirrhosis (Chen 2005, Chang 2007).

Fortunately, in the 1980s, a vaccine was developed for the primary prevention of HBV infections and by extension, HCC for those not previously infected with HBV. The World Health Organization considers the HBV vaccine as the first vaccine against a sexually transmissible disease and the American Cancer Society considers the HBV vaccine as the first effective "anti-cancer" vaccine (Chen 2005). In many countries, universal administration of the first dose of the HBV vaccine at birth and following it with two subsequent dosages represents one of the most effective, long-term public health strategies to reduce the incidence and prevalence of this infection.

Universal infant vaccination was first started in the United States in the 1990s. In the long run, vaccination may spare subsequent generations from HBV but will not alter the course of HBV infections or HCC onset in previously infected adults. Other primary prevention strategies include health education to avoid unsafe sexual behavior and the promotion of abstinence. Secondary prevention in the form of screening of individuals who are at high risk of infection is encouraged and would be the basis of initiating prompt treatment if appropriate or vaccination if not infected.

About 3% of the world's population (or more than 170 million) is infected with HCV. HCV is often acquired through intravenous injections and other blood-borne means (Kuper, Adami, Trichopoulos 2000). While cirrhosis and HCC may be outcomes of HCV infection, unfortunately, no vaccine currently exists to prevent this disease. HCV-infected individuals should be advised to avoid donating blood or sharing toothbrushes or razors, and to cover any cuts. Screening for HCV should be considered for high-risk individuals as symptoms for HCV may be absent or variable.

Disparities

Racial/ethnic differences in the occurrence of HCC are amenable to change by applying appropriate prevention and control measures, see Figure 10.2. Disproportionate representation of people of color who are infected with HBV and related risk factors lead to higher numbers in these populations that experience liver cancer. However, a different pattern of HCC attributed to hepatitis C viral infections occurs, as noted below.

HBV-induced HCC. HBV infections account for about 80% of HCC cases worldwide. In the United States, HBV-induced liver cancer is most common among APIs and people of color and is least common among non-Hispanic whites

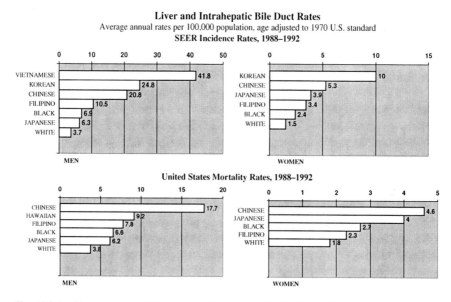

Fig. 10.2 Incidence and mortality rates of liver cancer in the United States

(Miller et al. 1996), although whites and Hispanics are experiencing the largest increase in HCC incidence. This disparity in liver cancer incidence and mortality is the most significant cancer health disparity affecting Asian Americans (Chen 2005) and certainly ranks in the "ten largest racial and ethnic health disparities" (Chang 2007, Keppel 2007a, b)

Specifically, the prevalence of chronic HBV infection is approximately 10% among APIs compared to less than 0.5% in the US population at-large and less than 0.2% among non-Hispanic whites. Due to the high prevalence of chronic hepatitis B infection, APIs living in the United States bear the largest burden of HCC, often unknowingly. APIs living in the United States have the highest age-adjusted incidence rate of HCC (7.0 per 100,000), compared to whites (1.5/ 100,000) and blacks (3.2/100,000) (Davila et al. 2003). In fact, the US SEER data indicate that HCC is the fourth most common cancer among Chinese and Korean males, second most common in Vietnamese males, and fifth most common among Filipino males (Miller et al. 2007). HCC is the second leading cause of cancer mortality among Chinese males and fourth leading cause of cancer mortality among Filipino males (Parker et al. 1998). In a recent review of HCC in API living in San Francisco (an area with the highest concentration of API in the continental United States), liver cancer was a leading cause of cancer incidence and death in API men, ranking among the five most common cancer sites for most Asian subgroups. The risk was highest in men, especially those of Chinese ancestry, followed by Vietnamese, Filipino, Korean, and Japanese (Miller et al. 2007). Moreover, Hawaii, the state with the highest concentration of API, has the highest age-adjusted incidence of liver cancer in the country, primarily due to high rates of chronic hepatitis B from its immigrant population. In particular, the prominence of liver cancer as a frequent cause of cancer deaths among APIs exemplifies the unusual cancer burden vis-à-vis whites. Americans born in Africa, who acquired hepatitis B as an infant during childbirth have a relatively high risk of developing liver cancer as well, with some developing cancer under the age of 30 (Kew and Macerollo 1988).

In contrast to other liver diseases, the development of HCC in patients with HBV can occur independently of the development of cirrhosis. In fact, 30–50% of HCC associated with HBV occurs in the absence of cirrhosis (Parkin et al. 2001) and has been reported even in those who have cleared hepatitis B surface antigen (Lin et al. 2007). In patients who develop cirrhosis due to HBV, the risk of developing HCC is estimated at 2.5% per year (Velazquez et al. 2003). In patients who obtained HBV during infancy and childhood, the development of HCC is strongly related to the characteristics of the virus and the host immune response. Patients who are hepatitis B e antigen positive have a risk of developing HCC six times higher than those who are surface antigen positive alone (Yang et al. 2002). In one of the largest prospective studies to date examining the risk of HCC in patients with chronic hepatitis B in Taiwan, patients with a high viral load (more than one million copies per milliliter) had the highest risk of developing HCC. Other risk factors included age, the development of cirrhosis, alcohol consumption, smoking, and a high ALT (alanine transaminase). However, even after adjusting for these factors, the risk of developing HCC decreased with lesser viral loads, suggesting a dose-response relationship.

HCV-induced HCC. Approximately 170 million people worldwide are infected with hepatitis C (Wasley and Alter 2000). The virus is transmitted primarily from infected blood transfusions and from the use of infected unsterile needles from intravenous drug abuse or medical procedures. Similar to hepatitis B, these rates vary geographically, primarily due to historical differences in the risk and mode of infection. In the United States, Australia, Canada, and most of Europe, hepatitis C was mainly transmitted by intravenous drug use among young adults during the mid-1980s to mid-1990s and is therefore found mostly in those aged 50–60 years old today. In Japan and southern Europe, hepatitis C was acquired mainly through non-sterilized devices (primarily needles) during medical care and folk medicine, and therefore is found primarily in today's elderly population. In developing countries, in contrast, hepatitis C is found among all age groups because of their risk for infection from unsterile medical devices, needles, and blood transfusions (Wasley and Alter 2000).

In the United States, men have higher rates of infection than women, and African Americans (Pyrsopoulos and Jeffers 2007) and Mexican Americans have higher rates of infection than their white counterparts (Rustgi 2007). Other populations at unusually high risk for infection include prisoners (with a reported infection rate of 15 to 25%), the homeless, Vietnam War veterans, health care workers, people with end-stage renal disease on hemodialysis, hemophiliacs, and those who received blood transfusions prior to 1991 (Rustgi 2007). Approximately 85% of those infected with hepatitis C eventually develop chronic hepatitis C, and of those 20% will develop cirrhosis (Strader et al. 2004). Despite a reduced number of new infections in the United States, the morbidity, mortality, and cost to the US health care system attributable to HCV infection is expected to continue to rise at least until 2019 (Wong et al. 2000, Kim 2002). These costs not only stem from the complications of cirrhosis (currently the most common indication for liver transplantation), but the development of liver cancer as well. It is estimated that 3–4 % of those with cirrhosis will develop liver cancer. In the United States, HCV-induced cirrhosis is the reason for the doubling prevalence of liver cancer in the United States from 1990 to 1998 and the increased occurrence in younger patients (El-Serag and Mason 1999).

Once patients infected with HCV develop cirrhosis, there are no obvious disparities among those who develop liver cancer; however, there are significant health care disparities among those who are at risk for infection with this virus, their access to care, and their risk of developing cirrhosis. At greatest risk are patients who are homeless, prisoners or current or past intravenous drug users, i.e., patients who are less likely to have access to health care than the general population. These at-risk patient populations are often identified late in their disease and are less likely to receive therapy with interferon and ribavirin, which is successful in eradicating the virus in about 50% of patients (Nyamathi et al. 2002, Reindollar 1999).

Another factor that may contribute to disparities among those who suffer from the complications of hepatitis C and cirrhosis are significant racial differences in response to therapy. African Americans are often infected with the more resistant hepatitis C genotype and respond less to treatment compared to their white counterparts (Muir et al. 2004, Reddy et al. 1999). Patients who are male over the age of 40, alcohol users, or co-infected with HIV and/or hepatitis B also have a high risk of developing cirrhosis and of not responding to therapy (Strader et al. 2004, Poynard et al. 2001).

Alcohol use. In the United States there are approximately 140 million people who suffer from alcohol dependency and they make up 40% of all cases of cirrhosis and 30% of all liver cancer patients (Kim et al. 2002). Alcohol use has a synergistic effect with viral hepatitis: heavy alcohol users have a higher risk of developing complications related to hepatitis B and C, including higher rates of cirrhosis and liver cancer. Independently, the risk of developing HCC from alcohol occurs only after the development of cirrhosis. Therefore most disparities that exist among heavy alcohol users are due to their higher risk of developing cirrhosis. Once alcoholic cirrhosis develops, the risk of hospitalization from HCC is approximately 8–9 of 100,000 (El-Serag and Mason 2000).

Alcohol use as a risk factor also underlies some of the racial and ethnic disparities in HCC. Although the rate of alcohol dependency appears to be highest in whites, African Americans and Latinos are at higher risk of dying or being hospitalized for excessive drinking (To 2007). In addition, many of these ethnic minorities, particularly those from a lower socioeconomic class, have less access to recovery programs and specialty care (Schmidt et al. 2007). Those of American Indian, Hispanic, or African descent, or with a relatively low SES or residence in urban areas have higher rates of alcoholic cirrhosis than other groups in the general population (Singh and Hoyert 2000). The highest mortality from alcoholic cirrhosis in the United States occurs in white Hispanic and African American men (Russo et al. 2004).

Diabetes, obesity, and non-alcoholic fatty liver disease. The roles of diabetes, obesity, and non-alcoholic fatty liver disease in HCC are being investigated intensively. Though all of these risk factors have been linked to the development of liver cancer, they often occur together in the same patient, and the precise relative roles of each factor are unclear (McGlynn and London 2005). Obesity, especially, appears to be an important risk factor. In a recent study of 800,000 people, men and women with a body mass index (BMI) >35 kg/m^2 had, respectively, a 4.52 and 1.68 higher relative risk of dying from liver cancer than those with a BMI of 18–24.9 kg/m^2 (Calle et al. 2003). This increase in relative risk among obese men was the highest compared to all other cancers studied. The explanation for this increase is unknown but may be due to the increase in non-alcoholic fatty liver disease and non-alcoholic steatohepatitis, which eventually leads to cirrhosis and liver cancer among these individuals. This is based on the observation that over 90% of obese patients and over 70% of all diabetics have fatty liver disease. About 25–30% of these fatty liver disease patients also have inflammation on liver biopsy that is consistent with non-alcoholic steatohepatitis, and 10% will have cirrhosis (Neuschwander-Tetri and Caldwell 2003). Most cases where the cause of cirrhosis is originally believed to be cryptogenic are later attributed to non-alcoholic steatohepatitis (Ayata et al. 2002). The association of cryptogenic cirrhosis and HCC has been reported as high as 29% of all HCC at one center (Marrero et al. 2002), although most data suggest it represents approximately 5% of all cases of HCC.

The groups that are at high risk of developing obesity, diabetes, and non-alcoholic fatty liver disease as risk factors for HCC are also those that typically have a poor diet and lack of exercise (Mokdad et al. 1999, Must et al. 1999). While this problem has affected most of the population, these health problems have particularly affected those of low SES and, in particular, some ethnic minorities. For example, in the United States, 38% of African Americans, 37% of Native Americans, and 27% of Hispanic Americans are obese, compared to only 21% of Caucasians (Liao et al. 2004). Those of lower SES have a higher rate of obesity compared to those of high SES, especially among women (Drewnowski and Specter 2004). Furthermore, African Americans suffer from the greatest amount of health-related conditions related to obesity compared to all other races (National Center for Health Statistics 2002).

Status of HCC Prevention, Detection, and Treatment

Preventing hepatitis B offers the potential for markedly reducing transmission and HCC for the next generation (Ni et al. 2007). In support of the American Cancer Society's declaration that the hepatitis B vaccine was the world's first successful "anti-cancer" vaccine, studies suggest that this approach could be prophylactically effective (Ni et al. 2007, Chen et al. 1987, 2004, Chang et al. 1997, 2005, Poland and Jacobson 2004) and cost-effective (Margolis et al. 1995, Zhou et al. 2003) in reducing infections, prevalence of HBV, and incidence of HCC. Pioneering epidemiological studies by Beasley (Beasley et al. 1982, Beasley 1988) first documented the etiologic relationships between HBV infections and HCC. Then, the world's first nationwide HBV vaccination program in Taiwan began, first in 1984 for infants born to mothers carrying hepatitis B surface antigen and later in 1986 to all infants (Chen et al. 1987, Chang et al. 1997). Two decades after nationwide implementation of universal birth-dose HBV vaccination, Taiwan has seen dramatic reductions in seropositive rates for hepatitis B surface antigens and other markers of HBV infections and increases in immunity against HBV. These indicators of reduced HBV infections have been consistent with the longitudinal tracking of the same birth cohorts in surveys previously conducted in 1984, 1989, 1994, and 1999 (Ni et al. 2007).

No such study has been conducted in the United States; however, the incidence of HBV transmission has declined due to the adoption of the Centers for Disease Control and Prevention (CDC)-recommended comprehensive strategy (MMWR 1991, 2002, 2004). Nevertheless, HBV continues to be an important cause of morbidity in the United States, particularly among foreign-born residents (Kim 2004) partly due to horizontal (or from mother to fetus) transmission (Franks et al. 1989).

Data from Hawaii, the state with the largest proportion of at-risk APIs, inidicate the effectiveness of the first three of CDC's recommended strategies among elementary school-aged children (Dilraj et al. 2003, Perz et al. 2006), namely, (1) universal vaccination of infants beginning at birth; (2) prevention of perinatal HBV infection through routine screening of all pregnant women for HBV infection and provision of immunoprophylaxis to infants born to infected women or to women of unknown infection status; and (3) routine vaccination of previously unvaccinated children and adolescents. The adoption of these three strategies has been facilitated by professional endorsement from various organizations such as the Advisory Committee on Immunization Practice, the passage of various state laws requiring evidence of HBV vaccination as prerequisites for school entry, and the provision of free or low-cost HBV vaccinations through the federally subsidized Vaccines for Children's program. However, increasing HBV vaccination rates have not yet measurably decreased liver cancer rates among APIs, since liver cancer occurs primarily in adults who were infected with HBV prior to the development of an effective vaccination program (Chen 2005). Also, preventing HBV infection does not guarantee prevention of HCC because of its links to HCV as well as non-viral risk factors (e.g., alcohol abuse, diabetes, and obesity).

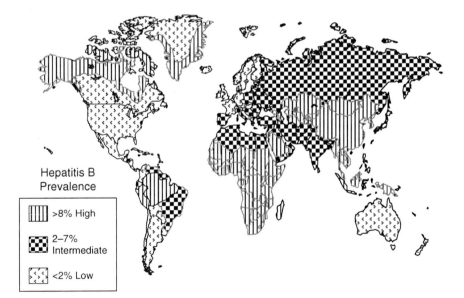

Fig. 10.3 Hepatitis B prevalence

Prevention of hepatitis C. There are no effective vaccinations for hepatitis C. Instead, the reduction in hepatitis C in the United States has come from an intense public health effort, including testing all blood products for the virus, viral inactivation of plasma-derived products, risk-reduction education for persons at risk, and routine practice of universal precautions in health care settings. These efforts represent a triumph for public health, which has seen the rates of new HCV infection since 1992 drop by 92% among those aged 25–39 years, the highest-risk age group. However, injection drug users remain at high risk, representing approximately 50% of all new infections (Wasley et al. 2007). Thus, continued efforts are needed to reduce the rate of infection among this group and provide access to health care for already infected populations. Current efforts are underway to provide education and health care to current and past injection drug users, prisoners, and the homeless (Des Jarlais et al. 2005, Birkhead et al. 2007, Klein et al. 2007, Roy et al. 2007).

Screening for viral hepatitis and alcohol abuse as a means to prevent liver cancer. Most patients who have been infected with viral hepatitis B and C have no symptoms, and often do not manifest them until over 30 years of chronic infection. Thus, there is a large population of patients at risk of developing liver cancer completely unaware of their situation. This is especially true among patients with chronic hepatitis B who have emigrated from areas of the world where hepatitis B is endemic. Among APIs born outside of the United States, approximately 10% are chronically infected with hepatitis B with up to two-thirds of them unaware of their infection (Lin et al. 2007). Current guidelines recommend that all patients born in countries where hepatitis B is endemic be screened for hepatitis B. In addition, anyone who may have been exposed to someone infected with hepatitis B, either through close household contacts or unprotected sex, should also be tested as well as those who have undergone renal dialysis and all pregnant patients (Lok and McMahon 2007).

Screening for HBV, particularly for Asian and Pacific Islander adults, and treating infected individuals and vaccinating close contacts, is likely to be highly cost-effective, resulting in about $36,000 to $40,000 per quality-adjusted life year (Hutton et al. 2007). Patients at risk for hepatitis C should also be screened in accordance with the guidelines set forth by the American Association of the Study of Liver Disease, which includes those who have ever used intravenous drugs or received a blood transfusion or organ donation prior to 1992, as well as children born to mothers who are HCV positive and patients on renal dialysis and/or who are HIV positive. Any health care worker who may have been exposed to a needle from or mucosal exposure of a hepatitis C-infected person, as well as current sexual partners of patients with hepatitis C should also be tested. Finally, anyone with a history of unexplained elevation in liver function tests should be evaluated for both hepatitis B and C (Strader et al. 2004).

Prevention by lifestyle modification. Once these patients who are at risk for liver cancer are identified, lifestyle modification may assist with reducing risk. This approach includes promoting the discontinuation of alcohol and tobacco, both of which act synergistically with viral hepatitis to increase risk of both cirrhosis and liver cancer (Yu and Yuan 2004). In addition, improved choices in diet and increased exercise reduce patients' risk of developing diabetes, obesity, and fatty liver disease (Cave et al. 2007). To reduce the spread of viral hepatitis and prevent others from being at risk for HCC, moreover, injection drug users should have access to treatment facilities and be taught the importance of not sharing needles or other devices exposed to blood. Prevention also involves abstinence for anyone chronically infected with hepatitis B.

Treatment of viral hepatitis. Theoretically, treating hepatitis B and C could be an avenue to prevent HCC, but this area is controversial. While therapies for both hepatitis B and C appear to reduce the risk of developing cirrhosis, only very limited data show a reduction in rates of liver cancer per se. In Asian patients with hepatitis B and cirrhosis, for example, there has been one randomized clinical trial to evaluate whether treatment reduces decompensation of liver disease along with liver cancer. In this trial of 651 patients with hepatitis B cirrhosis randomized to lamivudine or placebo, after a median duration of 3 years, 17 patients in the placebo group and 16 in the lamivudine group developed liver cancer, representing a hazard ratio of 0.49 with a *p*-value of 0.047 (Liaw et al. 2004). Similarly with hepatitis C, the data are primarily from retrospective data or secondary analysis. These favor treatment with pegylated interferon and ribavirin to prevent the development of liver cancer (Wright 2007).

On the other hand, in addition to the lack of data demonstrating prevention of liver cancer through treatment of viral hepatitis, therapies for both hepatitis B and C are expensive and, for hepatitis B, the duration of therapy can be lifelong. Many patients lack the means of obtaining these treatments and, for patients with hepatitis B, rates of resistance are high after prolonged treatment. Therapies for hepatitis C, moreover, often result in severe side effects, and patients with any psychiatric or substance abuse issues are usually poor candidates for therapy (Mehta et al. 2005).

Screening for HCC. Some have advocated for screening for HCC using abdominal ultrasound and a serum AFP every 6 months to identify patients at an early stage. This method is imperfect, however. For one thing, the ultrasound has limitations in accuracy, with sensitivity ranges between only 65–80% while specificity is approximately 90% and its accuracy is highly variable based on the operator (Bolondi et al. 2001). Serum AFP is also imperfect, with a sensitivity of only 60% and specificity of 76–94% when set at a cutoff of 20 ng/ml (Daniele et al. 2004). Combined, however, these two approaches have a better sensitivity and specificity than either alone (Tremolda et al. 1989). Consequently, the American Association for the Study of Liver Disease (AASLD) has advocated screening for HCC all patients with cirrhosis and chronic carriers of hepatitis B starting at age 40 in men and at age 50 in women, or earlier if they were born on the continent of Africa, or have a family history of liver cancer (Bruix and Sherman 2005). However the National Cancer Institute currently does not recommend screening, although the AASLD's recommended screening practice has been quickly adopted by many hepatologists (Leykum et al. 2007).

Of note, there has been only one randomized clinical trial that showed improved mortality with screening for HCC using serum AFP and abdominal ultrasound. This trial was specifically done in patients with chronic hepatitis B (Zhang et al. 2004). For patients with cirrhosis due to hepatitis C, alcohol, and non-alcoholic fatty liver disease (NAFLD), furthermore, the data are based on retrospective studies, which suffer from both lead and length-time biases (Bruix and Sherman 2005). In terms of cost-effectiveness, moreover, most data do not support this practice in patients with hepatitis C, alcohol, or NAFLD, due to the low prevalence of HCC among this patient population and frequent inability of therapy to improve overall mortality (Di Bisceglie 2004). In contrast, most cost-effectiveness models do support screening for HCC among chronic carriers of hepatitis B, who are often times excellent candidates for therapy if HCC is discovered at an early stage (Liaw et al. 2004).

Treatment of HCC. The only proven treatment for HCC is liver transplantation and resection. To qualify for these therapies the tumor must be identified at an early stage, and patients must be good candidates for surgery, based not only on their clinical condition but also on the stability of their social system and their financial means. These constraints keep many patients from receiving these potentially life-saving therapies. Many minorities also appear to be under-represented among those receiving these treatments (Reid et al. 2004), and more research and interventions are needed in order to improve their access to care.

Future Directions with Respect to Interventions

Reducing and eventually eliminating HCC-related disparities requires pursuing HCC prevention, control, and early detection. In the long run, prevention—as exemplified by universal hepatitis B vaccinations of uninfected individuals, beginning with the birth dose and extending through vaccination of young adults—should be pursued. These efforts have already been demonstrated effective in dramatically reducing viral loads and infection rates. For those residing in endemic areas, specifically in Eastern Asia, Africa, and a number of Pacific Islands or who have migrated from endemic areas, individuals should be screened for hepatitis B prior to vaccination. Hence, research into earlier detection strategies is essential.

Increased outreach among those at greatest risk, particularly those from endemic areas and those who are outside mainstream populations such as English-limited groups, is needed as well. In 2006 the National Cancer Institute and the National Center on Minority Health and Health Disparities funded a community-based program project "Liver Cancer Control Interventions for Asian Americans" that should yield both theoretical and pragmatic findings and insights on how to better reach these populations (Chen et al. 2007). Preliminary studies to address disparities in HBV-induced liver cancer among Asian Americans include assessments of the prevalence of HBV knowledge, vaccination rates, and screening rates among specific Asian groups (Bastani et al. 2007, Butler et al. 2005, Coronado et al. 2007, Nguyen et al. 2007). All of these studies point toward the need for greater tailoring of interventions. Through the culturally sensitive education, investigators hope to improve screening for hepatitis B and thereby reduce the prevalence of liver cancer among APIs living in the United States. Equally vital are policy interventions to assure that all those who test positive to the hepatitis B surface antigen receive appropriate medical care regardless of their means. This approach must also be used to assist populations who are vulnerable to infection with hepatitis C.

More effective and less-expensive therapies for both hepatitis B and C need to be developed as well. Once identified, patients must be counseled about maintaining a healthy lifestyle and about controlling or curtailing use of alcohol, tobacco, and high-fat foods. Those who have developed cirrhosis, are hepatitis B carriers with a family history, and who reach the critical ages (40 in men, 50 in women) should also be screened for liver cancer through abdominal ultrasound and an AFP test every 6 months. At the same time, we must pursue breakthroughs in treatment and interventions to bring these treatments to all patient populations, especially those who are disproportionately affected by liver cancer.

Ultimately, of course, the best hope of eliminating HCC will be through an effective and intensive vaccination effort for those without the disease and encouraging positive lifestyle health habits such as exercise and healthful eating. In the meantime, aggressive case finding and earlier detection with improved treatment is the blueprint for eliminating HCC-induced disparities.

References

Ayata G, Gordon FD, Lewis WD, Pomfret E, Pomposelli JJ, Jenkins RL, Khettry U. Cryptogenic cirrhosis: clinicopathologic findings at and after liver transplantation. Hum Pathol 2002;33:1098–104.

Bastani R, Maxwell AM, Jo AM. Hepatitis B testing for liver cancer control among Korean Americans. Ethnicity and Disease 2007;17:359–67.

Beasley RP, Lin CC, Chien CS, Chen CJ, Hwang LY. Geographic distribution of HBsAg carriers in China. Hepatology 1982;2:553–6.

Beasley RP. Hepatitis B virus. The major etiology of hepatocellular carcinoma. Cancer 1988;61:1942–56.

Birkhead GS, Klein SJ, Candelas AR, O'Connell DA, Rothman JR, Feldman IS, Tsui DS, Cotroneo RA, Flanigan CA. Integrating multiple programme and policy approaches to hepatitis C prevention and care for injection drug users: a comprehensive approach. Int J Drug Policy 2007;18:417–25.

Bolondi L, Sofia S, Siringo S, Gaiani S, Casali A, Zironi G, Piscaglia F, Gramantieri L, Zanetti M, Sherman M. Surveillance programme of cirrhotic patients for early diagnosis and treatment of hepatocellular carcinoma: a cost effectiveness analysis. Gut 2001;48: 251–9.

Bruix J, Sherman M. Management of hepatocellular carcinoma. Hepatology 2005;42: 1208–36.

Butler LM, Mills PK, Yang RC, Chen MS, Jr. Hepatitis B knowledge and vaccination levels in California Hmong youth: implications for liver cancer prevention strategies. Asian Pac J Cancer Prev 2005;6:401–3.

Byrd KM, Wilson DC, Hoyler SS, Peck GL. Advanced presentation of melanoma in African Americans. J Am Acad Dermatol 2004;50:21–4; discussion 142–3.

Calle EE, Rodriguez C, Walker-Thurmond K, Thun MJ. Overweight, obesity, and mortality from cancer in a prospectively studied cohort of U.S. adults. N Engl J Med 2003;348: 1625–38.

Cave M, Deaciuc I, Mendez C, Song Z, Joshi-Barve S, Barve S, McClain C. Nonalcoholic fatty liver disease: predisposing factors and the role of nutrition. J Nutr Biochem 2007;18:184–95.

Chang MH, Chen CJ, Lai MS, Hsu HM, Wu TC, Kong MS, Liang DC, Shau WY, Chen DS. Universal hepatitis B vaccination in Taiwan and the incidence of hepatocellular carcinoma in children. Taiwan Childhood Hepatoma Study Group. N Engl J Med 1997;336:1855–9.

Chang MH, Chen TH, Hsu HM, Wu TC, Kong MS, Liang DC, Ni YH, Chen CJ, Chen DS. Prevention of hepatocellular carcinoma by universal vaccination against hepatitis B virus: the effect and problems. Clin Cancer Res 2005;11:7953–7.

Chang SS. Ten largest racial and ethnic health disparities in the United States based on Healthy People 2010 objectives (Letter) 2007:1106–1107.

Chen DS, Hsu NH, Sung JL, Hsu TC, Hsu ST, Kuo YT, Lo KJ, Shih YT. A mass vaccination program in Taiwan against hepatitis B virus infection in infants of hepatitis B surface antigen-carrier mothers. JAMA 1987;257:2597–603.

Chen HL, Chang CJ, Kong MS, Huang FC, Lee HC, Lin CC, Liu CC, Lee IH, Wu TC, Wu SF, Ni YH, Hsu HY, Chen DS, Chang MH. Pediatric fulminant hepatic failure in endemic areas of hepatitis B infection: 15 years after universal hepatitis B vaccination. Hepatology 2004;39:58–63.

Chen MS Jr. NT, Bastani R, Stewart S, Maxwell AM, Ly M. Liver cancer control interventions for Asian Americans. Proceedings of the Science of Cancer Health Disparities 2007:120–121.

Chen MS, Jr. Cancer health disparities among Asian Americans: what we do and what we need to do. Cancer 2005;104:2895–902.

Cockburn MG, Zadnick J, Deapen D. Developing epidemic of melanoma in the Hispanic population of California. Cancer 2006;106:1162–8.

Cohen C EA, London WT, Block J, Conti M, Block T. Underestimation of chronic hepatitis B virus infection in the United States of American. Journal of Viral Hepatitis 2007: 1365–2893.

Cohn-Cedermark G, Mansson-Brahme E, Rutqvist LE, Larsson O, Johansson H, Ringborg U. Trends in mortality from malignant melanoma in Sweden, 1970–1996. Cancer 2000;89:348–55.

Coronado GD, Taylor VM, Tu SP, Yasui Y, Acorda E, Woodall E, Yip MP, Li L, Hislop TG. Correlates of hepatitis B testing among Chinese Americans. J Community Health 2007; 32:379–90.

Cress RD, Holly EA. Incidence of cutaneous melanoma among non-Hispanic whites, Hispanics, Asians, and blacks: an analysis of California Cancer registry data, 1988–93. Cancer Causes Control 1997;8:246–52.

Crocetti E, Capocaccia R, Casella C, Guzzinati S, Ferretti S, Rosso S, Sacchettini C, Spitale A, Stracci F, Tumino R. Population-based incidence and mortality cancer trends (1986–1997) from the network of Italian cancer registries. Eur J Cancer Prev 2004;13:287–95.

Daniele B, Bencivenga A, Megna AS, Tinessa V. Alpha-fetoprotein and ultrasonography screening for hepatocellular carcinoma. Gastroenterology 2004;127:S108–12.

Davila JA, Petersena NJ, Nelson HA, El-Serag HB. Geographic variation within the United States in the incidence of hepatocellular carcinoma. J Clin Epidemiol 2003;56:487–93.

de Vries E, Bray FI, Coebergh JW, Parkin DM. Changing epidemiology of malignant cutaneous melanoma in Europe 1953–1997: rising trends in incidence and mortality but recent stabilizations in western Europe and decreases in Scandinavia. Int J Cancer 2003;107:119–26.

Demierre MF, Chung C, Miller DR, Geller AC. Early detection of thick melanomas in the United States: beware of the nodular subtype. Arch Dermatol 2005;141:745–50.

Des Jarlais DC, Perlis T, Arasteh K, Torian LV, Hagan H, Beatrice S, Smith L, Wethers J, Milliken J, Mildvan D, Yancovitz S, Friedman SR. Reductions in hepatitis C virus and HIV infections among injecting drug users in New York City, 1990–2001. Aids 2005;19 Suppl 3:S20–5.

Di Bisceglie AM. Issues in screening and surveillance for hepatocellular carcinoma. Gastroenterology 2004;127:S104–7.

Di Quinzio ML, Dewar RA, Burge FI, Veugelers PJ. Family physician visits and early recognition of melanoma. Can J Public Health 2005;96:136–9.

Diepgen TL, Mahler V. The epidemiology of skin cancer. Br J Dermatol 2002;146 Suppl 61:1–6.

Dilraj A, Strait-Jones J, Nagao M, Cui K, Terrell-Perica S, Effler PV. A statewide hepatitis B vaccination program for school children in Hawaii: vaccination series completion and participation rates over consecutive school years. Public Health Rep 2003;118:127–33.

Drewnowski A, Specter SE. Poverty and obesity: the role of energy density and energy costs. Am J Clin Nutr 2004;79:6–16.

Eide MJ, Weinstock MA. Association of UV index, latitude, and melanoma incidence in nonwhite populations – US Surveillance, Epidemiology, and End Results (SEER) Program, 1992 to 2001. Arch Dermatol 2005;141:477–81.

El-Serag HB, Mason AC. Rising incidence of hepatocellular carcinoma in the United States. N Engl J Med 1999;340:745–50.

El-Serag HB, Mason AC. Risk factors for the rising rates of primary liver cancer in the United States. Arch Intern Med 2000;160:3227–30.

El-Serag HB. Epidemiology of hepatocellular carcinoma in USA. Hepatol Res 2007;37 Suppl 2:S88–94.

El-Serag HB. Hepatocellular carcinoma: an epidemiologic view. J Clin Gastroenterol 2002; 35:S72–8.

Ferlay J BF, Pisani P and D.M. Parkin. GLOBOCAN 2002. Cancer Incidence, Mortality and Prevalence Worldwide. IARC Press, 2004.

Franks AL, Berg CJ, Kane MA, Browne BB, Sikes RK, Elsea WR, Burton AH. Hepatitis B virus infection among children born in the United States to Southeast Asian refugees. N Engl J Med 1989;321:1301–5.

Freeman HP. Patient navigation: a community centered approach to reducing cancer mortality. J Cancer Educ 2006;21:S11–4.

Geller AC, Swetter SM, Elwood M, Brooks DR, Youl P, Demierrre MF, Aitken J. Risk factors and presentation of thin and thick nodular melanoma in Queensland Australia. Cancer 2009 (in press).

Geller AC, Koh HK, Miller DR, Clapp RW, Mercer MB, Lew RA. Use of health services before the diagnosis of melanoma: implications for early detection and screening. J Gen Intern Med 1992;7:154–7.

Geller AC, Miller DR, Annas GD, Demierre MF, Gilchrest BA, Koh HK. Melanoma incidence and mortality among US whites, 1969–1999. JAMA 2002;288:1719–20.

Geller AC, Miller DR, Lew RA, Clapp RW, Wenneker MB, Koh HK. Cutaneous melanoma mortality among the socioeconomically disadvantaged in Massachusetts. Am J Public Health 1996;86:538–43.

Geller AC, Miller DR, Swetter SM, Demierre MF, Gilchrest BA. A call for the development and implementation of a targeted national melanoma screening program. Arch Dermatol 2006;142:504–7.

Geller AC, Swetter SM, Brooks K, Demierre MF, Yaroch AL. Screening, early detection, and trends for melanoma: current status (2000–2006) and future directions. J Am Acad Dermatol 2007;57:555–72; quiz 573–6.

Gerbert B, Bronstone A, Maurer T, Berger T, McPhee SJ, Caspers N. The effectiveness of an Internet-based tutorial in improving primary care physicians' skin cancer triage skills. J Cancer Educ 2002;17:7–11.

Girgis A, Campbell EM, Redman S, Sanson-Fisher RW. Screening for melanoma: a community survey of prevalence and predictors. Med J Aust 1991;154:338–43.

Harris JM, Salasche SJ, Harris RB. Can Internet-based continuing medical education improve physicians' skin cancer knowledge and skills? J Gen Intern Med 2001; 16:50–6.

Hemmings DE, Johnson DS, Tominaga GT, Wong JH. Cutaneous melanoma in a multiethnic population: is this a different disease? Arch Surg 2004;139:968–72; discussion 972–3.

Hepatitis B vaccination – United States, 1982–2002. MMWR 2002;51:549–52, 563.

Hu S, Ma F, Collado-Mesa F, Kirsner RS. UV radiation, latitude, and melanoma in US Hispanics and blacks. Arch Dermatol 2004;140:819–24.

Hu S, Soza-Vento RM, Parker DF, Kirsner RS. Comparison of stage at diagnosis of melanoma among Hispanic, black, and white patients in Miami-Dade County, Florida. Arch Dermatol 2006;142:704–8.

Hutton DW, Tan D, So SK, Brandeau ML. Cost-effectiveness of screening and vaccinating Asian and Pacific Islander adults for hepatitis B. Ann Intern Med 2007;147:460–9.

Incidence of acute hepatitis B – United States, 1990–2002. MMWR 2004;52:1252–4.

Investigators TC. A new prognostic system for hepatocellular carcinoma: a retrospective study of 435 patients: the Cancer of the Liver Italian Program (CLIP) investigators. Hepatology 1998;28:751–5.

Jemal A, Siegel R, Ward E, Hao Y, Xu J, Murray T, Thun MJ. Cancer statistics, 2008. CA Cancer J Clin 2008;58:71–96.

Jemal A, Siegel R, Ward E, Murray T, Xu J, Thun MJ. Cancer statistics, 2007. CA Cancer J Clin 2007;57:43–66.

Keppel KG. (Author replies) Ten largest racial and ethnic health disparities in the United States based on Healthy People 2010 objectives. Am J Epidemiol 2007b:1106–1107.

Keppel KG. Ten largest racial and ethnic health disparities in the United States based on Healthy People 2010 Objectives. Am J Epidemiol 2007a;166:97–103.

Kew MC, Macerollo P. Effect of age on the etiologic role of the hepatitis B virus in hepatocellular carcinoma in blacks. Gastroenterology 1988;94:439–42.

Kim WR, Benson JT, Therneau TM, Torgerson HA, Yawn BP, Melton LJ, 3rd. Changing epidemiology of hepatitis B in a U.S. community. Hepatology 2004;39:811–6.

Kim WR, Brown RS, Jr., Terrault NA, El-Serag H. Burden of liver disease in the United States: summary of a workshop. Hepatology 2002;36:227–42.

Kim WR. The burden of hepatitis C in the United States. Hepatology 2002;36:S30–4.

Kirkpatrick CS, Lee JA, White E. Melanoma risk by age and socio-economic status. Int J Cancer 1990;46:1–4.

Kirsner RS, Wilkinson JD, Ma F, Pacheco H, Federman DG. The association of Medicare health care delivery systems with stage at diagnosis and survival for patients with melanoma. Arch Dermatol 2005;141:753–7.

Klein SJ, Wright LN, Birkhead GS, Mojica BA, Klopf LC, Klein LA, Tanner EL, Feldman IS, Fraley EJ. Promoting HCV treatment completion for prison inmates: New York State's hepatitis C continuity program. Public Health Rep 2007;122 Suppl 2:83–8.

Koh HK, Geller AC, Miller DR, Caruso A, Gage I, Lew RA. Who is being screened for melanoma/skin cancer? Characteristics of persons screened in Massachusetts. J Am Acad Dermatol 1991;24:271–7.

Koh HK. Cutaneous melanoma. N Engl J Med 1991;325:171–82.

Kuper H, Adami HO, Trichopoulous D. Infections as a major preventable cause of human cancer. J Int Med 2000;248:171–183.

Leykum LK, El-Serag HB, Cornell J, Papadopoulos KP. Screening for hepatocellular carcinoma among veterans with hepatitis C on disease stage, treatment received, and survival. Clin Gastroenterol Hepatol 2007;5:508–12.

Liao Y, Tucker P, Okoro CA, Giles WH, Mokdad AH, Harris VB. REACH 2010 Surveillance for Health Status in Minority Communities – United States, 2001–2002. MMWR Surveill Summ 2004;53:1–36.

Liaw YF, Sung JJ, Chow WC, Farrell G, Lee CZ, Yuen H, Tanwandee T, Tao QM, Shue K, Keene ON, Dixon JS, Gray DF, Sabbat J. Lamivudine for patients with chronic hepatitis B and advanced liver disease. N Engl J Med 2004;351:1521–31.

Lin SY, Chang ET, So SK. Why we should routinely screen Asian American adults for hepatitis B: A cross-sectional study of Asians in California. Hepatology 2007;46:1034–1040.

Llovet JM, Bru C, Bruix J. Prognosis of hepatocellular carcinoma: the BCLC staging classification. Semin Liver Dis 1999;19:329–38.

Lok AS, McMahon BJ. Chronic hepatitis B. Hepatology 2007;45:507–39.

Margolis HS, Coleman PJ, Brown RE, Mast EE, Sheingold SH, Arevalo JA. Prevention of hepatitis B virus transmission by immunization. An economic analysis of current recommendations. JAMA 1995;274:1201–8.

Institute of Medicine Extending Medicare Coverage for Preventive and Other Services. National Academy Press, 2000.

Marrero JA, Fontana RJ, Su GL, Conjeevaram HS, Emick DM, Lok AS. NAFLD may be a common underlying liver disease in patients with hepatocellular carcinoma in the United States. Hepatology 2002;36:1349–54.

McGlynn KA, London WT. Epidemiology and natural history of hepatocellular carcinoma. Best Pract Res Clin Gastroenterol 2005;19:3–23.

McGlynn KA, Tsao L, Hsing AW, Devesa SS, Fraumeni JF, Jr. International trends and patterns of primary liver cancer. Int J Cancer 2001;94:290–6.

Mehta SH, Thomas DL, Sulkowski MS, Safaein M, Vlahov D, Strathdee SA. A framework for understanding factors that affect access and utilization of treatment for hepatitis C virus infection among HCV-mono-infected and HIV/HCV-co-infected injection drug users. Aids 2005;19 Suppl 3:S179–89.

Miller BA KL, Bernstein et al., eds. Racial/ethnic patterns of cancer in the United States, 1988–1992. In: Institute NC, ed, 1996.

Miller BA, Chu KC, Hankey BF, Ries LA. Cancer incidence and mortality patterns among specific Asian and Pacific Islander populations in the U.S. Cancer Causes Control 2007.

Miller DR, Geller AC, Wyatt SW, Halpern A, Howell JB, Cockerell C, Reilley BA, Bewerse BA, Rigel D, Rosenthal L, Amonette R, Sun T, Grossbart T, Lew RA, Koh HK. Melanoma awareness and self-examination practices: results of a United States survey. J Am Acad Dermatol 1996;34:962–70.

Mokdad AH, Serdula MK, Dietz WH, Bowman BA, Marks JS, Koplan JP. The spread of the obesity epidemic in the United States, 1991–1998. JAMA 1999;282:1519–22.

Muir AJ, Bornstein JD, Killenberg PG. Peginterferon alfa-2b and ribavirin for the treatment of chronic hepatitis C in blacks and non-Hispanic whites. N Engl J Med 2004; 350:2265–71.

Must A, Spadano J, Coakley EH, Field AE, Colditz G, Dietz WH. The disease burden associated with overweight and obesity. JAMA 1999;282:1523–9.

National Cancer Institute Fact Book 2006, 2007.

National Center for Health Statistics. In: Health, ed: Government Printing Office, 2002.

Neuschwander-Tetri BA, Caldwell SH. Nonalcoholic steatohepatitis: summary of an AASLD Single Topic Conference. Hepatology 2003;37:1202–19.

Nguyen TT, Taylor V, Chen MS, Jr., Bastani R, Maxwell AE, McPhee SJ. Hepatitis B awareness, knowledge, and screening among asian americans. J Cancer Educ 2007;22:266–72.

Ni YH, Huang LM, Chang MH, Yen CJ, Lu CY, You SL, Kao JH, Lin YC, Chen HL, Hsu HY, Chen DS. Two decades of universal hepatitis B vaccination in taiwan: impact and implication for future strategies. Gastroenterology 2007;132:1287–93.

Nyamathi AM, Dixon EL, Robbins W, Smith C, Wiley D, Leake B, Longshore D, Gelberg L. Risk factors for hepatitis C virus infection among homeless adults. J Gen Intern Med 2002;17:134–43.

Parker SL, Davis KJ, Wingo PA, Ries LA, Heath CW, Jr. Cancer statistics by race and ethnicity. CA Cancer J Clin 1998;48:31–48.

Parkin DM, Bray F, Ferlay J, Pisani P. Estimating the world cancer burden: Globocan 2000. Int J Cancer 2001;94:153–6.

Parkin DM. Global cancer statistics in the year 2000. Lancet Oncol 2001;2:533–43.

Pennie ML, Soon SL, Risser JB, Veledar E, Culler SD, Chen SC. Melanoma outcomes for Medicare patients: association of stage and survival with detection by a dermatologist vs a nondermatologist. Arch Dermatol 2007;143:488–94.

Perz JF, Elm JL, Jr., Fiore AE, Huggler JI, Kuhnert WL, Effler PV. Near elimination of hepatitis B virus infections among Hawaii elementary school children after universal infant hepatitis B vaccination. Pediatrics 2006;118:1403–8.

Poland GA, Jacobson RM. Clinical practice: prevention of hepatitis B with the hepatitis B vaccine. N Engl J Med 2004;351:2832–8.

Poynard T, Ratziu V, Charlotte F, Goodman Z, McHutchison J, Albrecht J. Rates and risk factors of liver fibrosis progression in patients with chronic hepatitis c. J Hepatol 2001;34:730–9.

Pyrsopoulos N, Jeffers L. Hepatitis C in African Americans. J Clin Gastroenterol 2007; 41:185–93.

Reddy KR, Hoofnagle JH, Tong MJ, Lee WM, Pockros P, Heathcote EJ, Albert D, Joh T. Racial differences in responses to therapy with interferon in chronic hepatitis C. Consensus Interferon Study Group. Hepatology 1999;30:787–93.

Reid AE, Resnick M, Chang Y, Buerstatte N, Weissman JS. Disparity in use of orthotopic liver transplantation among blacks and whites. Liver Transpl 2004;10:834–41.

Reindollar RW. Hepatitis C and the correctional population. Am J Med 1999;107:100S–103S.

Resneck JS, Jr., Isenstein A, Kimball AB. Few Medicaid and uninsured patients are accessing dermatologists. J Am Acad Dermatol 2006;55:1084–8.

Reyes Ortiz CA, Freeman JL, Kuo YF, Goodwin JS. The influence of marital status on stage at diagnosis and survival of older persons with melanoma. J Gerontol A Biol Sci Med Sci 2007;62:892–8.

Reyes-Ortiz CA, Goodwin JS, Freeman JL, Kuo YF. Socioeconomic status and survival in older patients with melanoma. J Am Geriatr Soc 2006;54:1758–64.

Rhodes AR, Weinstock MA, Fitzpatrick TB, Mihm MC, Jr., Sober AJ. Risk factors for cutaneous melanoma. A practical method of recognizing predisposed individuals. JAMA 1987;258:3146–54.

Ries LAG EM, Kosary CL, et al. SEER Cancer Statistics Review, 1975–2002.

Roetzheim RG, Pal N, Tennant C, Voti L, Ayanian JZ, Schwabe A, Krischer JP. Effects of health insurance and race on early detection of cancer. J Natl Cancer Inst 1999;91: 1409–15.

Roetzheim RG, Pal N, van Durme DJ, Wathington D, Ferrante JM, Gonzalez EC, Krischer JP. Increasing supplies of dermatologists and family physicians are associated with earlier stage of melanoma detection. J Am Acad Dermatol 2000;43:211–8.

Roy E, Nonn E, Haley N, Cox J. Hepatitis C meanings and preventive strategies among street-involved young injection drug users in Montreal. Int J Drug Policy 2007;18:397–405.

Russo D, Purohit V, Foudin L, Salin M. Workshop on Alcohol Use and Health Disparities 2002: a call to arms. Alcohol 2004;32:37–43.

Rustgi VK. The epidemiology of hepatitis C infection in the United States. J Gastroenterol 2007;42:513–21.

Santmyire BR, Feldman SR, Fleischer AB, Jr. Lifestyle high-risk behaviors and demographics may predict the level of participation in sun-protection behaviors and skin cancer primary prevention in the United States: results of the 1998 National Health Interview Survey. Cancer 2001;92:1315–24.

Saraiya M, Hall HI, Thompson T, Hartman A, Glanz K, Rimer B, Rose D. Skin cancer screening among U.S. adults from 1992, 1998, and 2000 National Health Interview Surveys. Prev Med 2004;39:308–14.

Schmidt LA, Ye Y, Greenfield TK, Bond J. Ethnic disparities in clinical severity and services for alcohol problems: results from the National Alcohol Survey. Alcohol Clin Exp Res 2007;31:48–56.

Screening for hepatitis B virus infection among refugees arriving in the United States, 1979–1991. MMWR 1991;40:784–6.

Severi G, Giles GG, Robertson C, Boyle P, Autier P. Mortality from cutaneous melanoma: evidence for contrasting trends between populations. Br J Cancer 2000;82:1887–91.

Singh GK, Hoyert DL. Social epidemiology of chronic liver disease and cirrhosis mortality in the United States, 1935–1997: trends and differentials by ethnicity, socioeconomic status, and alcohol consumption. Hum Biol 2000;72:801–20.

Stitzenberg KB, Thomas NE, Dalton K, Brier SE, Ollila DW, Berwick M, Mattingly D, Millikan RC. Distance to diagnosing provider as a measure of access for patients with melanoma. Arch Dermatol 2007;143:991–8.

Strader DB, Wright T, Thomas DL, Seeff LB. Diagnosis, management, and treatment of hepatitis C. Hepatology 2004;39:1147–71.

Swetter SM, Miller DR, Layton CJ, Brooks KR, Geller AC. Melanoma in Middle-Aged and Older Men: a multi-institutional survey study of factors related to tumor thickness. Archives of Dermatology 2009 (in press).

To SE. Alcohol dependence patterns and their impact on New York City. MedGenMed 2007;9:23.

Tremolda F, Benevegnu L, Drago C, Casarin C, Cechetto A, Realdi G, Ruol A. Early detection of hepatocellular carcinoma in patients with cirrhosis by alphafetoprotein, ultrasound and fine-needle biopsy. Hepatogastroenterology 1989;36:519–21.

U.S. Department of Health and Human Services. Report on Carcinogens. 11 ed, 2004.

US Preventive Services Task Force. Guide to Clinical Preventive Services. 2nd ed. Baltimore: Williams Wilkins, 1996.

US Preventive Services Task Force. Screening for skin cancer: recommendations and rationale. Am J Prev Med 2001;20:44–6.

Velazquez RF RM, Navascues CA et al. Prospective analysis of risk factors for hepatocellular carcinoma in patients with liver cirrhosis. Hepatology 2003:520–527.

Wasley A, Alter MJ. Epidemiology of hepatitis C: geographic differences and temporal trends. Semin Liver Dis 2000;20:1–16.

Wasley A, Miller JT, Finelli L. Surveillance for acute viral hepatitis – United States, 2005. MMWR Surveill Summ 2007;56:1–24.

Wong JB, McQuillan GM, McHutchison JG, Poynard T. Estimating future hepatitis C morbidity, mortality, and costs in the United States. Am J Public Health 2000;90:1562–9.

Wright TL. Antiviral therapy and primary and secondary prevention of hepatocellular carcinoma. Hepatol Res 2007;37 Suppl 2:S294–8.

Yang HI, Lu SN, Liaw YF, You SL, Sun CA, Wang LY, Hsiao CK, Chen PJ, Chen DS, Chen CJ. Hepatitis B e antigen and the risk of hepatocellular carcinoma. N Engl J Med 2002;347:168–74.

Yu MC, Yuan JM. Environmental factors and risk for hepatocellular carcinoma. Gastroenterology 2004;127:S72–8.

Zamolo G, Gruber F, Jonjic A, Cabrijan L, Palle M, Grubisic-Greblo H. A 20-year epidemiological study of cutaneous melanoma in the Rijeka district of Croatia. Clin Exp Dermatol 2000;25:77–81.

Zhang BH, Yang BH, Tang ZY. Randomized controlled trial of screening for hepatocellular carcinoma. J Cancer Res Clin Oncol 2004;130:417–22.
Zhou F, Euler GL, McPhee SJ, Nguyen T, Lam T, Wong C, Mock J. Economic analysis of promotion of hepatitis B vaccinations among Vietnamese-American children and adolescents in Houston and Dallas. Pediatrics 2003;111:1289–96.

Part III
Some Avenues to Address Cancer Disparities

Chapter 11
Interventions, Policy, and Advocacy

Deborah Klein Walker and Christine M. Judge

I. Context and Framework for Action

Background

In the broadest sense, health disparities are inequities or inequalities in environment, access and utilization of care, health status, and health outcomes (Carter-Pokras and Baquet 2002). These inequalities can occur at any stage of the cancer continuum (prevention, incidence, etiology, screening, diagnosis, access to clinical trials, treatment, survival, morbidity, and mortality) (Krieger 2005). Another chapter in this monograph (Chapter 14) addresses community-based approaches for cancer disparities. This chapter reviews current knowledge about effective interventions to reduce cancer disparities, particularly with respect to policy and advocacy, and recommends strategies for implementing and sustaining these interventions. While there may be some necessary overlap in the approaches described in the two chapters, they complement one another to provide an array of possible interventions.

During the past two decades there has been a growing recognition of disparities in health—including those in the prevention, treatment, and outcomes of cancer—by individuals, families, clinicians, community-based organizations, and government agencies. In the past decade too, many national, state, and local initiatives have addressed these disparities throughout the full range of the cancer continuum. These include two major efforts from the Department of Health and Human Services (HHS): the national 2010 Healthy People goals for the nation (U.S. Department of Health and Human Services 2000), as well as the National Healthcare Disparities Report (Agency for Healthcare Research and Quality 2006). In addition, in 2004 a trans-HHS progress review group on cancer health disparities released a call to action with specific recommendations, following the Institute of Medicine's 2002 landmark report, *Unequal Treatment*, which drew attention to

D.K. Walker (✉)
Vice President and Public Health Practice Leader, Health Division, Abt Associates, Inc., Cambridge, MA, USA
e-mail: deborah_walker@abtassoc.com

H.K. Koh (ed.), *Toward the Elimination of Cancer Disparities*,
DOI 10.1007/978-0-387-89443-0_11, © Springer Science+Business Media, LLC 2009

racial and ethnic disparities in health care. The IOM report stated that differences in quality of health care between minority and non-minority populations are due to clinical appropriateness and need, operation of the health care system (including the legal and regulatory climate), and discrimination expressed by biases, stereotyping, and uncertainty (IOM 2002). Another IOM commissioned report, *The Unequal Burden of Cancer* (1999), reviewed the state of cancer research related to minority and medically underserved groups and provided recommendations to the National Institutes of Health (NIH) to further disparities research in the US. In addition, two major programs of the federal Department of Health and Human Services—REACH 2010 and Steps—have fostered community action to eliminate health disparities as well. In particular, REACH 2010, begun in 1999, by The Centers for Disease Control and Prevention addressed breast and cervical cancer screening as one of its six priority disparity areas (CDC 2007).

In addition to these national efforts, various state level initiatives are now in place. The Massachusetts legislature, for example, has supported a Commission to End Racial and Ethnic Health Disparities (Koutoujian and Wilkerson 2007) along with mandating universal health care reform. California has also launched a major campaign to end health disparities—the California Campaign to Eliminate Racial and Ethnic Disparities—led by the American Public Health Association, the California Health and Human Services Agency, and the Prevention Institute, and funded by the California Endowment, the California Wellness Foundation, and Kaiser Permanente (Horowitz and Lawlor 2008).

Principles and Model for Reducing Cancer Disparities

In the late 1990s, to evaluate prevention, screening, and treatment strategies, the Massachusetts Department of Public Health adopted a framework and logic model for addressing cancer disparities through a comprehensive state plan (Koh and Walker 2003). Used throughout this chapter to assess what we know about effective interventions for reducing cancer disparities, this framework is based on a social determinants or social ecological model of health (Evans and Stoddart 1990; Dahlgren and Whitehead 1991) (Fig. 11.1). The framework acknowledges the many basic life issues associated with cancer health outcomes in a particular community and assumes that root causes of inequalities, such as employment, education, and discrimination, must be addressed along with access to, and quality of, the health care system. This model also recognizes that targeting the medical care system, and health care financing, is necessary but not sufficient to address cancer disparities.

More specifically, effective strategies in this framework include a continuum of issues. *Healthy People 2010* estimates that medical services contribute 10% to health outcomes, compared with 20% for the environment, 20% for genetic endowment, and 50% for health behaviors (US Department of Health and Human Services 2000; McGinnis and Foege 1993). Thus, the Massachusetts logic model outlines three aspects of short-term outcomes, including cultural as well as systemic factors: health risk/behavior, screening and health system, and environmental/occupational health (Koh and Walker 2003). To design programmatic and policy strategies to reduce cancer and cancer disparities, this

A Model of the Determinants of Health

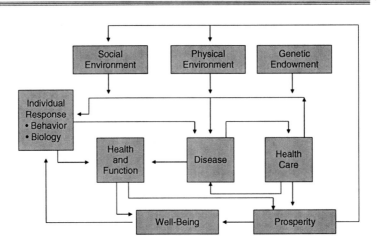

Fig. 11.1 A model of the social determinants of health (Evans and Stoddart, 1990)
Source: R.G. Evans and G.L. Stoddart, 1990. *Social Science and Medicine* 31:1347-1363; used
with permission from Elsevier Science Ltd.

framework also requires understanding which modifiable risk factors have been
associated with incidence and prevalence, as well as treatment and survival outcomes. Koh and Walker (2003) display the modifiable risk factors common to
different cancers, which include nutrition, physical activity, tobacco use, alcohol,
UV radiation, health seeking/promoting behavior, and environment/occupation
(Fig. 11.2). Although some of the risk factors relate to only one cancer (e.g.,
exposure to UV radiation for skin cancer), many of the risk factors relate to
several (e.g., tobacco use for cervical, colorectal, lung, and oral cancers).

Understanding the complex network of relationships among the possible
modifiable and non-modifiable factors linked to cancer applies to reducing
cancer disparities as well. We hypothesize that this basic framework of associations can be tailored for each of the populations with cancer disparities. In other
words, modifying a risk behavior such as exercise or increasing screening for a
particular cancer requires working within the context of a given population's
culture, attitudes, and knowledge.

This framework for addressing cancer disparities must be tailored to a specific
population and cancer disparity (Adler and Newman 2002, Freeman 2004, Powe
2006). Robinson (2005) argues for the critical role of community-level factors in
addressing health disparities—community development should become the
broad framework for implementing change. Also, although perceptions of racial
discrimination have been linked to health behavior (and to both mental and
physical health), Williams et al. (2003) note that the specific mechanism depicting
the way discrimination translates into physical or behavioral outcomes via stress
or other pathways is less empirically established.

Finally, these assumptions about a model for reducing cancer disparities imply
the need for multiple component, multiple sector strategies. In other words, a

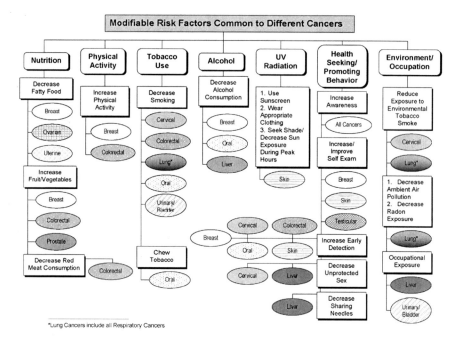

Fig. 11.2 Framework of modifiable risk factors as developed by the Massachusetts Comprehensive Cancer Control Program in 2003 for use in developing effective cancer prevention interventions (Koh and Walker 2003)

single solution or single sector activity is rarely enough to change and sustain positive behaviors. Instead, activities to reduce cancer disparities must occur simultaneously in a variety of sectors (e.g., schools, health provider offices, workplace, community, social marketing campaign, etc.). This multiple approach strategy was the framework used successfully in state level tobacco control programs such as the Massachusetts Tobacco Control Program (Koh et al. 2005).

According to Richmond and Kotelchuck (1983), making policy and program changes requires three elements: a knowledge base, social strategies, and political will. The next section of this chapter will present the current knowledge base concerning effective interventions that reduce cancer disparities; this will be followed by a discussion of the social strategies needed to generate the political will to develop and implement policies to reduce disparities.

II. Interventions to Reduce Cancer Disparities: Current Knowledge Base

Using the definition, assumptions, and framework for understanding cancer disparities outlined in the previous section, we conducted a literature search of PubMed to locate interventions with some evidence of effectiveness in reducing cancer disparities, including the treatment and outcomes of cancer as well as risk factors associated with the onset of cancers. Given the breadth and depth of cancer prevention intervention research literature and our goal to survey the literature for tested approaches to reducing cancer disparities for any cancer or cancer risk factor or among any special population, we focused on literature in which the term "cancer disparities" or the term "disparities" was named as a central theme or purpose.

Knowledge About the Existence of Cancer Disparities

Improvements in cancer outcomes in the overall population mask differences for selected populations; in fact, gaps or disparities in incidence and mortality by racial/ethnic groups often persist as rates in prevalence and incidence decline (Powe 2006). Many other chapters in this book document the dimensions of cancer disparities (particularly Chapters 1, 2, 3, 4). Recent national reports and studies in the US also indicate that disparities from prevention to palliative care exist by race/ethnicity, socio-economic status, health insurance status, and geography and amplify previous reviews published for breast cancer (Bigby and Holmes 2005), prostate cancer (Gilligan 2005), colorectal cancer (Palmer and Schneider 2005), and cervical cancer (Newman and Garner 2005).

Overall, more research has focused on racial, ethnic, and socio-economic disparities than on those related to geography, sexual preference, and disability. In all the reviews, African Americans tend to have a disproportionate share of the health inequalities across the cancer continuum. Briefly, and as noted elsewhere throughout this monograph, African Americans continue to have the highest overall cancer incidence and mortality rates among all racial/ethnic groups, and for most specific cancer sites. Whites have the second highest overall cancer burden, while Hispanics and Asians suffer disproportionately from cancers associated with infections, such as cervical cancer, which occurs disproportionately in Hispanic and Vietnamese women. American Indians and Alaska Natives have the highest rates of kidney cancer incidence and mortality (American Cancer Society 2008). People who live in poorer areas also suffer from relatively high cancer mortality and low cancer survival (Ward et al. 2004), and this disparity has widened since the 1970s (Singh et al. 2003). People who are less educated also experience worse cancer outcomes. For instance, black and white men with at least 12 years of education have half the overall cancer death rates of their less-educated counterparts (ACS 2008).

Recent studies on the impact of health insurance on cancer have also found that those who are uninsured are more likely not to receive recommended cancer screening (e.g., breast and colorectal screenings) and to be diagnosed at more advanced stages of cancer (Halpern et al. 2008, Ward et al. 2004). Analyzing 2005 NHIS data, Ward et al. found that having health insurance is an important predictor of cancer screening across all racial/ethnic groups and educational levels. While Ward et al. also reported consistently higher stage of diagnosis and lower survival rates for uninsured or Medicaid insured individuals across all racial/ethnic groups and educational levels, they documented that African Americans are more likely to be diagnosed at later stages of cancer and to have lower survival than whites. Halpern et al. also reported increased risk of diagnosis at late stage (stages III or IV) for black and Hispanic patients comparerd with white patients, regardless of insurance status. Perhaps not surprisingly given the documented lower survival rates for African Americans, a recent literature review also found descriptive evidence of lower quality of life for African American cancer survivors than for white cancer survivors, but mostly found inadequate research in this area (Powe et al. 2007).

Knowledge About Reducing Disparities in the Major Risk Factors Related to Cancer

We investigated the current state-of-the-science on effective approaches to reducing cancer disparities through reductions in risk factor disparities (e.g., tobacco use, physical activity, nutrition, sun exposure, access to screening, etc.). The majority of studies we identified, summarized below, focused on cancer screening and tobacco control.

Interventions to Reduce Disparities in Cancer Screening

Numerous studies have investigated a variety of approaches to addressing cancer screening disparities. These include studies testing the adaptation of a breast and cervical cancer screening education model from an African American community to a Latina community (Erwin et al. 2007); analyzing the impact of the National Breast and Cervical Cancer Early Detection Program on mammography and Pap test use across multiple racial/ethnic groups (Adams et al. 2007); examining the relationship between health and cultural beliefs and stage of mammography screening adoption (Russell et al. 2007); evaluating a model that uses primary care physicians to provide routine screening colonoscopy in a black community (Lloyd et al. 2007); and assessing a patient navigator program to improve follow-up of abnormal breast cancer screening among inner-city women (Battaglia et al. 2007). Other studies cited in a recent review of interventions to reduce cancer screening disparities among women (Loerzel and Busby 2005) tackled such subjects as risk factors associated with low screening (low SES, no health insurance, and no primary source of health care) (Sambamoorthi and McAlpine 2003), cultural influence on health beliefs; barriers to screening (system-level and human-level), and effectiveness of specific strategies to increase adherence to breast cancer screening guidelines at the patient level (e.g., telephone counseling) (Rimer et al. 1999).

Many of these studies reported positive findings for the effectiveness of their interventions. For the large-scale National Breast and Cervical Cancer Early Detection Program, which provides free breast and cervical cancer screening to low-income and uninsured women, Adams et al. (2007) found evidence that the program had helped to close the gap in screening between African American and white women (but not between Hispanic and white women) (see also Chapter 9). A patient navigator program in an urban, hospital-based setting increased timely follow-up for poor and minority women from abnormal breast screening finding to diagnostic evaluation from 64% to 78% (Battaglia et al. 2007). (See also Chapter 13 for a dedicated review of navigator programs in addressing disparities.) A review by Masi, Blackman, and Peek (2007) of interventions to improve breast cancer screening adherence for minority women found that cultural tailoring and addressing economic and logistical barriers with patients worked, as did chart reminders with providers (for mammography). A combination of provider prompts, printed tailored materials, and tailored telephone counseling increased Pap test scheduling among a community health center patient population of low-income black women (Rimer et al. 1999).

Other successful models include the use of community health advisors, or lay health advisors, to increase cancer screening in communities (Martin 2005). Martin defines community health advisors as "trusted natural helpers from within the community who provide emotional support, advice, and tangible aid to members of their social network" and reports evidence that programs using these advisors have increased cancer screening. A recent literature review defines lay health advisors as "community members who work almost exclusively in community settings and serve to connect healthcare consumers to providers in order to promote health and prevent diseases among groups that have traditionally lacked access to adequate care" and recognizes the emergence of this role over the last 25 years as an effort to address racial and ethnic health disparities (Rhodes et al. 2007). Another study found success in adapting a proven outreach intervention model using lay health workers to increase breast and cervical cancer screening in African-American communities to Latina communities, some of which have experience with Latina lay health workers called "promotoras" (Erwin et al. 2007). Citing the unique cancer burden of many Asian American ethnic groups, Chen (2005) has also called for interventions using approaches such as media, lay health workers, provider education, and Hepatitis B vaccinations to overcome low screening rates and other barriers to reducing cancer disparities in these populations (see also Chapter 10 of this monograph).

Interventions to Reduce Disparities in Tobacco Control

Chapter 5 in this book offers a detailed analysis of disparities in tobacco use and lung cancer. In addition, a recent NIH consensus statement summarizes currently known effective interventions to help people quit smoking and particularly addresses implementation in diverse populations (NIH 2006). The statement first describes effective strategies for increasing consumer demand for and use of cessation services in all populations including mass media education campaigns combined with other interventions (e.g., telephone-based support); provider advice combined with pharmacological and educational interventions; increasing prices of tobacco products; and reducing out-of-pocket costs for cessation therapy. The report recognizes that more work must be done to tailor these interventions to specific groups (e.g., defined by racial/ethnic status, immigrant status, and income) to reduce disparities. For example, a recent randomized clinical trial demonstrated the efficacy of a culturally tailored media and counseling dose to increase the use of a Spanish language smoking cessation counseling service provided by the National Cancer Institute's Cancer Information Service among a low-SES, immigrant Latino community (Wetter et al. 2007).

We know more about the effectiveness of cessation interventions in controlled clinical settings such as clinics and hospitals (i.e., clinical health care settings) than about those implemented at the broader community level (e.g., cities or colleges). In health care settings, certain financial incentives, such as lowering costs to patients for cessation services or reimbursing providers, have been successful, although whether insurance premium discounts would entice smokers to quit remains to be studied. Health care institutions that create dedicated staff positions for providing tobacco cessation services also appear to be particularly effective (National Institutes of Health 2006). The above-mentioned Spanish-language smoking counseling service for low-SES smokers using increased media promotion and cultural tailoring offers promise for improving uptake of cessation interventions and reducing disparities in tobacco use among hard-to-reach populations (Wetter et al. 2007). National tobacco control experts looking to future research opportunities highlight disparities in tobacco use and tobacco-related cancer outcomes among vulnerable and underserved populations in a variety of settings as one of the most important upcoming research areas (Morgan et al. 2007). A more detailed overview of disparities related to tobacco use is found in Chapter 5 of this monograph.

Promising Individual and Community Interventions for Reducing Disparities

Our review of the literature revealed many studies that tested prevention and screening interventions on different types of cancer with different racial/ethnic minority or low-SEP populations in different clinical settings (community health center, hospital, etc.) but again we found few evidence-based interventions at the individual or community level that framed the question in terms of reducing cancer disparities specifically (see also Chapter 14 of this book). Beyond the information summarized in the previous two sections on approaches to screening and tobacco control, moreover, there was a paucity of information about interventions to address the other risk factors for cancer or about interventions in schools, workplaces, and the media.

Interestingly, however, a number of multi-component programs are currently being funded by federal, state, and foundation resources. These programs hold some promise for reducing cancer disparities since they target culturally appropriate interventions in the multiple-component framework needed to address cancer disparities. The largest number of community interventions are funded by the Centers for Disease Control and Prevention (CDC) (2007) and the National Cancer Institute (NCI) (2007) in the NIH. The CDC, for example, has funded cancer disparities programs via the REACH 2010 and Steps to a Healthier US (i.e., Steps) programs and the Comprehensive Cancer Control Program.

These national programs funded to reduce health disparities highlight the general need for broad, multi-faceted approaches. Recognizing that disparities are created within a complex context of biological, social, and environmental factors over time, they affirm that solutions must also necessarily target these various levels of health determinants. Therefore, some researchers advocate a paradigm in disparities reduction and elimination efforts that addresses multiple factors at multiple levels (e.g., patient, provider, health care system, cultural) (Powe 2006, Chin et al. 2007). As summarized by Powe, "there is no single answer, no single intervention, no single person, entity, or organization that can fix, reduce or eliminate cancer disparities in isolation (p. 346)." While focusing more broadly on interventions to reduce racial/ethnic health disparities in health care, Chin et al. similarly suggest that effective interventions are those that are multifactorial, or that address multiple barriers at the same time (Chin et al. 2007).

Powe (2006) also raises the need for partnership approaches to reducing cancer disparities. Many community-academic partnership programs in this area are currently funded and in progress (e.g., the NCI Center to Reduce Cancer Health Disparities' Community Networks Program). Furthermore, community participation in identifying, designing, and implementing research-based strategies (i.e., community-based participatory research) to address health disparities is now recognized as a vital component to translating evidence-based interventions into successful community programs (Israel et al. 1998, 2003, Minkler et al. 2003, Viswanathan et al. 2004).

Hayes et al. (2005) present an overview of resulting approaches that various cancer control programs are using to address disparities. For example, Georgia is using a coordinated care approach linked to clinical research. The Pacific Island Nations associated with the US are leveraging resources for geographically dispersed populations. The Native American tribes in the Northwest are using community-based participatory research and training tools. Finally, Maryland's Department of Health and Mental Hygiene published a chapter on cancer-related disparities in the 2004–2008 Maryland Comprehensive Cancer Plan as a Call to Action that resulted in legislation and statewide change. In another article, Koh and Walker (2003) review the way in which the Massachusetts Cancer Control Program is implementing the CDC comprehensive cancer control program grant by using a public health approach and a social determinants logic model.

In 2007, the Institute of Medicine of the National Academies convened a group of professionals representing community-based organizations, health care, government, foundations, and academia, called the Roundtable on Racial and Ethnic Health Disparities, to bring attention and action to solving racial and ethnic health disparities in the US. In its recently published monograph, the IOM (2008) summarizes the findings and conclusions of the Roundtable regarding the effectiveness and challenges of these clinical and community-based programs. The monograph decries the "silo" approach that creates the conditions that separate community-based and clinically-based initiatives. Instead it advocates a "hybrid" approach that incorporates the strengths of both the clinical and community approaches. The authors argue that the hybrid approach simultaneously addresses both the biological and social determinants of health, maximizes the resources and increases the capacity of each sector, and ultimately creates the sustainability currently lacking in the siloed approach. Furthermore, the IOM Roundtable authors argue that the hybrid approach must also include the implementation of CBPR (community-based participatory research) principles, which provide "an opportunity for health leaders to listen and learn from and with community members ... to discover the power, wisdom, and ideas that minority groups in the community, or people directly affected by illnesses, have to offer (IOM 2008, p. 52)." Establishing strong, working, equitable relationships between community and clinical partners, and building on each other's strengths, particularly the community's assets, holds the potential for real change and sustainability.

Examples of successful hybrid approaches described in the IOM report are the above-mentioned CDC REACH (Racial and Ethnic Approaches to Community Health) and Steps to a Healthier US programs. REACH 2010 is a $34 million initiative of the CDC and, since its inception in 1999, has funded 40 communities to create and implement plans to address particular health issues in their communities. Steps to a Healthier US Cooperative Agreement Program has awarded over $100 million to 40 communities to conduct local chronic disease prevention programs since 2003. Funded initiatives have tackled improving nutrition, increasing physical activity, and reducing smoking in their communities—all risk factors for cancer. For example, The Healthy Nation Program of the Cherokee Nation in Oklahoma, funded through both REACH and Steps programs, implemented tobacco control programs across schools, worksites, health care settings, and broader community venues (such as a community-wide 2005 promotion of the Oklahoma Tobacco Quit Line that resulted in 59 of 191 initial participants quitting (31%), and subsequent significant reductions in smoking among Native American community members). Program leaders highlight the importance of an integrated approach to "saturate all levels of the social structure" (IOM 2008, p. 86).

Finally, national partners for cancer control planning and implementation frequently use three resources (*Cancer Control P.L.A.N.E.T., the Guide to Community Preventive Services, and CancerPlan.org*) that are summarized below (Hayes et al. 2005):

Cancer Control P.L.A.N.E.T. (Plan, Link, Act, Network with Evidence-Based Tools) is a web portal (http://cancercontrolplanet.cancer.gov/) that provides links to comprehensive cancer control (CCC) planning for public health professionals. It was developed by the NCI with assistance from the CDC, the American Cancer Society, the Substance Abuse and Mental Health Administration, the Agency for Healthcare Research and Quality, and the Commission on Cancer. The portal provides community groups, public health program planners, and researchers with the tools needed to bridge the gap between research on interventions that work and dissemination of such interventions in communities. The goal is for users to be able to design, implement, and evaluate evidence-based cancer control projects. This tool presents a unique opportunity to bring together and utilize the expertise of national cancer prevention organizations providing free easily accessible data and planning tools, the expertise of communities and community-based organizations providing information about social and environmental context of their communities, and the expertise and resources of local and state government agencies, non-profits, and academic institutions to galvanize resources and help ensure scientific and programmatic feasibility in adapting and implementing evidence-based interventions in communities.

The Guide to Community Preventive Services (http://www.thecommunityguide.org/) provides systematic reviews of and recommendations for program interventions related to cancer. The information in the Guide comes from the work of the Task Force on Community Preventive Services (2005), an independent, non-governmental volunteer group comprising top public health and prevention scientists and administrators. The Task Force carefully reviews and summarizes the work of researchers who conduct systematic reviews of particular public health diseases and risk factors (e.g., obesity, cancer, violence, and tobacco) and then makes calls for further research, or makes recommendations for interventions that "work," based on the latest scientific evidence. The Guide thus represents another valuable compendium of synthesized scientific evidence on "what works" to reduce cancer disparities that communities, academics, and public health practitioners can easily access.

CancerPlan.org is an interactive website for cancer control planners and implementers in states, tribes, territories, or communities to share resources that helps them develop and implement effective CCC plans. The site was developed by the American Cancer Society, the CDC, and the NCI. Among the tools available on the site are information about CCC plans and best practices for their development and implementation, such as sample planning models or needs assessments, and links to the Cancer Control P.L.A.N.E.T. site to access descriptions of evidence-based interventions to address particular cancers. The site also provides professional and project management support through information on leadership institutes in which cancer control planners can participate around the US, as well as a "workbook," or private online space, for individual CCC coalitions (representing different geographic or community groups designing CCC plans) to post and store documents, keep calendars and planning documents, and communicate via a message board.

Several local communities across the country are also making efforts to reduce cancer disparities using a combination of local, state, federal, and private resources. The Applied Research Center and Northwest Federation of Community Organizations, for example, outlines some promising solutions to race-based health disparities in their report, entitled *Closing the Gap* (2005). The report highlights various promising approaches within the overall socioecological model hypothesized as necessary to reduce cancer disparities. Among these are the focus on integrating primary care with urgent and hospital care for the Alaska Native and Native American populations in Anchorage, Alaska; the language and interpreter services at Bellevue Hospital in New York City; the approaches to improving quality health care access in Washington, DC and Santa Clara County, California; and the community-based services outside of the health care system in Sells, Arizona, and Berkeley, California.

III. Social Strategies Needed to Implement Current Knowledge

General Approach for Pursuing Policy Changes and Interventions

Given the limited evidence base for interventions that work to reduce cancer disparities, continuing to advocate for research and evaluation to build the knowledge base clearly remains just as important as building the social strategies and political will to implement this knowledge base as it evolves. We must therefore continue to invest in local and state-based programs so that individuals and communities alike can focus on cancer disparities reduction at all points on the cancer continuum.

The public health approach offers a framework and platform for action in this regard. As noted earlier, reducing cancer disparities will take a sustained multi-disciplinary and multi-pronged approach to implementing effective policies and interventions at both the individual and community levels. In particular, effective policy changes will require the active engagement of partnerships among consumers, health care providers, researchers, the media, public health, and other government agencies, as well as private insurance and health providers, community-based organizations, cancer advocacy groups, and the legislators at the state and federal levels.

The public health approach uses the three core public health functions—assessment, policy development, and assurance—to reduce cancer disparities within a multi-component social determinants model of health (Institute of Medicine 1988, 1997, 2003). This approach necessitates addressing all determinants of health, including "access to care, behavior, social and physical environments, and overriding policies of universal access to care, physical education in schools, and restricted exposure to toxic substances" (Satcher and Higginbotham 2008). The public health approach also requires good data to track progress on all these determinants, cancer prevalence and incidence, and cancer mortality and morbidity over time at the community level. Furthermore, this assessment function of public health must be supported at all levels of government to assure that public health surveillance systems available today are maintained and improved (Koh et al. 2005).

The framework for addressing cancer disparities developed by the Massachusetts Comprehensive Cancer Control Program (Koh and Walker 2003) exemplifies this approach. This framework specifies key indicators for the risk factors and cancer outcomes that must be tracked over time and embraces both individual clinical interventions and community-based population-based interventions. Both levels of interventions must be tailored for the populations who experience cancer disparities and work together at all parts of the cancer continuum (Horowitz and Lawlor 2008). Given the lack of proven interventions to reduce cancer disparities, many researchers and policy advocates have recommended focusing solutions on determining the concerns and needs of various affected populations, as well as local knowledge about community context and best practices (Underwood et al. 2004, Yabroff et al. 2005). Acquiring an in-depth knowledge about the specific population and community setting can assist practitioners and researchers in tailoring interventions to specific groups (Loerzel and Busky 2005) and this approach can be effective even in the absence of health professionals (Haynes 2006).

Finally, taking successful interventions to scale will require sustained public health funding so that the approaches that are successful for reducing cancer disparities can be maintained and tracked over time at the local and state levels. The few interventions found to be effective to date have not been implemented on a large-scale basis nor maintained consistently in one area over time. Public health initiatives such as REACH 2010 and the CDC Comprehensive Cancer Control Program, for example, are a necessary and important step in supporting local activities to address cancer disparities, but neither of these programs is currently funded sufficiently to support individual and community interventions for every community and state facing cancer disparities. These approaches are very similar to those recommended by the Institute of Medicine (1997) for improving community health and those adopted by the Healthy Cities and Healthy Communities movement (Norris and Pittman 2000, Twiss et al. 2000). Incorporating the reduction of cancer disparities into these ongoing public health efforts may prove to be a better approach than funding isolated community-based cancer reduction initiatives.

IV. Current Recommendations

While our knowledge base regarding effective intervention strategies remains limited, it is already clear that a sustained, adequately funded public health population-based approach promises to make a difference in reducing future cancer disparities. Our challenge now is to develop and implement social strategies to assure that the political will is available to make this approach a reality. Once a broad-based coalition of interested parties committed to the goal of reducing cancer disparities has adopted a set of principles and agenda for reducing cancer disparities, we will be able to determine the most pressing policies and priorities for a cancer disparities reduction advocacy agenda and campaign. In the meantime, the following are some suggested recommendations for reducing cancer disparities worth considering at this point.

- Strengthen the capacity of the public health system at all levels of government (federal, state, and local) to monitor outcomes over time and implement known effective strategies and policies.
- Create incentives for health care providers and stakeholders to "do the right thing" and implement effective strategies for individual and population health.
- Create partnerships at federal, state, and local levels to implement successful interventions and policies.
- Create an advisory committee that reports to Congress and the Executive Branch (e.g., MedPac for Medicare, Immunization Advisory Committee, etc.) to monitor research and evaluate and assure incorporation of known effective strategies into clinical and public health practice to reduce cancer disparities.
- Support community-based participatory and population-based research and evaluation efforts to document best practices to reduce cancer disparities at both the individual and community levels.

Finally, the most effective improvements in cancer disparities will entail enduring systemic changes to maintain better outcomes for all populations and reduce cancer disparities for vulnerable populations across the lifespan. Policymakers need to identify the most effective ways to make local, state, and federal systemic changes that will lead to a comprehensive, coordinated, quality, culturally competent, family-centered, and community-based system of care. Such a vision using an adequately funded, public health, population-based approach will support policies that assist in the design and implementation of these systems of care for every local community in the nation.

References

Adams, E.K., Breen, N., and Joski, P.J. Impact of the National Breast and Cervical Cancer Early Detection Program on mammography and Pap test utilization among white, Hispanic, and African American women: 1996–2000. Cancer. 2007;109(2 Suppl):348–358.

Adler, N.E. and Newman, K. Socioeconomic disparities in health: pathways and policies. Health Affairs. 2002;21(2):60–76.

Agency for Healthcare Research and Quality. National Healthcare Disparities Report. Rockville, MD: AHRQ, DHHS, 2006.

American Cancer Society. Cancer Facts and Figures. Atlanta: American Cancer Society, 2008.

Applied Research Center and Northwest Federation of Community Organizations. *Closing the Gap: Solutions to Race-based Health Disparities.* Seattle, WA: Northwest Federation of Community Organizations, 2005.

Battaglia, T.A., Roloff, K., Posner, M.A., and Freund, K.M. Improving follow-up to abnormal breast cancer screening in an urban population: A patient navigation intervention. Cancer. 2007;109 Suppl:359–367.

Bigby, J., and Holmes, M.D. Disparities across the breast cancer continuum. Cancer Causes and Control. 2005;16:35–44.

Carter-Pokras, O., and Baquet, C. What is a "health disparity?" Public Health Reports. 2002;117:426–434.

Center for Disease Prevention and Control. Health Disparities in Cancer. 2007. Available at: http://www.cdc.gov/cancer/healthdisparities/ and http://www.cdc.gov/cancer/healthdisparities/basic_info/disparities.htm. Accessed May 1, 2008.

Chen, M.S. Cancer health disparities among Asian Americans: what we do and what we need to do. Cancer. 2005;104 Suppl:2895–2902.

Chin, M.H., Walters, A.E., Cook, S.C., and Huanges. Interventions to reduce racial and ethnic disparities in healthcare. Medical Care Research and Review. 2007;64(5 suppl):7s–28s.

Dahlgren, G., and Whitehead, M. Policies and Strategies to Promote Social Equity in Health. Stockholm, Sweden: Institute for Futures Studies, 1991.

Erwin, D.O., Johnson, V.A., Trevino, M., Duke, K., Feliciano, L., and Jandorf, L. A comparison of African American and Latina social networks as indicators for culturally tailoring a breast and cervical cancer education intervention. Cancer. 2007;109 Suppl:368–377.

Evans, R.G., and Stoddart, G.L. Producing health, consuming health care. Social Science and Medicine. 1990;31:1347–1363.

Freeman, H.P. Poverty, culture, and social injustice: Determinants of cancer disparities. CA: A Cancer Journal for Clinicians. 2004;54:72–77.

Gilligan, T. Social disparities and prostate cancer: mapping the gaps in knowledge. Cancer Causes and Control. 2005;16:45–53.

Halpern, M.T., Ward, E.M., Pavluck, A.L., Schrag, N.M., Bian, J., and Chen, A.Y. Association of insurance status and ethnicity with cancer stage at diagnosis for 12 cancer sites: a retrospective analysis. Lancet Oncology. 2008;9(3):222–231.

Haynes, N.A. Reflections on programs designed to reduce cancer disparities. Cancer. 2006;107 Suppl:1936s–1938s.

Hayes, N., Rollins, R., Weinberg, A., Brawley, O., Baquet, C., Kaur, J.S., and Palafox, N.A. Cancer-related disparities: weathering the perfect storm through comprehensive cancer control approaches. Cancer Control and Causes. 2005;16(suppl 1):41–50.

Horowitz, C. and Lawlor, E.F. Community approaches to addressing health disparities. In Challenges and successes in reducing health disparities: Workshop summary. Washington, DC: The National Academies Press, 2008, pp. 161–192.

Institute of Medicine. The Future of Public Health. Washington, DC: National Academies Press, 1988.

Institute of Medicine. Improving Health in the Community: A Role for Performance Monitoring. Washington, DC: National Academy Press, 1997.

Institute of Medicine. The Unequal Burden of Cancer. Washington, DC: National Academies Press, 1999.

Institute of Medicine. Unequal Treatment: Confronting Racial and Ethnic Disparities in Health Care. Washington, DC: National Academies Press, 2002.

Institute of Medicine. The Future of the Public's Health in the 21st Century. Washington, DC: National Academies Press, 2003.

Institute of Medicine. Challenges and Successes in Reducing Health Disparities: Workshop Summary. Washington, DC: The National Academies Press, 2008.

Israel, B.A., Schulz, A.J., Parker, E.A., Becker, A.B., et al. Critical issues in developing and following community-based participatory research principles. In M. Minkler and N. Wallerstain (eds.). Community-based Participatory Research for Health. San Francisco, CA: Jossey-Bass, 2003, pp. 53–76.

Israel, B.A., Shultz, A.J., Parker, E.A., and Becker, A.B. Review of community-based research: assessing partnerships approaches to improving public health. Annual Review of Public Health. 1998;19:173–202.

Koh, H.K. and Walker, D.K. The role of state health agencies in cancer prevention and control: lessons learned from Massachusetts. Cancer Epidemiology, Biomarkers and Prevention. 2003;12:261s–268s.

Koh, H.K., Judge, C., Robbins, H., Celebucki, C., Walker, D.K., and Connolly, G. The first decade of the Massachusetts Tobacco Control Program. Public Health Reports. 2005;120(5):482–495.

Koh, H.K., Judge, C., Ferrer, B., and Gershman, S.T. Using public health data systems to understand and eliminate cancer disparities. Cancer Causes and Control. 2005; 16:15–26.

Koutoujian, P.J. and Wilkerson, D. (eds.). Commission to End Racial and Ethnic Health Disparities: Final Report. 2007. Available at: http://www.hcfama.org/_data/global/resources/live/Disparities%20Comission%20Full%20Report.pdf. Accessed January 15, 2008.

Krieger, N. Defining and investigating social disparities in cancer: critical issues. Cancer Causes and Control. 2005;16:5–14.

Lloyd, S.C., Harvey, N.R., Hebert, J.R., Daguise, V., Williams, D., and Scott, D.B. Racial disparities in colon cancer: primary care endoscopy as a tool to increase screening rates among minority patients. Cancer. 2007;109 Suppl:378–385.

Loerzel, V.W. and Busby, A. Interventions that address cancer health disparities in women. Family and Community Health. 2005;28:79–89.

Martin, M.Y. Community health advisors effectively promote cancer screening. Ethnicity and Disease. 2005;15(Suppl 2):14s–16s.

Masi, C.M., Blackman, D.J., and Peek, M.E. Interventions to enhance breast cancer screening, diagnosis, and treatment among racial and ethnic minority women. Medical Care Research and Review. 2007;64(5 Suppl):195s–242s.

McGinnis, J.M. and Foege, W.H. Actual causes of death in the United States. JAMA. 1993;270(18):2207–2212.

Minkler, M., Blackwell, A.G., Thompson, M., et al. Community-based participatory research: implications for public health funding. American Journal of Public Health. 2003;93:1672–1679.

Morgan, G.D., Backinger, C.L., and Leischow, S.J. The future of tobacco-control research. Cancer Epidemiol Biomarkers Prevention. 2007;16:1077–1080.

National Cancer Institute. Cancer health disparities. 2007. Available at: http://www.cancer.gov/cancertopics/types/disparities and http://crchd.cancer.gov/. Accessed February 12, 2008.

National Institutes of Health. NIH State-of-the-Science conference on tobacco use: prevention, cessation, and control. Annals of Internal Medicine. 2006;145:839–844.

Newman, S.J. and Garner, E.O. Social inequities along the cervical cancer continuum: a structured review. Cancer Causes and Control. 2005;16:63–70.

Norris, T. and Pittman, M. The Healthy Communities movement and the Coalition for Healthier Cities and Communities. Public Health Reports. 2000;115:118–124.

Palmer, R.C. and Schneider, E.C. Social disparities across the continuum of colorectal cancer: a systematic review. Cancer Causes and Control. 2005;16:5–61.

Powe, B.D. Eliminating cancer disparities. Cancer. 2006;109 Suppl:345–347.

Powe, B.D., Hamilton, J., Hancock, N., Johnson, N., Finnie, R., Ko, J., Brooks, P., and Boggan, M. Quality of life of African American cancer survivors: a review of the literature. Cancer. 2007;109 Suppl:435–445.

Rhodes, S.D., Foley, K.L., Zometa, C.S., and Bloom, F.R. Lay health advisor interventions among Hispanics/Latinos: a qualitative systematic review. The American Journal of Preventive Medicine. 2007;33(5):418–427.

Richmond, J.B. and Kotelchuck, M. The effect of the political process on the delivery of health services. In C.H. McGuire, R. Foley, A. Gorr and R.W. Richards (eds.). Handbook of Health Professions Education. San Francisco, CA: Jossey-Bass, 1983, pp. 386–404.

Rimer, B.K., Conaway, M., Lyna, P., Glassman, B., Yarnall, K.S.H., Lipkus, I., and Barber, L.T. The impact of tailored interventions on a community health center population. Patient Education and Counseling. 1999;7:125–140.

Robinson, R.G. Community development model for public health applications: overview of a model to eliminate population disparities. Health Promotion Practice. 2005;6:338–346.

Russell, K.M., Monahan, P., Wagle, A., and Champion, V. Differences in health and cultural beliefs by stage of mammography screening adoption in African American women. Cancer. 2007;109(2 Suppl):386–395.

Sambamoorthi, U. and McAlpine, D.D. Racial, ethnic, socioeconomic, and access disparities in the use of preventive services among women. Preventive Medicine. 2003;37:475–484.

Satcher, D. and Higginbotham, E.J. The public health approach to eliminating disparities in health. American Journal of Public Health. 2008;98:400–403.

Singh, G.K., Miller, B.A., Hankey, B.F., and Edwards, B.K. Area Socioeconomic Variations in U.S. Cancer Incidence, Mortality, Stage, Treatment, and Survival, 1975–1999. Bethesda, MD: National Cancer Institute, 2003.

Task Force on Community Preventive Services. Guide to Community Preventive Services: What Works to Promote Health? New York: Oxford University Press, 2005.

Twiss, J.M., Duma, S., Look, V., Shaffer, G.S., and Watkins, A.C. Twelve years and counting: California healthy cities and communities. Public Health Reports. 2000;115:125–133.

Underwood, S.M., Buseh, A.G., Canales, M.K., Powe, B., Dockery, B., Kather, T., and Kent, N. Nursing contributions to the elimination of health disparities among African-Americans: review and critique of a decade of research. Journal of National Black Nurses' Association. 2004;12:48–62.

U.S. Department of Health and Human Services. Healthy People 2010. Washington, DC, DHHS, 2000.

U.S. Department of Health and Human Services. Making Health Disparities History: Report of the Trans-HHS Cancer Disparities Progress. Washington, DC: DHHS, 2004.

U.S. Department of Health and Human Services. Healthy People 2010 Mid-Course Review. 2003. Available at: http://www.healthypeople.gov/data/midcourse/default.htm#pubs Accessed May 1, 2008.

Viswanathan, M.A.A., Eng, E., Gartlehner, G., Lohr, K.N., et al. Community-based Participatory Research: Assessing the Evidence: Summary. Evidence Report/Technology Assessment, No. 99. Rockville, MD: Agency for Healthcare Research and Quality, 2004.

Ward, E., Jemal, A., Cokkinides, V., Singh, G.K., Cardinez, C., Ghafoor, A., et al. Cancer disparities by race/ethnicity and socioeconomic status. CA: A Cancer Journal for Clinicians. 2004;54(2):78–93.

Wetter, D.W., Mazas, C., Daza, P., Nguyen, L., Fouladi, R.T., Li, Y., and Cofta-Woerpel, L. Reaching and treating Spanish-speaking smokers through the National Cancer Institute's Cancer Information Service: a randomized controlled trial. Cancer. 2007;109 Suppl:406–413.

Williams, D.R., Neighbors, H.W., and Jackson, J.S. Racial/ethnic discrimination health: findings from community studies. American Journal of Public Health. 2003; 93:200–208.

Yabroff, K.R., Lawrence, W.F., King, J.C., Mangan, P., Washington, K.S., Yi, B., Kerner, J.F., and Mandelblatt, J.W. Geographic disparities in cervical cancer mortality: what are the roles of risk factor prevalence, screening, and use of recommended treatment? The Journal of Rural Health. 2005;21:149–157.

Chapter 12
Health Communication and Communication Inequalities in Addressing Cancer Disparities

K. Viswanath and Karen M. Emmons

Introduction

The advances in knowledge about the causes of and treatments for cancer underscores the need for understanding how to disseminate this knowledge widely and effectively. Dissemination maximizes the chances for appropriate and timely actions in cancer prevention that can lead to considerable savings in lives as well as costs associated with medical care of cancer patients (Warren et al. 2008). Adoption of preventive health behaviors is more likely when individuals have knowledge about why those behaviors are important and have the skills and the *means* to adopt them. Further, treatment advances often take some time to become widely available in practice, and thus an individual's ability to take advantage of them requires knowledge and resources.

This presents a dilemma given the cancer-related morbidity and mortality disproportionately faced by members of minority groups and those from lower socioeconomic status (or SES) (Kawachi & Kroenke 2006), documented throughout this book. Researchers have identified a variety of factors, "social determinants," spanning the prevention, treatment, and survivorship/end-of-life continuum that are potentially linked to and exacerbate health disparities (Kawachi & Kroenke 2006; Krieger 2007; Paltoo & Chu 2004; Ries et al. 2004). As noted throughout this monograph, these social determinants include social class or SES, race/ethnicity, social networks, work environment and life transition events, neighborhood and residential conditions, and social policies (Galea & Vilahov 2005; Kaplan 2004; Kawachi & Berkman 2000; Krieger et al. 2005; Phelan et al. 2004) Although many studies have documented the role of these factors on health disparities, the precise mechanisms through which different levels of social determinants influence individual health remain little understood (Kaplan 2004).

K. Viswanath (✉)
Harvard School of Public Health, Dana-Farber Cancer Institute, Boston, MA, USA
e-mail: Vish_viswanath@dfci.harvard.edu

H.K. Koh (ed.), *Toward the Elimination of Cancer Disparities*,
DOI 10.1007/978-0-387-89443-0_12, © Springer Science+Business Media, LLC 2009

A fundamental thesis of this chapter is that communication, more specifically *inequalities in communication*, is a critical social determinant that contributes to existing disparities across the cancer continuum. Unlike other social determinants listed above, communication inequalities are a more readily modifiable and addressable factor. As a result, addressing inequalities in communication could have particularly important influences on the trajectory of cancer incidence, prevalence, and mortality.

The goal of this chapter is to review the role of communication, especially, mass media and health communication, in addressing cancer disparities. Many of these themes are also addressed elsewhere in this book, especially Chapters 5, 11, 13, and 14. We will briefly review major dimensions of communication inequality and selectively review key factors that are important in understanding how health communication strategies can contribute to reducing disparities.

Communication and the Cancer Control Continuum

Despite the rapid advances in molecular biology and genetics, cancer control requires a multilevel strategy that intervenes at different stages of the disease (Hiatt & Rimer 1999; Stein & Colditz 2004). The promise of cancer communication runs through the cancer control continuum: prevention, detection, diagnosis and treatment, survivorship, and end-of-life (EOL) (Viswanath 2005). Communication campaigns have been successful in reducing youth smoking (see also Chapter 5 of this book) (Center for Disease Control 2008; Davis et al. 2007; Farrelly et al. 2005). Communication facilitates patients' involvement in their own health care, reduces distress, improves adherence to treatment regimes, and increases the patient's sense of control (Mills & Sullivan 1999). Some communication interventions can influence patient's knowledge and recall, satisfaction, and ability to manage symptoms (Hack et al. 1999; Johnson 1982; McPherson et al. 2001; Mohide et al. 1996). Preparing patients ahead of time for the clinical visit by providing practical information may also have a beneficial effect (Cegala 2003; Huchcroft et al. 1984).

Communication is equally important at survivorship and EOL stages (Cherlin et al. 2005; Earle 2007). There are almost ten million cancer survivors in the US today, a number that is expected to increase with the growing success of treatment options, early disease detection, and drug developments (Twombly 2004). Survivors in the post-treatment phase need information on the probability of disease recurrence, tertiary prevention, long-term side effects of treatment, and quality of life and personal finances, among other topics. Studies show that interventions could potentially reduce uncertainty about the future and associated distress, improve outlook, and help patients develop a problem-solving approach. Greater patient–physician communication has also been linked to greater satisfaction with care and a sense of involvement with the treatment decisions (Liang et al. 2002). The Internet has changed the way cancer survivors seek support and communicate with each other as well (Rimer et al. 2005; Sharp 1999). A number of online listserves (that is, electronic discussion forums) and support groups now cater to an increasing number of patients and survivors.

Similarly, EOL conversations between advanced cancer patients and their oncologists can provide substantial benefits for patients and, potentially, society. Communications about prognosis have been associated with advance care planning, greater use of palliative care services, and lower use of expensive, burdensome, and futile EOL care.

At the same time, the information environment—in the mass media, the Internet, and other media—is rife with cancer information that continues to grow. One study showed that the word "cancer" generates millions of hits on Google and thousands of stories in the news media (Viswanath 2005). Advances in medicine are routinely covered in the media and on the Internet, and are widely available to some audiences. The challenge, however, is that the sheer amount and complexity of information place considerable demands on people who may not be able to easily access and/or comprehend it. Despite the vast information available to patients, survivors, and family members, there are several questions concerning how accurately, equitably, and effectively this information is being accessed and applied.

To begin addressing these questions, we will start by describing the information environment on cancer and how the way information is constructed may influence cognition and behavior, i.e., "message effects." We will then delineate communication inequalities and how they may contribute to health disparities. Next, we will briefly discuss how emerging communication technologies such as the Internet, often discussed under the topic of *e-health*, may influence health. We will conclude the chapter with a brief summary of why paying attention to inequalities in communication can pay dividends in addressing health disparities.

Representation of Health and Cancer in the Media and the Internet

Health is a topic of considerable attention and interest in a variety of media and other communication channels. Health coverage cuts across a variety of genres—advertising, television, and movies among them—and has an impact on knowledge, beliefs, and behaviors of those exposed to the messages. The number of Internet sites and people seeking health information on the Internet has also been increasing in recent years (Pew 2005; Viswanath 2006).

Not all of this coverage is positive in intent or effect. Depiction of smoking in entertainment media, particularly movies, is widely documented (Worth et al. 2006), for example, and exposure to smoking in movies is known to influence smoking behavior among youth (see also Chapter 5) (Dalton et al. 2003). Despite the many studies documenting the relationship between exposure to smoking and movies, few have focused on this relationship among minority and low-SES groups, a critical gap in the literature. It is conceivable that the mechanisms that link exposure in movies to smoking and smoking behavior differ by racial/ethnic and SES groups.

Health has also received considerable attention in the news media, and this attention has been increasing over the last 25 years (Viswanath 2006). News coverage may influence not only what the public learns about specific health issues but also may influence perceptions of a topic's importance and the priority placed on it, depending on the how the topic was framed in the media (Iyengar 1991; Reese et al. 2001; Stryker 2003; Viswanath & Finnegan 1996). In terms of cancer, ideal reporting would be related to prevalence and preventability of different cancers. However, this is not typically the case. For example, one recent analysis found limited coverage of skin cancer and sun protection in US newspapers from 2002 to 2003 and virtually no coverage on television news programs, despite the continually increasing prevalence of skin cancer in the US (Viswanath et al. 2006).

Mainstream vs. Ethnic Media

Notable variations among media exist when catering to different ethnic and racial groups. These differences can be quite important, particularly in light of polling data showing that 45% of racial/ethnic minority adults prefer ethnic media to mainstream media, and an additional 35% used ethnic media on a regular basis (New California Media Partnership 2005). Stryker et al.'s 2006 study of the way in which mainstream (MSN) vs. ethnic (EN) newspapers cover cancer news was intriguing in this regard. First, although the reading grade level of stories in both types of newspapers was relatively high, it was significantly higher in mainstream than in ethnic newspapers (11.99 vs. 10.1, respectively). Of note, the National Cancer Institute recommends a fifth-grade reading level for cancer information prepared for the general public (Davis et al. 2002). Both types of newspapers were similar in the types of stories they included (e.g., scientific news, fund-raising/benefits, stories on affected individuals), but EN were more likely to profile local, non-celebrity individuals, while MSN were more likely to profile celebrities.

The most striking difference between the two types of newspaper was the greater likelihood of EN to publish general awareness stories. Coverage of breast cancer was disproportionately high in both newspaper types, relative to coverage of other cancers and to incidence. However, the reported types of cancers differed. Ethnic news media were more likely to report on the cancers for which there are larger disparities (e.g., breast, prostate, colorectal, and reproductive cancers) (see also Chapters 5, 6, 7, 8, and 9). Primary prevention did not receive much attention in either type of paper, although it was significantly higher in ethnic media (33% of stories mentioned prevention) vs. MSN (20%). This difference was likely a function of the higher prevalence of general awareness stories in EN, as these stories were most likely to include preventive information. Cancer screening information was also more common in ethnic than in mainstream media (35% vs. 18.8% of stories, respectively).

In both types of papers, treatment was the most commonly discussed aspect of the cancer continuum, with about 60% of stories in MSN focused on treatment, and 52% in EN. There were important differences in the framing of treatment-related stories, particularly related to clinical trials, with EN being much more likely to frame such stories in a neutral tone (70% vs. 39.7%), and MSN being more likely to use a positive tone (50.5% vs. 26.7%). These data illustrate the EN may be a very important channel for narrowing the knowledge gap among racial/ethnic minority communities. Although the balance of reporting is still focused on treatment, ethnic news media have made a greater commitment to general and prevention-related knowledge than have mainstream media.

Finally, this study's findings affirmed the importance of finding better ways to work with media to align the level of coverage of specific cancer topics with the corresponding prevalence of that cancer. The disproportionate coverage of breast cancer, and relative inattention to some more prevalent cancers, for example, may contribute to the general public's significant overestimation of the likelihood of developing breast cancer, and simultaneously reduce concern about more common, more preventable cancers.

Health Journalists, Occupational Practices, and Disparities

The unbalanced coverage in the news media described above can be traced to occupational practices of reporters, a topic that has received considerable attention in media studies. Health journalists, however, represent a specific subgroup that has received much less attention. A recent study of national survey of health journalists has found that they primarily relied on news sources, press conferences, or press releases for initial ideas on the story (Viswanath et al. 2008). Moreover, the "potential for public impact" and "new information or development" are the major newsworthiness criteria cited by the health journalists. These findings offer a possible opening to work with news media to educate the public about cancer.

More relevant to disparities, however, is the finding that minorities are severely under-represented among health journalists. The national survey found that 93% of the health journalists were white and 97% non-Hispanic. When asked about the topics likely to attract attention in the "next 2–3 years," moreover, only 11.5% of the reporters mentioned cost/access to health care as an important topic and rated obesity, stem/cell, genetics, and cancer as more attractive topics than disparities.

Potentiating Inequalities

In summary, media, whether through advertising, entertainment, or news, has a profound influence on public knowledge, beliefs, and behaviors and could be engaged to bring about changes in cancer-related behaviors and put disparities on the public agenda. At present, however, it remains an untapped channel to influence the public. Ironically, the sheer glut in health information and the proliferation of channels serve as an advantage of the few over many, an idea at the heart of communication inequalities.

Message Construction, Communication Effects, and Disparities

Media representations about cancer are sometimes straightforward facts. More often, however, they come in the form of executional elements—format, structure, and construction—that are aligned in different ways to increase audience exposure and attract attention, a prerequisite to communication effects (Hornik 2002). The body of work concerning "message effects" explores how different formats may ultimately influence health cognitions, beliefs, and behaviors (Capella 2006; Viswanath & Emmons 2006). We argue that the construction of the messages has influence on how audiences receive and react to messages, with preferences for and reactions to different formats varying by social determinants such as race/ethnicity, education, and income.

A variety of message formats and elements that could potentially help improve audience attention, processing, and learning include humor, fear, sex, narratives or stories, sensation seeking, and exemplars. A more extensive overview of message formats and their relevance to cancer control is discussed in a special issue of *Journal of Communication* (2006). Here we provide a selective review of two formats that are more proximally linked to social determinants: framing and narratives.

Framing is a rhetorical device that attempts to define an issue for the audience with the intention of influencing their cognition and behavior. In cancer control, frames have either emphasized benefits (gain) of taking an action or disadvantages (loss) of not taking an action. This technique has been extensively used in promoting cancer screening and treatment decisions (Banks et al. 1995; Davey et al. 2003; Finney & Iannotti 2002; Lauver & Rubin 1990; Lewis et al. 2003; Llewellyn-Thomas et al. 1995; Meyerowitz & Chaiken 1987; Salovey & Williams-Piehota 2004; Schneider et al. 2001). The way media frames an issue may also influence how audience perceives a "problem" and its potential "solution" (Gamson 2001). For example, restrictions on secondhand smoke may either be "framed," or portrayed, as unfair infringement on the rights of smokers or legitimate protection of the health of non-smokers.

A way an issue is framed and the metaphors used to frame it (e.g., "epidemic of obesity") may generate sustained coverage in the media and attract audience attention. Publicity and appropriate framing of obesity as an "epidemic" might spur actions from government, funding agencies, and the scientific establishment that in turn will influence the audience behaviors, a phenomenon documented for heart disease (Hornik 2002; Viswanath & Emmons 2006; Viswanath & Finnegan 2002).

Activist groups have also successfully used framing to draw public and media attention to policy changes in AIDS, vaccination, binge drinking, drunk driving, or tobacco use (Edelman 1977; Gamson & Modigliani 1987; Hilgartner & Bosk 1988; Olien et al. 1983; Tichenor et al. 1980). In theory, framing health disparities has similar potential to attract media attention, particularly in terms of the moral clarity and outrage regarding social justice and American ideals of equality of opportunity.

Narratives or messages in the form of stories draw on cultural traditions of storytelling and are a standard fare of media genres, particularly in entertainment and advertising. Narratives are constructed with a persuasive intent, but not explicitly. Stories influence the audience through effects of "transportation" to a new reality and by minimizing counter-arguments to the messages (Green 2006; Green & Brock 2000). Narratives have been used extensively to promote "pro-social" behaviors in *telenovelas*, television shows such as *Sesame Street*, and, in developing countries, even flip charts (Slater 2002). Within public health, narratives have been used to promote family planning, AIDS education, and cancer screening (Kreuter & McClure 2004; Slater 2002), premised on the belief that public health approaches that are culturally compatible with the intended audience are more effective. The Institute of Medicine's report on health communication, *Speaking of Health*, in fact, calls for public health approaches that are culturally compatible with the intended audience (Institute of Medicine & Committee on Communication for Behavior Change in the 21st Century: Improving the Health of Diverse Populations 2002). Culture—a system of beliefs, norms, values, and practices—interacts with socioeconomic position in a complex pattern potentially influencing health behavior (Sorensen et al. 2003) (See also Chapter 4), though it is often mistakenly equated with race and ethnicity (Kreuter & McClure 2004). The difficulty in using culture in health communication, however, stems from the fact that much work remains to be done on how to operationalize and measure the role of culture in research (Kreuter & McClure 2004).

Communication Inequalities and Cancer Disparities

Social factors, such as socioeconomic position, not only have a profound effect on life course (see Chapter 1), influencing an individual's access to material and intellectual resources, social support, and living conditions (Krieger 2001; Lynch & Kaplan 2000; Lynch et al. 2000) but also affect communication inequalities. Just as with wealth and other material resources, advantages accruing from communication and information are also unequally distributed. We define communication inequalities as differences among social groups in the generation, manipulation, and distribution of information at the group level, and differences in access, use, and holding of relevant information, as well as the capacity to take advantage of it at the individual level.

Communication inequality, a structural property, requires consideration of the individual within the structural context. Some key dimensions of communication inequality include access to and use of information channels, as well as capacity to actively seek, process, and act on information. Though the picture is more complex, two indicators, formal schooling or education and income, are often used as proxies for socioeconomic position, while a third, race/ethnicity, is often part of the context of SES.

The Structural Influence Model (SIM)

Communication inequalities, one critical pathway explaining the relationship between social determinants and health outcomes, is diagrammatically offered in our framework *The Structural Influence Model (SIM) of Health*

Social Determinants	*Mediating/ Moderating Conditions*	*Health Communication Outcomes*	*Health Outcomes*
Socioeconomic position • Education • Income • Employment • Occupation **Place** • Neighborhood • Urban versus rural	**Sociodemographics** • Age • Gender • Race • Ethnicity **Social Networks** • Social capital • Resources	• Health media use and exposure • Information seeking • Attention • Information processing • Knowledge • Comprehension • Capacity for action	• Health beliefs • Incidence • Health behaviors • Prevention • Screening • Treatment • Survivorship • End-of-life care

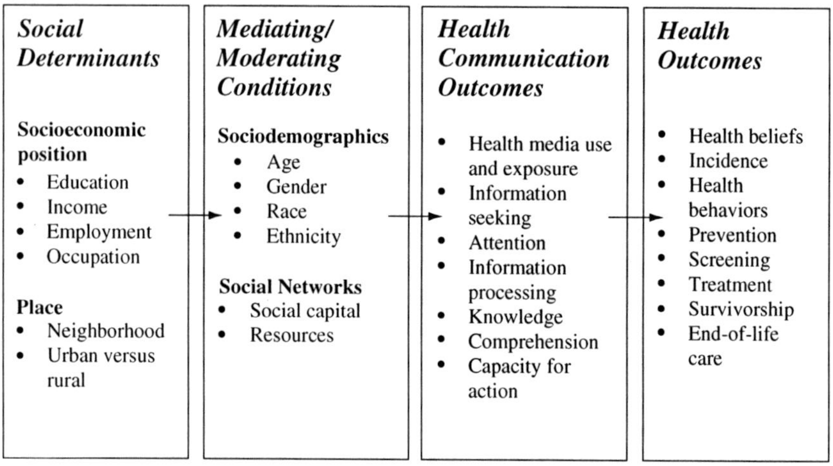

Fig. 12.1 The Structural Influence Model (SIM) of health communication

Communication (see Fig. 12.1) (Kontos et al. 2007; Viswanath & Kreuter 2007). This model is based on the premise that control of communication is power and that whoever has the capacity to generate, access, use, and distribute information enjoys social power and advantages that accrue from it (Tichenor et al. 1980; Viswanath & Demers 1999). Our model posits that health disparities can at least in part be explained by understanding how structural determinants (e.g., SES and race) lead to differential communication outcomes (such as access to and use of information channels, attention to health content, recall of information, knowledge and comprehension, and a capacity to act on relevant information).

Access to and Use of Channels of Information

Differences in access to communication services can occur across such dimensions as ease of availability of information, use of different media channels, and affordability in subscription to communications services among different SES groups. In fact, the data from National Cancer Institute's Health Information National Trends Survey (HINTS) demonstrate differential access and exposure to information services among different social groups. Income, education, and employment are positively associated with subscription to cable or satellite TV and the Internet, services that allows for access to diverse information sources. Similarly, income and education are associated with daily readership of newspapers (Viswanath 2006).

Attention to and Processing of Health Information

We argue that SES influences attention to health information and the ability to process that information. For example, various socioeconomic groups differ in the degree of attention they pay to health, with education and income positively influencing media attention (Finnegan et al. 1993; Viswanath et al. 2007). Similarly, people from low-SES groups are more likely to agree that they are so overwhelmed with the recommendations about cancer that they do not know which ones to follow.

The sheer complexity of the subject matter of health poses a significant challenge to those trying to learn, understand, and act on information. Health recommendations, of course, are often conflicting, contradictory, and/or complicated. Recommendations for infectious diseases may differ from recommendations for cardiovascular disease or for cancer. Cancer itself is many diseases with different causes, and prevention and treatment recommendations vary by type, with recommendations for diagnoses and treatment, a complex subject matter, disease and stage specific. For example, recommendation about breast cancer screening may vary depending on age and family history. Adding to this cognitive burden, screening recommendations for cancer differ from recommendations for cardiovascular disease such as blood pressure and cholesterol screening. Issues in treatment require adherence to complex drug regimens and compliance with detailed recommendations. Lastly, the recommendations and instructions change with age and life course. Such a lack of consensus and scientific disagreements on screening recommendations, and the nuanced discussions within the scientific community, only serve to reinforce public confusion on what recommendations to follow (e.g., cites for mammography) (Meissner et al. 2003a).

The confusion is greater among low-SES groups (Meissner et al. 2003b). Information on prevention for different chronic diseases is broad and varied (e.g., tobacco use or cessation for CVD or cancer prevention vs. recommendation for nutrition primarily for CVD). Furthermore, issues such as language, culture, and social status may undermine their experience with the system (Cooper & Roter 2003), placing special burdens when trying to navigate the health system.

Information Seeking Inequalities and Cancer

Information seeking has gained critical importance in health communication as patients, advocates, and scholars move away from the paternalistic model of patient-provider communication to more informed or shared decision making (IDM & SDM) (Johnson 1997; Rimer et al. 2004). This trend rests on the assumption that when people make a health-related decision, they actively look for health information, weigh the pros and cons of options, and consider their values and preferences before actively engaging in decision making with their providers (Balint & Shelton 1996; Charles et al. 2003; Rimer et al. 2004).

Despite recent reports about increased interest in health information by the general public, and the assumed importance of information seeking, not all individuals diagnosed with a serious condition actively seek information from sources other than their health care providers (Czaja et al. 2003; Leydon et al. 2000; Rees & Bath 2001). Some, in fact, intentionally avoid information that may cause them anxiety or stress, a behavior characterized as "blunting" (Folkman & Lazarus 1980; Miller 1987; Rees & Bath 2001).

Information seeking impacts cancer outcomes in a number of ways. Informed patients participate more fully in decision making (Epstein et al. 2004) and report greater satisfaction with treatment approaches (Walker 2007), which in turn is significantly associated with higher levels of emotional, social, and cognitive functioning. They also demonstrate closer adherence to treatment protocols, as well as lower reports of side effects (Schou et al. 2005). Well-informed patients are better able to cope with the diagnosis, treatment, and survivorship phases of their diseases, as well as with the effects of these phases on quality of life (Rutten et al. 2005).

Patients and their families often cite physicians and friends as their preferred sources of information (Chalmers et al. 2003; Norum et al. 2003; Rees & Bath 2000). However, various studies show that patients are also paying attention to cancer information provided by professional societies, libraries, others in their social networks, and the Internet, although the choice of sources is mediated by gender, age, and education (Carlsson 2000; Rutten et al. 2005). A review of published research from 1980 to 2003 found that preferred sources varied by stage in the treatment process as well. Patients in the diagnosis and treatment phases tended to rely on print media and information from health professionals, whereas those in the "post-treatment" phase relied more on providers and interpersonal contacts for information (Rutten et al. 2005).

So far, most of the attention on information seeking has focused on individual-level factors. For example, trust in health information gained from a variety of sources is an important driver of information seeking. As with other aspects of the patient-provider relationship, trust in the provider impacts the information exchange greatly. An environment allowing for participatory decision making and information sharing is often accompanied by, and may depend upon, high levels of trust between the patient and provider (Kraetschmer et al. 2004). Trust is also one reason that patients often turn to individuals in their social networks for information, an observation widely discussed in the social capital literature (Berkman & Glass 2000; Kawachi et al. 2004; Viswanath 2008). We also know that cancer patients are interested in gaining information from the Internet, provided that the source is a reputable website (LaCoursiere et al. 2005).

Other important drivers of information seeking regarding cancer are the beliefs the individual has about cancer diagnosis, treatment, and survivorship. For example, fatalism is often cited as a barrier to diagnosis and treatment, particularly among many African Americans and Hispanics (Reynolds 2004; Wolff et al. 2003). A recent study of African Americans' perceptions of colorectal cancer (CRC) found the disturbing theme that screening and treatment procedures may be wasted efforts and that surgery may result in the spread of the cancer (Greiner et al. 2005). One would expect that individuals who perceive action in this area to be futile would not be motivated to seek health information. Other studies have focused on individual behaviors such as "blunting" and "monitoring" (Case et al. 2005; Folkman & Lazarus 1980; Miller 1987; Rees & Bath 2001).

Despite the extensive focus on individual drivers of information seeking, more recent work has demonstrated that education is a key determinant (Ramanadhan & Viswanath 2006). More educated individuals are more likely to seek information—whether they are cancer patients or not—than the less educated. More educated people are also likely to report fewer difficulties in obtaining the information they are seeking (Arora et al. 2008).

Learning from Communication Channels

Although there is an abundance, and perhaps in some cases an overload, of health-related information available today, it is not equally distributed. This situation may have serious implications for some social groups. It has been hypothesized that one mechanism for the well-known cancer morbidity and mortality disparities between certain social and racial/ethnic groups may be differential access to, and knowledge of, cancer-relevant information (Viswanath 2005). Individuals from higher SES groups typically have higher knowledge about health than those from lower SES groups, a "knowledge gap" (Tichenor et al. 1970; Viswanath & Finnegan 1996) hypothesized to be a critical contributor to persistent health disparities.

The problem, again, is not always lack of information. The news media have paid considerable attention over the years to scientific discoveries related to a range of topics, including, in recent years, increasing attention to genetics, treatment, and cancer screening (Viswanath 2006). Mass media are a viable way for the general public to learn about health-related topics, and such knowledge clearly influences both individual and institutional behavior. However, as work in the knowledge gap has demonstrated, this increased knowledge disseminated through mass media has not had equal effects across population groups. Paradoxically, in fact, increasing information flow can widen the knowledge gap because of differential speed of information flow to various social groups. Too much information flow can also contribute to disparities because depending on educational levels, different social groups may become overwhelmed with sorting through a high volume of information, some of which may be conflicting and/or otherwise confusing.

Acting on Information

The ability to act on obtained health information depends on opportunity structure, particularly the built environment. For example, it is difficult to act on information on obesity prevention when one does not have access to decent neighborhood grocery stores, fruits and vegetables at reasonable prices, or safe neighborhoods in which to engage in physical activity. It is difficult to quit smoking if there is a lack of access to cessation aids. Lack of insurance may deter people from acting on screening recommendations. *Any effort to bridge this inequality requires efforts to offer information on possible resources that allow people to act on that information.*

Structural antecedents such as social class, race and ethnicity, and geography influence both the information environment and resources for consumption, leading to differential communication behaviors that in turn may affect actions along the public health continuum, including knowledge, prevention, detection and treatment, survivorship, and quality of life. Health disparities, therefore, could potentially be explained by inequalities in the ability to act on information, however well that information might otherwise be provided.

E-Health and Communication Technology

The proliferation of electronic communication technologies today, ranging from the Internet, mobile computing devices, and advanced cell phone technology, contribute to a broad range of venues for dissemination and "communication functionality." A growing body of scientific evidence demonstrates the potential of these communication technologies—sometimes termed "e-health"—to promote healthy behavior change. E-health applications may be deployed through any number of interactive mediums, including telephones, handheld computers, personal computers, and kiosks. A key aspect of e-health systems is their ability to be tailored to any number of personal characteristics, ranging from individual efficacy with such technology, to literacy levels, and learning style. The IOM report, *Speaking of Health* (Institute of Medicine & Committee on Communication for Behavior Change in the 21st Century: Improving the Health of Diverse Populations 2002), noted that e-health might improve adherence to behavior change efforts by providing motivation, social support, and guidance during the early phases of change.

Despite the considerable potential of new media technologies, Bonfadelli (2002) drew attention to the inequality in their diffusion and adoption, a fact that was widely reported in several earlier studies (Bonfadelli 2002; Ettema 1984; Finnegan et al. 1988; Katzman 1974; Scherer 1989; Tomita 1989; US Department of Commerce, National Telecommunications and Information Administration, & Economic and Statistics Administration 2000). The most recent data from HINTS suggest that disparities in access to media technology remain: while gaps by race/ethnicity appear to be narrowing, gaps by education remain large. As technologies become more affordable, differences in ownership that only require a one-time investment may disappear, but differences in services that require recurring expenditures (e.g., monthly fees) may endure.

In addition to unequal access to technology contributing to disparities, there are concerns about the effectiveness of e-health tools with different population groups. Despite the demonstrated empirical success of such technologies, their evaluation has rarely been extended to traditionally underserved, lower income, and ethnic minority populations (Institute of Medicine & Committee on Communication for Behavior Change in the 21st Century: Improving the Health of Diverse Populations 2002). To evaluate the extent to which such systems might be differentially efficacious, it is therefore critical to test e-health systems among sociodemographically diverse populations alone or in combination with additional supports (Viswanath & Kreuter 2007).

Inaccessibility of Web-Based Information

Accessibility of health information on the Web has also been an area of significant concern. Regardless of the assessment tool, research uniformly points out the gap between the increasing number of low SEP online users and Web content that matches their interests and needs (Pew 2005). For example, understanding most health websites requires a reading ability associated with completing at least 2 years of college (a reading level of 10th–14th grade), despite the fact that the average US adult reads only at an eighth-grade reading level (Berland et al. 2001; Croft & Peterson 2002; D'Alessandro et al. 2001; Graber et al. 2002; Kaphingst et al. 2006; Lazarus 2002). The mismatch between the average literacy skills of US adults and the literacy levels of health websites has been well documented and frequently cited as one of the main barriers to utilization of information on the Web among lower SEP groups.

One recent study evaluated the accessibility of information available on the Internet about colorectal cancer screening (CRC) screening (Kaphingst et al. 2006). Both the SMOG readability formula and the Suitability Assessment of Materials (SAM) instrument were used to assess accessibility in terms of both reading level and presentation style. The SAM instrument examines 22 factors related to reading difficulty, which are organized into six categories (i.e., content, literacy demand, graphics, layout and typography, learning stimulation and motivation, and cultural appropriateness) (Doak et al. 1996). Nineteen websites focusing on CRC screening were evaluated. The average SMOG reading grade level was 12.8. Twelve of the websites (63%) required college-level reading ability. The SAM results overall indicated that ten sites (53%) were "not suitable" for limited literacy audiences, and nine (47%) were "adequate," meaning that they would likely require some assistance to use. Specific problems with the sites included (1) lack of review of key ideas, (2) insufficient use of illustrations for key messages, (3) crowded layout and long line lengths, (4) small type size and lack of cues to highlight key content, and (5) lack of interactive features. This study confirmed that many websites providing CRC information may be too difficult for the average American adult and much too difficult for adults with limited literacy. These sites were also not utilizing unique features of the Internet that could support learning.

Importance of Other Technology-Based Approaches to Address Disparities

Health technology interventions are increasingly being considered as a strategy for increasing dissemination of effective interventions. Although the Internet has received the most attention as a "new" communication technology, efforts to address disparities must also consider new applications of existing technologies. For example, use of automated phone systems for disease management has been found to be acceptable and effective in low-income populations

(Piette 2000; Piette et al. 1999; Piette et al. 2000). Practical tools increase access to information and promote behavior changes that will simultaneously work to prevent multiple diseases across a broad range of communities. If designed appropriately in collaboration with the community, such tools could have real potential to address disparities.

Conclusion

Reduction of behavioral risk factors can lower a substantial proportion of the national cancer burden (Colditz et al. 1997). Using conservative assumptions, Byers predicted that by 2015 overall cancer incidence and mortality could be reduced by 13% and 21%, respectively, compared to 1990 baseline rates (Byers et al. 1999). To accomplish these goals, however, it is imperative that we translate our research findings about cancer risk reduction to community-based settings that have the potential to affect population health. Unfortunately, to date there has been relatively little adoption of evidence-based practices (Ellis et al. 2005; Kerner et al. 2005; Mankoff et al. 2004; Marincola 2003; National Cancer Institute of Canada Working Group on Translation), and as a result, the potential of risk reduction efforts for cancer prevention have largely been unrealized. Crowley (Crowley et al. 2004) recently characterized the field as at a crossroads, and called for the fundamental restructuring of the way in which research moves from basic science through clinical trials, as well as for the development of more effective services to improve public health.

Concomitant with this call for fundamental changes to how we move knowledge from bench to bedside and the community is the urgent moral imperative of tackling the profound disparities among different social classes and racial and ethnic groups. As has been so starkly demonstrated throughout this book, these disparities are persistent, pervasive, and seemingly intractable. The role of social determinants—including social and economic policies, neighborhoods, institutional racism, and social class—is now clear. Without a radical alteration of social structure, they will continue to perpetuate disparities at a time of radical innovations in science and medicine.

This chapter documented the profound inequalities in communication—from generating, manipulating, and disseminating information, to accessing and using that information—between different classes and races/ethnicities. It also showed that these inequalities in communication are *one* important pathway possibly linking social determinants and disparate health outcomes. Our hypothesis of the role of communication inequalities and their relationship to cancer disparities, and our review of empirical evidence, also make a third point: communication inequalities are readily modifiable and possibly less intractable than many other determinants, given the right actions at individual, institutional, and policy levels. Identifying, defining, and documenting communication inequalities, and designing appropriate interventions, thus have promise in helping to resolve disparities. At the same time, if we fail to address inequities in communication, we will effectively shut the door on addressing these longstanding inequities.

References

Arora N. K., Hesse B. W., Rimer B. K., Viswanath K., Clayman M. L., Croyle R. T. Frustrated and Confused: The American Public Rates its Cancer-Related Information-Seeking Experiences. *J Gen Intern Med.* 2008;23(3):223–228.

Balint J., Shelton W. Regaining the initiative. Forging a new model of the patient-physician relationship. *JAMA.* 1996;275(11):887–891.

Banks S. M., Salovey P., Greener S., Rothman A. J., Moyer A., Beauvais J., et al. The effects of message framing on mammography utilization. *Health Psychol.* 1995;14(2):178–184.

Berkman L, Glass T. Social integration, social networks, social support, and health. In *Social Epidemiology.* L. Berkman & I. Kawachi, eds. New York: Oxford University Press, 2000.

Berland G. K., Elliott M. N., Morales L. S., Algazy J. I., Kravitz R. L., Broder M. S., et al. Health information on the Internet: accessibility, quality, and readability in English and Spanish. *JAMA.* 2001;285(20):2612–2621.

Bonfadelli H. The Internet and knowledge gaps: A theoretical and empirical investigation. Euro *J Commun.* 2002;17:65–84.

Byers T., Mouchawar J., Marks J., Cady B., Lins N., Swanson G., et al. The American Cancer Society challenge goals: How far can cancer rates decline in the U.S. by the year 2015? *Cancer.* 1999;86:715–727.

Capella J. Integrating message effects and behavior change theories: Organizing comments and unanswered questions. *J Commun.* 2006; 56 (suppl):S265–S278.

Carlsson M. Cancer patients seeking information from sources outside the health care system. *Support Care Cancer.* 2000;8(6):453–457.

Case D. O., Andrews J. E., Johnson J. D., Allard S. L. Avoiding versus seeking: the relationship of information seeking to avoidance, blunting, coping, dissonance, and related concepts. *J Med Lib Assoc.* 2005;93(3):353–362.

Cegala D. J. Patient communication skills training: a review with implications for cancer patients. *Patient Educ Couns.* 2003:50(1):91–94.

Center for Disease Control. Cigarette Use Among High School Students—United States, 1991–2007. MMWR. 2008;57(25):686–688.

Chalmers K., Marles S., Tataryn D., Scott-Findlay S., Serfas K. Reports of information and support needs of daughters and sisters of women with breast cancer. *Eur J Cancer Care.* 2003:12(1):81–90.

Charles C. A., Whelan T., Gafni A., Willan A., Farrell S. Shared treatment in decision making: what does it mean to physicians? *J Clin Oncol.* 2003; 21(5):932–936.

Cherlin E., Fried T., Prigerson H. G., Schulman-Green D., Johnson-Hurzeler R., Bradley E. H. Communication between physicians and family caregivers about care at the end of life: when do discussions occur and what is said? *J Palliat Med.* 2005;8(6):1176–1185.

Colditz G., DeJong D., Emmons K., Hunter D., Mueller N., Sorensen G. Harvard report on cancer prevention: prevention of human cancer, volume 2. *Cancer Causes Control.* 1997;8(suppl 1).

Cooper L., Roter D. Patient-provider communication: The effect of race and ethnicity on process and outcomes of healthcare. In *Unequal Treatment: Confronting Racial and Ethnic Disparities in Healthcare.* B. Smedley A. Stith & A. Nelson, eds. Washington, DC: The National Academies Press, 2003.

Croft D. R., Peterson M. W. An evaluation of the quality and contents of asthma education on the World Wide Web. *Chest.* 2002;121(4):1301–1307.

Crowley W. F., Jr., Sherwood L., Salber P., Scheinberg D., Slavkin H., Tilson H., et al. Clinical research in the United States at a crossroads: proposal for a novel public-private partnership to establish a national clinical research enterprise. *JAMA*. 2004;291(9):1120–1126.

Czaja R., Manfredi C., Price J. The determinants and consequences of information seeking among cancer patients. *J Health Commun*. 2003; 8 (6):529–562.

D'Alessandro D. M., Kingsley P., Johnson-West J. The readability of pediatric patient education materials on the World Wide Web. *Arch Pediatr Adolesc* Med. 2001;155(7):807–812.

Dalton M. A., Sargent J. D., Beach M. L., Titus-Ernstoff L., Gibson J. J., Ahrens M. B., et al. Effect of viewing smoking in movies on adolescent smoking initiation: a cohort study. *Lancet*. 2003;362(9380):281–285.

Davey H. M., Butow P. N., Armstrong B. K. Cancer patients' preferences for written prognostic information provided outside the clinical context. *Br J Cancer*. 2003:89(8):1450–1456.

Davis K. C., Nonnemaker J. M., Farrelly M. C. Association between national smoking prevention campaigns and perceived smoking prevalence among youth in the United States. *J Adol Health*. 2007;41(5):430–436.

Davis T. C., Williams M. V., Marin E., Parker R. M., Glass J. Health literacy and cancer communication. *CA Cancer J Clin*. 2002:52(3):134–149.

Doak C. C., Doak L. G., Root J. H. *Teaching Patients with Low Literacy Skills*. Philadelphia: Lippincott Company, 1996.

Earle C. C. Cancer survivorship research and guidelines: maybe the cart should be beside the horse. *J Clin Oncol*. 2007;25(25):3800–3801.

Edelman M. *Political Language*. New York: Academic Press, 1977.

Ellis P., Robinson P., Ciliska D., Armour T., Brouwers M., O'Brien M. A., et al. A systematic review of studies evaluating diffusion and dissemination of selected cancer control interventions. *Health Psychol*. 2005;24(5):488–500.

Epstein R. M., Alper B. S., Quill T. E. Communicating evidence for participatory decision making. *JAMA*. 2004;291(19):2359–2366.

Ettema J. S. Three phases in the creation of information inequities: an empirical campaign. *J Broadcasting*. 1984;28(4):383–395.

Farrelly M. C., Davis K. C., Haviland M. L., Messeri P., Healton C. G. Evidence of a dose-response relationship between "truth" antismoking ads and youth smoking prevalence. *Am J Public Health*. 2005;95(3):425–431.

Finnegan J. R., Viswanath K., Kahn E., Hannan P. Exposure to the sources of heart disease prevention information: community type and social group differences. *Journal Q*. 1993;70(3):569–584.

Finnegan J. R., Viswanath K., Loken B. Predictors of cardiovascular health knowledge among suburban cable TV subscribers and non-subscribers. *Health Educ Res*. 1988;3:141–151.

Finney L. J., Iannotti R. J. Message framing and mammography screening: a theory-driven intervention. *Behav Med*. 2002;28(1):5–14.

Folkman S., Lazarus R. S. An analysis of coping in a middle-aged community sample. *J Health Soc Behav*. 1980;21(3):219–239.

Galea S., Vilahov D. *Handbook of Urban Health: Populations, Methods, and Practice*. New York: Sprinter, 2005.

Gamson W. A. Foreword. In *Framing Public Life: Perspectives on our Understanding of the Social World*. S. D. Reese J. R. Gandy & A. E. Grant, eds. Mahwah NJ: Lawrence Erlbaum Associates, 2001.

Gamson W. A., Modigliani A. The changing culture of affirmative action. In *Research in Political Sociology*. Vol. 3. R. D. Braungart, ed. Greenwich CT: JAI Press, 1987, pp. 137–177.

Graber M. A., D'Alessandro D. M., Johnson-West J. Reading level of privacy policies on Internet health Web sites. *J Fam Pract*. 2002;51(7):642–645.

Green M. Narratives and cancer communication. *J Commun*. 2006; 56 suppl:S163–S183.

Green M., Brock T. C. The role of transportation in the persuasiveness of public narratives. *J Pers Soc Psychol.* 2000;79(5):701–721.

Greiner K. A., Born W., Nollen N., Ahluwalia J. S. Knowledge and perceptions of colorectal cancer screening among urban African Americans. *J Gen Int Med.* 2005;20(11):977–983.

Hack T. F., Pickles T., Bultz B. D., Denger L. F., Katz A. K., Davison B. J. Feasibility of an audiotape intervention for patients with cancer: a multicenter, randomized controlled pilot study. *J Psycosoc Oncol.* 1999;17(2):1–15.

Hiatt R. A., Rimer B. K. A new strategy for cancer control research. Cancer, Epidemiol, *Biomarkers Prev.* 1999;8(11):957–964.

Hilgartner S., Bosk C. L. The rise and fall of social problems—A public arenas model. Am *J Soc.* 1988;94(1):53–78.

Hornik R. (ed.). *Public Health Communication: Evidence for Behavior Change.* New York: Lawrence Erlbaum, 2002.

Huchcroft S., Snodgrass T., Troyan S. Testing the effectiveness of an information booklet for cancer patients. *J Psychosoc Oncol.* 1984;2(2), 73–83.

Institute of Medicine, & Committee on Communication for Behavior Change in the 21st Century: Improving the Health of Diverse Populations. *Speaking of Health: Assessing Health Communication Strategies for Diverse Populations.* Washington, DC: National Academies Press, 2002.

Iyengar S. Is Anyone Responsible?: *How Television Frames Public Issues.* Chicago: University of Chicago Press, 1991.

Johnson J. The effects of a patient education course on persons with a chronic illness. *Cancer Nurs.* 1982;5(2):117–123.

Johnson J. D. *Cancer-related information seeking.* Cresskill, New Jersey: Hampton Press, Inc., 1997.

Kaphingst K., Zanfini C., Emmons K. Accessibility of web sites containing colorectal cancer information to adults with limited literacy. *Cancer Causes Control.* 2006;17(2):147–151.

Kaplan GA. What's wrong with social epidemiology, and how can we make it better? *Epidemiol Rev.* 2004;26:124–135.

Katzman N. The impact of communication technology. *J Commun.* 1974;24(4):47–58.

Kawachi I., Berkman L. Social cohesion, social capital, and health. In *Social Epidemiology.* L. Berkman & I. Kawachi, eds. New York: Oxford University Press, 2000, pp. 174–190.

Kawachi I., Kim D., Coutts A., Subramanian S. V. Commentary: Reconciling the three accounts of social capital. Int *J Epidemiol.* 2004;33(4):682–690; discussion 700–684.

Kawachi I., Kroenke C. Socioeconomic disparities in cancer incidence and mortality. In *Cancer Epidemiology and Prevention.* 3rd ed. D. Schottenfeld & J. F. J. Fraumeni. eds. Oxford: Oxford University Press, 2006.

Kerner J., Rimer B., Emmons K. M. Dissemination research and research dissemination: How can we close the gap? *Health Psychol.* 2005;24(5):443–446.

Kontos E. Z., Bennett G. G., Viswanath K. Barriers and facilitators to home computer and Internet use among urban novice computer users of low socioeconomic position. *J Med Internet Res.* 2007;9(4):e31.

Kraetschmer N., Sharpe N., Urowitz S., Deber R. B. How does trust affect patient preferences for participation in decision-making? *Health Expect.* 2004;7(4):17–326.

Kreuter M. W., McClure S. The role of culture in health communication. *Ann Rev Pub Health.* 2004;25:439–455.

Krieger N. Historical roots of social epidemiology: socioeconomic gradients in health and contextual analysis. *Intl J Epidemiol.* 2001;30(4):899–900.

Krieger N. Why epidemiologists cannot afford to ignore poverty. *Epidemiology.* 2007;18(6):658–663.

Krieger N., Chen J. T., Waterman P. D., Rehkopf D. H., Subramanian S. V. Painting a truer picture of US socioeconomic and racial/ethnic health inequalities: the Public Health Disparities Geocoding Project. *Am J Pub Health.* 2005;95(2):312–323.

LaCoursiere S. P., Knobf M. T., McCorkle R. Cancer patients' self-reported attitudes about the Internet. *J Med Internet Res.* 2005;7(3):e22.

Lauver D., Rubin M. Message framing, dispositional optimism, and follow-up for abnormal Papanicolaou tests. *Res Nurs Health.* 1990;13(3):199–207.

Lazarus W. *Online Content for low-income and under served Americans: the digital divide's new frontier: a strategic audit of activities and opportunities.* Santa Monica: Children's Partnership, 2002.

Lewis C. L., Pignone M. P., Sheridan S. L., Downs S. M., Kinsinger L. S. A randomized trial of three videos that differ in the framing of information about mammography in women 40 to 49 years old. *J Gen Intern Med.* 2003;18(11):875–883.

Leydon G. M., Boulton M., Moynihan C., Jones A., Mossman J., Boudioni M., et al. Cancer patients' information needs and information seeking behaviour: in depth interview study. *Brit Med J.* 2000;320(7239):909–913.

Liang W., Burnett C. B., Rowland J. H., Meropol N. J., Eggert L., Hwang Y. T., et al. Communication between physicians and older women with localized breast cancer: implications for treatment and patient satisfaction. *J Clin OncoL.* 2002;20(4):1008–1016.

Llewellyn-Thomas H. A., McGreal M. J., Thiel E. C. Cancer patients' decision making and trial-entry preferences: the effects of "framing" information about short-term toxicity and long-term survival. *Med Decis Making.* 1995;15(1):4–12.

Lynch J., Kaplan G. Socioeconomic position. In *Social Epidemiology.* L. Berkman & I. Kawachi, eds. New York: Oxford University Press, 2000, pp. 13–35.

Lynch J., Smith G. D., Kaplan G. A., House J. S. Income inequality and mortality: importance to health of individual income, psychosocial environment, or material conditions. *Brit Med J.* 2000;320(7243):1200–1204.

Mankoff S. P., Brander C., Ferrone S., Marincola F. M. Lost in translation: obstacles to translational medicine. J Transl Med. 2004;2(1):14.

Marincola F. M. Translational medicine: a two-way road. *J Transl Med.* 2003;1(1):1.

McPherson C. J., Higginson I. J., Hearn J. Effective methods of giving information in cancer: a systematic literature review of randomized controlled trials. *J Public Health Med.* 2001;23(3);227–234.

Meissner H. I., Rimer B. K., Davis W. W., Eisner E. J., Siegler I. C. Another round in the mammography controversy. J. Women's Health (Larchmt) 2003a; 12(3): 261–74.

Meissner H. I., Breen N., Yabroff K. R. Whatever happened to clinical breast examinations? *Am J Prev Med.* 2003b;25(3):259–263.

Meyerowitz B. E., Chaiken S. The effect of message framing on breast self-examination attitudes, intentions, and behavior. *J Pers Soc Psychol.* 1987;52(3):500–510.

Miller S. M. Monitoring and blunting: validation of a questionnaire to assess styles of information seeking under threat. *J Pers Social Psych.* 1987;52(2):345–353.

Mills M. E., Sullivan K. The importance of information giving for patients newly diagnosed with cancer: a review of the literature. *J Clin Nurs.* 1999;8(6):631–642.

Mohide E. A., Whelan T. J., Rath D., Gafni A., Willan A. R., Czukar D., et al. A randomized trial of two information packages distributed to new cancer patients before their initial appointment at a regional cancer center. Br J Cancer. 1996;73(12):1588–1593.

National Cancer Institute of Canada Working Group on Translation The language and logic of research transfer – finding common ground. Presentation Conducted by Bendixen and Associates, NCM Poll., Posted June 07, 2005.

New California Media Partnership (2005). New California Media partnership, The Ethnic Media in America: The Giant Hidden in Plain Sight.

Norum J., Grev A., Moen M. A., Balteskard L., Holthe K. Information and communication technology (ICT) in oncology. Patients' and relatives' experiences and suggestions. *Supportive Care in Cancer.* 2003;11(5):286–293.

Olien C. N., Donohue G. A., Tichenor P. J. Structure, communication, and social power: evolution of the knowledge gap hypothesis. In *Mass Communication Review Yearbook 4.* E. Wartella & D. C. Whitney, eds. Beverly Hills, CA: Sage, 1983, pp. 455–462.

Paltoo D. N., Chu K. C. Patterns in cancer incidence among American Indians/Alaska natives, United States, 1992–1999. *Pub Health Reports.* 2004;119(4):443–451.

Pew.Digital Divisions. www.pewinternet.org. 2005. Accessed October 2005.

Phelan J. C., Link B. G., Diez-Roux A., Kawachi I., Levin B. "Fundamental causes" of social inequalities in mortality: a test of the theory. *J Health Soc Behav.* 2004;45(3):265–285.

Piette J. D. Satisfaction with automated telephone disease management calls and its relationship to their use. *Diabetes Educ.* 2000;26(6):1003–1010.

Piette J. D., McPhee S. J., Weinberger M., Mah C. A., Kraemer F. B. Use of automated telephone disease management calls in an ethnically diverse sample of low-income patients with diabetes. *Diabetes Care.* 1999;22(8):1302–1309.

Piette J. D., Weinberger M., McPhee S. J., Mah C. A., Kraemer F. B., Crapo L. M. Do automated calls with nurse follow-up improve self-care and glycemic control among vulnerable patients with diabetes? *Am J Med.* 2000;108(1):20–27.

Ramanadhan S.,Viswanath K. Health and the information non-seekers: a profile. *Health Commun.* 2006;20(2):131–139.

Rees C. E., Bath P. A. The information needs and source preferences of women with breast cancer and their family members: a review of the literature published between 1988 and 1998. *J Adv Nurs.* 2000;31(4):833–841.

Rees C. E., Bath P. A. Information-seeking behaviors of women with breast cancer. *Oncol Nurs Forum.* 2001;28(5):899–907.

Reese S. D., Gandy O. H., Grant A. E., eds. Framing Public Life: Perspectives on Media and *Our Understanding of the Social World.* Mahwah, NJ: Lawrence Erlbaum Associates, 2001.

Reynolds D. Cervical cancer in Hispanic/Latino women. *Clinical J Oncology Nurs.* 2004;8(2):146–150.

Ries L. A. G., Eisner M. P., Kosary C. L., Hankey B. F., Miller B. A., Clegg L., et al., eds. *SEER Cancer Statistics Review*, 1975–2001. Bethesda, MD: National Cancer Institute, 2004.

Rimer B. K., Briss P. A., Zeller P. K., Chan E. C., Woolf S. H. Informed decision making: what is its role in cancer screening? *Cancer.* 2004;101(5 suppl):1214–1228.

Rimer B. K., Lyons E. J., Ribisl K. M., Bowling J. M., Golin C. E., Forlenza M. J., et al. How new subscribers use cancer-related online mailing lists. *J Med Internet Res.* 2005;7(3):e32.

Rutten L. J., Arora N. K., Bakos A. D., Aziz N., Rowland J. Information needs and sources of information among cancer patients: a systematic review of research (1980–2003). *Patient Educ Couns.* 2005;57(3):250–261.

Salovey P., Williams-Piehota P. Field experiments in social psychology: Message framing and the promotion of health protective behaviors. *Am Behav Scientist.* 2004;47(5):488–505.

Scherer C. W. The videocassette recorder and the information inequity. *J Commun.* 1989;39(3):94–109.

Schneider T. R., Salovey P., Apanovitch A. M., Pizarro J., McCarthy D., Zullo J., et al. The effects of message framing and ethnic targeting on mammography use among low-income women. *Health Psychol.* 2001;20(4):256–266.

Schou I., Ekeberg O., Sandvik L., Hjermstad M. J., Ruland C. M. Multiple predictors of health-related quality of life in early stage breast cancer. Data from a year follow-up study compared with the general population. *Qual Health Res.* 2005;14(8):1813–1823.

Sharp J. W. The Internet. Changing the way cancer survivors obtain information. *Cancer Pract.* 1999;7(5):266–269.

Slater M. D. Entertainment education and the persuasive impact of narratives. In Narrative Impact: *Social and Cognitive Foundations.* M. C. Green, J. F. Strange, & T. C. Brock, eds. Mahwah, NJ: Lawrence Erlbaum, 2002, pp. 157–181.

Sorensen G., Emmons K., Hunt M. K., Barbeau E., Goldman R., Peterson K., et al. Model for incorporating social context in health behavior interventions: applications for cancer prevention for working-class, multiethnic populations. *Prev Med.* 2003;37:188–197.

Stein C. J., Colditz G. A. Modifiable risk factors for cancer. *Brit J Cancer.* 2004;90(2):299–303.

Stryker J. E. Media and marijuana: A longitudinal analysis of news media effects on adolescents' marijuana use and related outcomes, 1977–1999. *J Health Comm.* 2003;8(4):305–328.

Stryker J. E., Emmons K. M., Viswanath K. (2006). Uncovering differences across the cancer control continuum: a comparison of ethnic and mainstream cancer newspaper stories. *Prev Med.* 2007;44(1):20–25.

Tichenor P. J., Donohue G. A., Olien C. N. Mass media flow and differential growth in knowledge. *Pub Opin Q.* 1970;34(2):159–170.

Tichenor P. J., Donohue G. A., Olien C. N. *Community Conflict and the Press.* Newbury Park, CA: Sage Publications, 1980.

Tomita M. R. *The role of cable television in providing information on world news: A test of the knowledge gap hypothesis.* Unpublished Doctoral Dissertation. University of Minnesota, Minneapolis, 1989.

Twombly R. Experts debate message sent by increased cancer survival rate. *J Natl Cancer Inst.* 2004;96(19):1412–1413.

US Department of Commerce, National Telecommunications and Information Administration, & Economic and Statistics Administration. Falling through the net: toward digital inclusion. http://www.ntia.doc.gov/ntiahome/digitaldivide/. 2000.

Viswanath K. The communications revolution and cancer control. *Nat Rev Cancer.* 2005;5(10):828–835.

Viswanath K. Public communications and its role in reducing and eliminating health disparities. In *Examining the Health Disparities Research Plan of the National Institutes of Health: Unfinished Business.* G. E. Thomson, F. Mitchell, M. B. Williams, eds. Washington, DC: Institute of Medicine, 2006, pp. 215–253.

Viswanath K. Social Capital and Health Communications. In *Social Capital and Health.* I. Kawachi, S. V. Subramanian, D. Kim, eds. New York: Springer, 2008.

Viswanath K., Blake K. D., Meissner H. I., Saiontz N. G., Mull C., Freeman C. S., et al. Occupational practices and the making of health news: a national survey of health and medical journalists in the United States. *J Health Comm.* 2008;13(8):759–777.

Viswanath K., Breen N., Meissner H., Moser R. P., Hesse B., Steele W. R., et al. Cancer knowledge and disparties in the information age. *J Health Comm.* 2006; 11 suppl 1:1–17.

Viswanath K., Demers D. Mass media from a macrosocial perspective. In *Mass Media, Social Control and Social Change: A Macrosocial Perspective.* D. Demers, K. Viswanath, eds. Ames, IA: Iowa State University Press, 1999, pp. 3–28.

Viswanath K., Emmons K. M. Message effects and social determinants of health: its application to cancer disparities. *J Comm.* 2006;56 suppl 1:S238–S264.

Viswanath K., Finnegan J. R. The knowledge gap hypothesis: twenty five years later. In *Communication Yearbook* 19. B. Burleson, ed. Thousand Oaks: Sage Publications, 1996, pp. 187–227.

Viswanath K., Finnegan J. R. Community health campaigns and secular trends: insights from the Minnesota Heart Health Program and Community Trials in Heart Disease Prevention. In *Public Health Communication: Evidence for Behavior Change.* R. Hornik, ed. New York: Lawrence Erlbaum, 2002, pp. 289–312.

Viswanath K., Kreuter M. W. Health disparities, communication inequalities, and eHealth. *Am J Prev Med.* 2007;32(5 suppl):S131–S133.

Viswanath K., Ramanadhan S., Kontos E. Z. Mass Media and Population Health: A Macrosocial View. In *Macrosocial Determinants of Population Health.* S. Galea, ed. New York: Springer, 2007, pp. 275–294.

Walker J. A. What is the effect of preoperative information on patient satisfaction? *Br J Nurs.* 2007;16(1):27–32.

Warren J. L., Yabroff K. R., Meekins A., Topor M., Lamont E. B., Brown M. L. Evaluation of trends in the cost of initial cancer treatment. *J Natl Cancer Inst.* 2008;100(12):888–897.

Wolff M., Bates T., Beck B., Young S., Ahmed S. M., Maurana C. Cancer prevention in underserved African American communities: barriers and effective strategies—a review of the literature. *Wisc Med J.* 2003;102(5):36–40.

Worth K. A., Dal Cin S., Sargent J. D. Prevalence of smoking among major movie characters: 1996–2004. *Tobacco Control.* 2006;15(6):442–446.

Chapter 13
Overcoming Barriers to Cancer Care: Patient and Public Perspectives

Karen Donelan

Introduction

A diagnosis of cancer thrusts patients and their loved ones into a sea of emotions, information, and life-altering decisions. A person with a frequently complex disease meets a complex health care system. The circumstances of diagnosis are variable. Some people feel completely healthy and are totally surprised by a positive cancer screening test. Others come to this moment following weeks or months of foreboding in which they either sought or even avoided a diagnosis.

The road people take to a cancer diagnosis, and the pathway they travel from that point forward, twists and turns under the influences of a host of individual and societal determinants. Variations in diagnosis, genetic makeup, age, gender, gender identity, social networks, interpersonal relationships, place of residence, travel, school, work, education, income, language, literacy, health insurance status, health service capacity, and faith, hope, and courage—all may influence what one faces throughout the cancer journey.

Added to this mix are the many disparities, described elsewhere in this volume, that exist along the cancer continuum. Substantial evidence shows numerous inequities between various groups with respect to prevention, detection, diagnosis, treatment, and follow-up. Our challenge as a society is to tailor solutions to those disparities that honor and recognize individual needs and preferences while assuring that people have access to an equal standard of care. This chapter reviews patient and public perspectives on barriers to health care that prevent us from meeting this challenge and describes the current state of research on programs and tools, including "patient navigation programs," that might reduce those barriers throughout the cancer continuum.

K. Donelan (✉)
ScD, MGH Cancer Center, Massachusetts General Hospital, Boston, MA 02114, USA
e-mail: kdonelan@partners.org

H.K. Koh (ed.), *Toward the Elimination of Cancer Disparities*,
DOI 10.1007/978-0-387-89443-0_13, © Springer Science+Business Media, LLC 2009

I. Measuring Public and Patient Perceptions of Cancer and Health

For many years, patients' voices were rarely heard in analysis of health systems and health services. Over the past two decades, however, efforts to develop patient-centered approaches to health care have taken root, with the importance of including patient perspectives in assessing health system performance and outcomes increasingly recognized. In recent years, surveys of the public about health issues have become increasingly common. In addition to periodic surveys conducted by federal agencies (e.g., the Behavioral Risk Factor Surveillance Survey (BRFSS), the National Health Interview Survey (NHIS), and the Medicare Current Beneficiaries Survey (MCBS)), various polling organizations, foundations, and disease information and advocacy organizations all conduct frequent public surveys about health care, health practices, and health outcomes. Patient surveys have also become widespread in health institutions, leading to the development of a variety of measures of patients' experience, satisfaction, and perception. The Consumer Assessment of Healthcare Providers and Systems (CAHPS) surveys are a notable example of a dedicated effort by the Agency for Healthcare Research and Quality to measure the consumer and patient experience of care.

Public Perceptions of Cancer

People view the public face of cancer on a daily basis. On any given day in the US, stories of people living with and dying of cancer can be heard everywhere. On one summer day in 2008, current media stories included Senator Ted Kennedy (D-Massachusetts) recently diagnosed with a brain tumor; Senator John McCain (R-Arizona), the Republican presidential nominee, in remission from a recurrent malignant melanoma; a well-loved professor at Carnegie Mellon University and a celebrity heartthrob movie star struggling with pancreatic cancer; and a young Olympic swimmer diagnosed with testicular cancer delaying treatment until after the Games. Indeed, the American Cancer Society indicates that approximately 1.5 million people are diagnosed with cancer each year, and approximately 550,000 will die of the disease (see also Chapter 2 of this book). Some ten million people currently alive in the US have ever had a cancer diagnosis (American Cancer Society 2007). For each patient, there is a web of family, friends, neighbors, coworkers, health professionals, and other contacts who are part of the cancer experience as well.

Cancer causes great concern and even fear. A series of national surveys probing the health concerns of the public found in each year from 2004 to 2007 that cancer was the health risk or problem that concerns Americans most. In 2007, 84% of Americans indicated that cancer is of concern to them, with 27% indicated that it was of greatest concern to them in a list of health issues (Greenberg et al. 2007).

Surveying Public Perceptions of Disadvantaged Populations

It is especially challenging to conduct surveys of the public and patients about health care in general, and about cancer more specifically—and to measure disparities related to age, race, ethnicity, insurance status, language, literacy, disability, or other populations—where access to health services may be limited. Chapter 12 of this book addresses many of these issues in detail. Even though cancer affects millions, fewer than 10% of Americans today have ever had cancer. The underserved are minorities within that minority of cancer patients. Surveys sufficiently powered to measure differences in experience and outcomes require special designs and methods. Accurate data collection can be expensive and difficult.

Designing surveys to measure disparities should include consideration of the following factors, which are discussed in the remainder of this section: key definitions, representativeness, sample size and design, questionnaire development, and response rate effort. Consideration of these factors, as well as best practices, in surveys will help to improve the quality of data collected from patients, consumers, and the public for the use of health institutions and professionals, policy makers, insurers, patients, and consumers attempting to reduce health disparities.

Definitions

Developing the capacity to monitor health outcomes among vulnerable populations requires careful attention to operational definitions of race, ethnicity, insurance, disability, language proficiency, literacy, and even cancer itself. Populations that experience diminished access to health services, and lesser quality of care once they do access the system, have been variously defined in multiple studies (e.g., Fiscella et al. 2002, Schneider et al. 2002, Asplin et al. 2005, Ponce et al. 2006).

We can illustrate the challenges of measurement by reviewing standards for measuring race and ethnicity, which are major criteria for assessing health disparities. Chapters 1 and 2 in this book also offer analyses on this topic. One common set of standards used in federal surveys—specified by the Office of Management and Budget (OMB) in 1997 and adopted by NIH for agency research in 2001—specifies five minimum race categories for data collection (American Indian or Alaska Native, Asian, Black or African American, Native Hawaiian or other Pacific Islander, and White) and two ethnicity categories (Hispanic or Latino and non-Hispanic or non-Latino). These categories are used in the US Census and are the most often used categories for health data collection (OMB 1997; NIH 2001, U.S. Census 2006). The OMB measures are commonly used, but disparities researchers use a range of measures that are not always consistent with them, further complicating measurement and analyses of racial and ethnic disparities. Other metrics include self-identification, assignment by others, vital statistics and hospital registration data, measures used in epidemiological and health services research, and even state and federal census protocols (Jones et al. 1991, Williams 1994:261, Oppenheimer 2001, Weinick et al. 2007).

Similar definitional issues exist in measuring the experience of other vulnerable or disadvantaged populations. Iezzoni and O'Day discuss the complexities of defining and measuring disability in detail in *More than Ramps: A Guide to Improving Health Care Quality and Access for People with Disabilities* (2006). Likewise, different definitions of insurance status, language proficiency, socioeconomic status, and other factors can change the measures used, the problem identified, and the solutions that can be developed to address those problems. It is essential for researchers to report definitions and measures with clarity as societal institutions try to meet federal goals to eliminate health disparities in the US.

Representativeness

Survey designs must take into account the population of interest and ask how surveys can be designed and conducted so that the data represent the population of interest. High quality surveys have well-defined populations, use a source of sample that allows for maximum coverage of that population without introducing bias, and sample the population to assure a known or equal probability of selection for people in that sample. Institutional surveys offer the opportunity to utilize list samples of patients or health professionals but may not be representative of individuals who do not seek care or who work outside of that setting. Community-based research offers the opportunity to collect data from people where they live and work, but, here too, ensuring representative sample development is more complex. This is because some survey designs may systematically under-represent or over-represent the underserved. Telephone surveys, for example, may systematically exclude people without insurance, people who live in poverty, or people with disabilities, while, at the same time, achieve better response from low literacy populations. Internet surveys will exclude people without computer access, thereby excluding disproportionate numbers of elderly, lower education, or low literacy populations. Mail surveys are inexpensive and appropriate with list samples, but will often have lower response rates, especially from people with language or literacy barriers. All of these factors must be carefully balanced to ensure representativeness.

Sample Size and Design

High-quality surveys have sample sizes sufficient to minimize sampling error and assure sufficient statistical power to analyze critical variables and outcome measures. Surveys that adequately represent the experience and views of cancer patients, especially cancer patients from underserved or vulnerable populations, often require complex sampling designs, including the use of disproportionate sampling techniques. Simple random samples are generally not sufficient to provide reliable estimates in these populations, unless they are so large as to be very costly, or unless the underlying population has high proportions of minorities. Before implementing a complex sampling design, moreover, a clear, operational definition of the variable or construct to be measured is essential.

Questionnaire Development

A particular challenge in the development of questionnaires in surveys to measure cancer disparities is the development of reliable and valid measures. As our society becomes more diverse, routine surveys will need to be conducted in multiple languages if they are to represent the diverse populations served by the US health care system. Translation is more easily accomplished with instruments that, from the outset, use plain language, omitting colloquialisms and achieving reading levels for lower literacy populations. The realities of reaching different populations in different modes also require questionnaires to be flexible enough to be administered in multiple modes whenever possible. Qualitative research to develop and test key concepts, terms, and constructs may be important as well, and pretesting is essential.

Response Rate Effort

Currently, many surveys suffer from declining response rates in all modes of data collection. Achieving desirable response rates has always been more challenging with many underserved populations, who may be hard to reach by traditional mail, telephone, and household surveys. People without insurance and with problems paying medical bills are also more likely to have problems paying housing or utilities expenses and may move more frequently or lose telephone coverage. Diligent efforts may be required to reach people whose life circumstances—cancer diagnosis, family structure, changing work habits, multiple jobs, health and disability issues, and language problems—render them difficult to reach. These same circumstances may make surveys a low priority, especially when people are undergoing cancer treatment or coping with a cancer diagnosis. High-quality surveys may thus require multiple and varied respondent contacts, multiple modes, extended data collection periods, efforts to convert non-responders and refusals, and, in some cases, incentives.

II. Unequal Access: Barriers Along the Cancer Continuum

Various major policy reports have summarized a variety of barriers faced by cancer patients that may result in disparities at many stages in the cancer continuum of care (Presidents Cancer Panel 2001, 2003, 2004, National Cancer

Institute 2008, Mead et al. 2008, Haynes and Smedley 1999, Smedley et al. 2003). These include information and education barriers (e.g., language, education, literacy, cultural competence, and communication), financial barriers (e.g., insurance, underinsurance, out-of-pocket costs, transportation costs, poverty), issues of real or perceived discrimination, including cultural sensitivity and bias, and multiple system barriers (e.g., fragmentation of care, medical record accessibility, medical appointment scheduling, interpreter capacity, transportation, and structural barriers for the disabled and frail elderly). These are not mutually exclusive factors, and disentangling their multiple effects can be complex. The cumulative effect of these barriers is unequal access to health care services in cancer prevention, detection, diagnosis, and treatment of cancers in affected populations.

Information and Education Barriers

Americans get information about cancer in many different ways (see also Chapter 12). Throughout the history of the delivery of health care services, patients and families have relied on the advice and counsel of a wide variety of professional, paraprofessional, administrative, and volunteer staff within health care organizations. Beyond the walls of health care organizations lies a complex of other health information sources as well. Print and broadcast media, community organizations, churches, friends and family, local libraries, employers, insurers, and government agencies form a large and complex web of places to turn when difficult health issues arise.

Despite the abundance of cancer information available to the public, factors such as illness or disability, literacy, numeracy, language, cognitive issues of aging, and education may all adversely impact the ability of some people to access or understand cancer information. In a 2006 Pew Internet and American Life survey, only 51% of Americans with a chronic illness and disability used the Internet, compared with 74% of Americans without a disability. However, 86% of Internet users with a health condition had looked online for information, compared with 79% of users without a disability (Pew Internet & American Life Project 2006). A 2007 Pew study reported that while 71% of non-Hispanic whites use the Internet vs. only 60% of non-Hispanic blacks and 56% of Hispanic/ Latino Americans. Only one in three (32%) of Hispanics whose dominant language is Spanish go online. The researchers concluded that most of the difference is accounted for by differences in educational attainment and English proficiency. In particular, Internet use is especially low among whites (32%), Hispanics (31%), and African Americans (25%) who have not completed high school (Pew Hispanic Center and Pew Internet Project 2007). These findings suggest that although the Internet has great promise as a provider of health information, at present not everyone in our society can use that resource.

There are comparatively few national studies about differential access to and use of cancer-specific information (see Chapter 12). In 2003 and 2005, the NCI-sponsored HINTS (Health Information National Trend Surveys) provided the public with data on popular sources of cancer information. The survey was repeated in 2007, but data are not yet public. Data from the 2005 survey, however, reveal that nearly half (48%) of American adults had looked for cancer information in the past year. More than half of those who looked for cancer information began their search on the Internet, while approximately one in four first consulted a health professional, and the remainder relied on a variety of print media and library resources. Health professionals are far preferred as trusted sources of information about cancer, although interactions with physicians are far more limited. Analyses of the HINTS survey also showed significant differences by race and ethnicity in the way Americans use this health information once it had been accessed. The survey also detected some disturbing differences in understanding of cancer screening guidelines, with Hispanics, African Americans, and American Indians/Alaska Natives all showing less knowledge about breast, cervical, and colorectal screening guidelines.

Communication within the health care system itself is also a particular problem in health systems for patients with limited English proficiency, as well as for people with impaired hearing or speech. Several patient surveys document lower patient satisfaction among patients with language barriers, as well as difficult communication with physicians resulting in unanswered questions and the feeling that their concerns were not understood (Fiscella 2002, Flores et al. 2005, 2008, Mead et al. 2008). The need for assistance from interpreters often creates delays for patients in many of their health interactions, adding a level of stress and aggravation for patients and health professionals that undermines positive communication (Iezzoni and O'Day 2006).

Financial Barriers, Financial Consequences

In March 2007, 46.5 million Americans were uninsured, and more than 60 million were underinsured. Insurance coverage in the US varies markedly by race and ethnicity—13% of non-elderly non-Latino whites were uninsured in 2006 compared with 36% of Latinos, 22% of African American, 33% of American Indian/Alaska Natives, and 17% of Asian/Pacific Islanders (Urban Institute and Kaiser Commission 2008). A study published in 2003 analyzed data from the late 1990s and concluded that while cancer patients tend to have slightly lower rates of uninsurance than the general public in the US, nearly one in ten was uninsured and one in five (20%) of Hispanic/Latino cancer patients were uninsured and incurred significantly higher out-of-pocket costs while using significantly fewer physician visits (Thorpe and Howard 2003).

Multiple studies have pointed to the hazards of being uninsured or underinsured for patients seeking cancer screening, diagnosis, treatment, and appropriate follow-up care in particular. A 2006 Kaiser Family Foundation survey of Americans who had experienced cancer personally or in their families showed that some 27% of uninsured cancer patients had at some time delayed or foregone care for their cancer because of costs. In a study published in March 2008, Halpern and colleagues found that uninsured patients are more likely to be diagnosed with colorectal, lung, melanoma, and breast cancers in stage III or IV vs. stage I cancers than are insured patients, even after controlling for age, sex, race/ethnicity, geography, and other socioeconomic factors. Finally, a recent American Cancer Society report looking at trends in insurance and underinsurance for cancer patients using data from the Medical Expenditure Panel Survey, a periodic survey of the US population, provides additional evidence that the uninsured and underinsured, especially racial and ethnic minorities, are at risk for inadequate screening and decreased survival after cancer diagnosis (American Cancer Society 2008).

Financial consequences are another burden for cancer patients who are uninsured, notably for people of color. In a national survey of households affected by cancer, patients who had ever been uninsured were significantly more likely to suffer any of several adverse consequences—46% had used up all or most of their savings, compared with 22% of insured persons, and 41% experienced problems paying for basic necessities such as food, housing, and heat, compared with 7% of the insured (USA Today/Kaiser Family Foundation 2006).

Discrimination and Bias

Health care is a microcosm of our society, and so it is both disappointing and perhaps not surprising that discrimination may find its way even into relationships where professional ethics require equal treatment. Studies have pointed to patients perceptions of bias or unfair treatment in the health care system (Saha et al. 2003, Institute of Medicine 2002). Patient perceptions of mistrust and of unfair treatment have been linked with diminished adherence to therapy and poor follow-up care.

Surveys of the public document a divide in the perception of the magnitude of this problem. A 2006 Kaiser Family Foundation survey asked the public about the quality of health care services available to whites, blacks, and Hispanic/Latino patients. While 62% of whites thought blacks and whites received the same quality of care, only 36% of blacks agreed. Conversely, the majority of blacks, 55%, indicated they thought blacks received lower quality care than whites. Latinos also indicated that they believe there is a disparity in the quality of care they receive compared to whites. While 26% of whites said Latinos get lower quality care than whites, 48% of Latinos thought this was true (Kaiser 2006).

System Barriers

The organization and capacity of our health care institutions often exacerbates the many barriers to accessible health care services for vulnerable populations. A 2006 study by the Commonwealth Fund underscores several problematic issues in health system organization. Minority and uninsured patients are less likely to have a usual source of care and more likely to rely on emergency rooms for care. These populations are more likely to receive care in community health centers and public health clinics with limited resources. Minority patients may also have more difficulty getting and keeping appointments, and African American patients are more likely to report leaving emergency rooms without getting needed care. Systematic differences in the care of minority patients with several different chronic and acute conditions within hospitals have been documented. In addition to cancer screening, other services, including vaccinations, dental visits, and mental health care, are less often provided to minority patients than to white patients (Commonwealth Fund 2006).

The time and costs of traveling to health care facilities may also be particular problems for cancer patients and their families, particularly when multiple visits are required over an extended period of time. Transportation barriers and issues of physical plant design may especially affect people with physical disabilities as they try to access the care they need, keep appointments, and avoid being skipped over when physical barriers cause delays. Iezzoni, McCarthy, and colleagues have described multiple disparities resulting in cancer patients with disabilities, including problems with access to screening, decreased use of breast conserving surgery and radiation in breast cancer patients with disabilities, and a lower rate of surgical procedures for patients with multiple cancers. Whether these differences arise from accessibility of services, patient preferences, or provider factors needs further examination (Iezzoni et al. 2008a,b, McCarthy et al. 2006, McCarthy et al. 2007).

III. Overcoming Barriers: Solutions to Reduce Cancer Disparities

Several consumer- and patient-directed initiatives have emerged in recent years as part of a national exhaustive effort to end health disparities. Activities in cancer screening, diagnosis, treatment, and follow-up have been widely developed and published. While our primary focus will be describing the opportunities and challenges of patient navigation programs, we also review several other activities representing areas of substantial progress.

Improving Consumer Health Information

We previously noted several challenges in making health information more widely available to and used by consumers. Several organizations have developed resources for patients with limited English proficiency (LEP) and made them available to the public. These include The 24 Languages Project at the University of Utah (http://library.med.utah.edu/24languages/), Ethnomed (http://ethnomed.org/) at the University of

Washington, the National Institutes of Health Medline Plus (http://www.nlm.nih.gov/medlineplus/languages/all_healthtopics.html), Healthy Roads Media (http://www.healthyroadsmedia.org/index.htm), and other websites that have been developed to try to expand the array of health information for all. Many of these sites offer materials that are downloadable for patients without Internet access.

Electronic Medical Records and Patient Access

The use of electronic medical records promises to expand the information base available for analysis of health outcomes by race and ethnicity. Such analyses are important for organizations who want to measure the quality of the care they provide to a diverse population of patients. Patient gateways in these systems may eventually provide an avenue through which patients and providers can exchange targeted information along the cancer continuum. Progress, albeit slow progress, is currently being made to expand the diffusion of these technologies: although fewer than 10% of patients currently report having access to their own records, as many as 23% of physicians have implemented basic record systems in their offices (DesRoches et al. 2008, Donelan and Miralles 2008).

Access to information technologies also appears to be expanding to open new avenues of communication with patients that might ultimately be linked with health records. A 2007 Pew study indicated that 58% of American adults have used a cell phone or personal digital assistant (PDA) to send text messages, e-mail, browse the Internet, or use other media, and 41% have logged on to the Internet away from work or home with a wireless laptop connection or handheld device. Although Internet use currently does not vary considerably by race or ethnicity, mobile connectivity varies dramatically by age, race, and ethnicity. While 53% of white respondents sent or received text messages, 68% of African Americans and 73% of Hispanic respondents had done so. While 18% of white respondents accessed the Internet on a mobile device, 27% of African American and 22% of Hispanics had done so (Health Care Association of New York State 2002, Hesse et al. 2005, Hiatt et al. 2001, Horrigan 2008).

Improving Cultural Competency of Health Providers

Multiple studies suggest that bias or implicit assumptions on the part of physicians may play a role in unequal treatment of patients in several diseases (Green et al. 2007, Sabin et al. 2008). A task force formed by the Society of General Internal Medicine recently put forth recommendations to address provider factors in health disparities. They recommend cultural competency curricula that address three areas of racial and ethnic health disparities and focus on the following specific learning objectives: (1) examining and understanding attitudes, such as mistrust, subconscious bias, and stereotyping, which practitioners and patients may bring to clinical encounters; (2) gaining knowledge of the existence and magnitude of health disparities, including the multifactorial causes of health disparities and the many solutions required to diminish or eliminate them; and (3) acquiring the skills to effectively communicate and negotiate across cultures, languages, and literacy levels, including the use of key tools to improve communication (Smith et al. 2007). Several model curricula have been developed to assist organizations in implementing cultural competency programs (see https://cccm.thinkculturalhealth.org/, http://www.hrsa.gov/culturalcompetence, http://www.aamc.org/meded/tacct/culturalcomped.pdf).

Medical interpreters have also begun efforts to create standardization and certification in their profession. Because improving communication assistance and technologies is a critical factor in patient-provider communication for patients with LEP or other sensory impairment, this is an essential step to quality improvement in health services where considerable variation exists in the provision of these critical services (Regenstein et al. 2008). New technologies, including video medical interpretation, remote medical interpretation by telephone, or Internet protocol, will enhance the ability of organizations to have qualified professional interpreters accessible in a timely way.

Improving Patient Navigation

Over the past two decades, a variety of programs have been developed to encourage cancer screening, diagnostic testing, and appropriate treatment and follow-up care among all cancer patients. "Patient navigation," a term coined by Dr. Harold P. Freeman when he established the nation's first such program in 1990 at Harlem Hospital Center, was developed as an approach to help patients overcome a variety of system barriers. The original program was intended to improve access to breast and cervical cancer screening, and results of a 5-year pilot showed improved follow-up of abnormal screening tests in patients who were "navigated" (Freeman HP et al. 1995; Freeman HP, 2004; 2006). In 2005, President Bush signed the Patient Navigator Outreach and Chronic Disease Prevention Act of 2005 (The Patient Navigator Act P. L. 109-18), authorizing $25 million from FY 2006 to FY 2010 to HRSA (Health Resources and Services Administration) to provide grants to eligible entities to recruit, assign, train, and employ patient navigators. The Act sets a priority on serving populations affected by health disparities by employing navigators with direct knowledge of the communities they serve to facilitate the care and improve health care outcomes for individuals with cancer or chronic disease.

As a result of public and private funding, patient navigator programs are now available in hundreds of health systems across the US and Canada. Several private and public sector organizations—including the Avon, Lance Armstong, Gillette, and other charitable foundations, the American Cancer Society, Pfizer, and federal and state agencies—have launched significant efforts to develop and fund similar programs in addition to the publicly funded programs.

Variations of patient navigator programs include an array of intermediaries such as health coaches, volunteers, and lay health advisors and outreach workers who guide patients who need assistance. Intermediaries may be paid or volunteer nurses, social workers, peer educators, community health workers, and others. Services are provided in person, by telephone, and by electronic communication. The patient navigator assists patients and their families through the cancer care continuum, providing services including the following: arranging various forms of financial support; arranging for transportation to, and childcare during, scheduled diagnosis and treatment appointments; identifying and scheduling appointments with culturally sensitive caregivers; coordinating care among providers (such as screening clinics, diagnosis centers, and treatment facilities); arranging for translation/interpretation services; ensuring coordination of services among medical personnel; ensuring that medical records are available at each scheduled appointment; and coordinating other services to overcome access barriers encountered during the cancer care process.

Patient navigation programs were first developed for breast and cervical cancer patients and have been reported effective in improving the timeliness of screening and abnormal follow-up appointments, enhancing access to genetic screening for high-risk patients, and improving adherence to therapy (Battaglia et al. 2007, Bickell and Young 2001, Burhansstipanov et al. 1998, Dignan et al. 2005, Dohan and Schrag 2005, Ferrante et al. 2008; Steinberg et al. 2006). Several studies, ranging from randomized trials to cohort studies, have found patient navigators helpful in improving adherence to screening colonoscopy as well (Christie et al. 2008, Chen et al. 2008, Jandorf 2005). In addition, patient navigation during radiation therapy significantly reduced interruptions in the course of treatment in a population of American Indians in South Dakota (Petereit et al. 2008) as well as in other diseases and settings (Rahm et al. 2007, Weinrich et al. 1998).

Several research challenges are posed by the proliferation of navigator programs, not the least of which is the vast array of interventions that are called by the same name. Effective evaluation of these programs will require addressing numerous issues, including defining the intervention, describing the training and role of the navigator, measuring navigator activities, tracking the use of services by patients, linking navigator activity to the medical record, differentiating whether outcomes genuinely result from activities performed or arranged by the navigator, mediating between the needs of the program to function flexibly and the need to do research in a setting with some standardization of the intervention, providing services in multiple languages, and determining whether racial/ethnic/linguistic concordance of navigator and patient is essential to effective navigation (Centers for Medicare and Medicaid Services 2003, Steinberg et al. 2006).

Recognizing the need for further research in the effectiveness of patient navigation, the National Cancer Institute (NCI) in October 2005 awarded a total of $25 million in grants as part of the Patient Navigator Research Program (PNRP). The 5-year grants are administered by NCI's Center to Reduce Cancer

Health Disparities (CRCHD). Proposals were solicited to test and evaluate navigator interventions designed to improve access to timely and appropriate cancer care and treatment following a cancer diagnosis, including improving screening, reducing time to diagnosis, increasing adherence to therapy, and improving follow-up care. These grants will focus on cancer patients from racial/ethnic minority groups, patients with low socioeconomic status, and patients from medically underserved areas.

All grantees will use several common measures including, but not limited to, the number of patients referred; type of cancer and stage at diagnosis; appointments kept/missed and reasons for missing them; number of patients accepting navigation; number of current dependents in the patient's family; reasons for accepting or not accepting navigation; baseline knowledge of cancer treatment alternatives; education/information materials provided to patient/family members; patient demographics (i.e., gender, race/ethnicity, age, socioeconomic status, primary language); patient-access barriers and time to resolve each barrier, including issues addressed in resolving access; distance of patient's home from diagnosis and treatment centers; recommended diagnostic procedures and adherence to schedule; patient's primary mode of transportation to diagnosis and treatment centers; recommended treatment procedures and adherence-to-treatment protocol; and other non-access-specific navigation services requested/provided.

IV. Conclusion

The challenges of our health care system are many, and the needs of cancer patients are as varied as their life circumstances. The demands of an increasingly diverse society are forcing constant change upon institutions that are trying to end health disparities even as the population ages, cancer care becomes more complex, and our global society presents seemingly endless possibilities in the detection, diagnosis, and treatment of cancer. New technologies that could potentially help facilitate these goals are available, but not widely disseminated. In the meantime, organizations desperate for solutions have turned to a unique approach to solving the problems of a fragmented health system: human assistance. Specifically, we look at all of the system failures that prevent us from leveraging our many societal advantages, and we ask family members, navigators, coaches, and lay advisors to step in to help. Patient navigation represents the promise of providing knowledgeable human support, timely reminders, transportation assistance, language tools, health information, and more to people who must learn to get the most out of a health system that does not provide equal access or equal outcomes to all. These programs are as plentiful as the problems they are designed to address and as varied as the populations they are designed to serve.

We need to assure that as solutions are developed and tested, they are also evaluated for effectiveness. Across the cancer care continuum, we need to assess the relative roles of human and technological assistance in overcoming system barriers. While we tailor programs and services at the local level, we need to develop some standards to assure that the methods being employed represent best practice to end disparities and relieve human suffering. Assessing the success of these programs requires that we include the voice and perspectives of patients and the public.

The barriers that patients and families face are multi-faceted. Some of those barriers exist because of disorganization of health care systems and services. The prescription for change must begin with the diagnosis of the problems and continued efforts to find workable solutions.

References

American Cancer Society. Cancer Facts and Figures, 2007. Atlanta: American Cancer Society, 2007.

American Cancer Society. Insurance and Cost Related Barriers to Cancer Care. Cancer Facts and Figures 2008. Available at: http://www.cancer.org/downloads/accesstocare/CFF2008_Special_Section.pdf. Accessed August 15, 2008.

Asplin BR, Rhodes KV, Levy H, et al. Insurance status and access to urgent ambulatory care follow-up appointments. JAMA. 2005;294(10):1248–1254.

Battaglia TA, Roloff K, Posner MA, Freund KM. Improving follow-up to abnormal breast cancer screening in an urban population. A patient navigation intervention. Cancer. 2007;109(2 Suppl):359–367.

Bickell NA, Young GJ. Coordination of care for early-stage breast cancer patients. J Gen Intern Med. 2001;16(11):737–742.

Burhansstipanov L, Wound DB, et al. Culturally relevant "Navigator" patient support. The Native sisters. Cancer Pract. 1998;6(3):191–194.

Cancer Care Nova Scotia. Cancer Patient Navigation Evaluation: Final Report. Halifax, Nova Scotia, Canada: Cancer Care Nova Scotia, 2004.

Chen LA, Santos S, Jandorf L, Christie J, Castillo A, Winkel G, Itzkowitz S. A program to enhance completion of screening colonoscopy among urban minorities. Clin Gastroenterol Hepatol. 2008;6(4):443–450. Epub 2008 Mar 4.

Centers for Medicare and Medicaid Services. Evidence report and evidence based recommendations: cancer prevention and treatment demonstration for ethnic and racial minorities. Prepared by Schneider Institute for Health Policy and the Heller School for Social Policy and Management, Brandeis University, Contract No. 500-00-0031. Baltimore: Centers for Medicare and Medicaid Services, 2003.

Christie J, Itzkowitz S, Lihau-Nkanza I, Castillo A, Redd W, Jandorf L. A randomized controlled trial using patient navigation to increase colonoscopy screening among low-income minorities. J Natl Med Assoc. 2008;100(3):278–284.

The Commonwealth Fund. 2006 Health Care Quality Survey. Available at: http://www.commonwealthfund.org/surveys/surveys_show.htm?doc_id=506847. Accessed August 15, 2008.

DesRoches CM, Campbell EG, Rao SR, Donelan K, Ferris TG, Jha A, Kaushal R, Levy DE, Rosenbaum S, Shields AE, Blumenthal D. Electronic health records in ambulatory care— A national survey of physicians. N Engl J Med 2008;359:50–60.

Dignan MB, Burhansstipanov L, Hariton J, Harjo L, Rattler T, Lee R, Mason M. A comparison of two Native American Navigator formats: face-to-face and telephone. Cancer Control. 2005;12 (Suppl 2):28–33.

Dohan D, Schrag D. Using navigators to improve care of underserved patients. Cancer. 2005;104(4):848–855.

Donelan K, Miralles P. Consumers, EHRs and PHRs: measures and measurement. In Blumenthal D, Desroches C, Donelan K, Ferris T, Jha A, Kaushal R, Rao S, Rosenbaum S, Shields A (eds). Health Information Technology in the United States: Where Do We Stand? Princeton NJ: Robert Wood Johnson Foundation, June 2008. Available from: http://www.rwjf.org/qualityequality/product.jsp?id = 31831 Accessed August 15, 2008.

Farber JM, Deschamps M, et al. Investigation and Assessment of the Navigator Role in Meeting the Information, Decisional and Educational Needs of Women with Breast Cancer in Canada. Ottawa, Canadian Breast Cancer Initiative, Centre for Chronic Disease Prevention and Control, Health Canada. 2002. http://www.hc-sc.gc.ca/pphb-dgspsp/ccdpc-cpcmc/cancer/publications/navigator_e.html Canadian Breast Cancer Initiative.

Ferrante JM, Chen PH, Kim S. The effect of patient navigation on time to diagnosis, anxiety, and satisfaction in urban minority women with abnormal mammograms: a randomized controlled trial. J Urban Health. 2008;85(1):114–124. Epub September 29, 2007. Available at: http://www.springerlink.com.ezp-prod1.hul.harvard.edu/content/16u877j728414512.

Fiscella K, Franks P, Doescher MP. Disparities in health care by race, ethnicity, and language among the insured: findings from a national sample. Med Care. 2002;40:52–59.

Flores G, Abreu M, Tomany-Korman SC. Limited English proficiency, primary language at home, and disparities in children's health care: how language barriers are measured matters. Public Health Rep. 2005;120(4):418–430.

Flores G, Tomany-Korman SC. The language spoken at home and disparities in medical and dental health, access to care, and use of services in US children. Pediatrics. 2008;121:e1703–e1714.

Freeman HP. Patient navigation: A community based strategy to reduce cancer disparities. J Urban Health. 2006;83(2):139–141.

Freeman HP. A model patient navigation program. Oncol Issues. 2004, Sept/Oct;19:44–46.

Freeman HP, Muth BJ, et al. Expanding access to cancer screening and clinical follow-up among the medically underserved. Cancer Pract. 1995;3(1):19–30.

Green AS, Carney DR, Pallin DJ, Ngo LH, Raymond KL, Iezzoni LI, Banaji MR. Implicit bias among physicians and its prediction of thrombolysis decisions for black and white patients. J Gen Intern Med. 2007 Sep;22(9):1231–1238. Epub June 27, 2007. Available at: http://www.pubmedcentral.nih.gov/articlerender.fcgi?tool = pubmed&pubmedid = 17594129

Greenberg Quinlan Rosner. 2007 Health Priorities Survey. Available at: http://healthyamericans.org/reports/files/2007HealthPriorities.pdf. Accessed August 15, 2008.

Halpern MT et al. Association of insurance status and ethnicity with cancer stage at diagnosis for 12 cancer sites: a retrospective analysis. Lancet Oncol. March 2008;9(3):222–231.

Haynes MA, Smedley BD (eds). The Unequal Burden of Cancer: An Assessment of Research and Program for Ethnic Minorities and the Medically Underserved. Washington, DC: Institute of Medicine, National Academy Press. 1999.

Health Care Association of New York State (HANYS) Breast Cancer Demonstration Project. Breast Health Patient Navigator Resource Kit. Rensselaer, NY: HANYS, 2002.

Hesse BW, Nelson DE, Kreps GL, Croyle RT, Arora NK, Rimer BK, Viswanath K. Trust and sources of health information: The impact of the Internet and its implications for health care providers. Arch Intern Med. 2005;165(22):2618–2624.

Hiatt RA, Pasick RJ, et al. Community-based cancer screening for underserved women: design and baseline findings from the Breast and Cervical Cancer Intervention Study. Prev Med. 2001;33(3):190–203.

Horrigan J. 62% of all Americans are part of a wireless, mobile population that participates in digital activities away from home or work. Pew Internet and American Life Project, March 2008.

Iezzoni LI, Ngo LH, Li D, Roetzheim RG, Drews RE, McCarthy EP. Early Stage Breast Cancer Treatments for Younger Medicare Beneficiaries with Different Disabilities. Health Serv Res. 2008a May 12. [Epub] Available at: http://www3.interscience.wiley.com/journal/120120491/abstract?CRETRY = 1&SRETRY = 0

Iezzoni LI, Ngo LH, Li D, Roetzheim RG, Drews RE, McCarthy EP. Treatment disparities for disabled Medicare beneficiaries with stage I non-small cell lung cancer. Arch Phys Med Rehabil. 2008b;89(4):595–601.

Iezzoni LI, O'Day B. More Than Ramps: A Guide to Improving Health Care Quality and Access for People with Disabilities. Oxford, New York: Oxford University Press, 2006.

Institute of Medicine, Board on Health Care Services, Care Without Coverage: Too Little, Too Late, Washington, DC: National Academy of Sciences, 2002

Institute of Medicine, Ensuring Quality Cancer Care, Washington DC: National Academy of Sciences, 2004.

Jandorf L, Gutierrez Y, Lopez J, Christie J, Itzkowitz SH. Use of a patient navigator to increase colorectal cancer screening in an urban neighborhood health clinic. J Urban Health. 2005;82(2):216–224. Epub May 11, 2005. Available at: http://www.springerlink.com.ezp-prod1.hul.harvard.edu/content/m6h4635852004x26

Jones C, LaVeist T, Lillie-Blanton M. "Race" in epidemiologic literature: an examination of the American Journal of Epidemiology, 1921–1990. Am J Epidemiol. 1991;134:1079–1084.

Kaiser Family Foundation, March/April 2006 Kaiser Health Poll Report Survey, April 2006

McCarthy EP, Ngo LH, Chirikos TN, Roetzheim RG, Li D, Drews RE, Iezzoni LI. Cancer stage at diagnosis and survival among persons with Social Security Disability Insurance on Medicare. Health Serv Res. 2007;42(2):611–628.

McCarthy EP, Ngo LH, Roetzheim RG, Chirikos TN, Li D, Drews RE, Iezzoni LI. Disparities in breast cancer treatment and survival for women with disabilities. Ann Intern Med. 2006;145(9):637–645.

Mead H, Cartwright-Smith L, Jones K, Ramos C, Woods K, Siegel B. Racial and Ethnic Disparities in U.S. Health Care: A Chartbook. The Commonwealth Fund, March 2008. Available at: http://www.commonwealthfund.org/publications/publications_show.htm?doc_id=672908. Accessed August 15, 2008.

National Cancer Institute. Health Information National Trends (HINTS) Surveys, 2003 and 2005. Available at: http://hints.cancer.gov/questions/qDisplay.jsp?specCase=0&qID=1317&dataset=2005 and http://hints.cancer.gov/questions/qDisplay.jsp?specCase=0&qID=1317&dataset=2005http://hints.cancer.gov/docs/HINTS_Brief070606.pdf. Accessed August 15, 2008.

National Cancer Institute. NCI Cancer Health Disparities Fact Sheet. Available at: http://www.nci.nih.gov/newscenter/healthdisparities. Accessed August 15, 2008.

National Cancer Institute. NCI Awards $25 Million for Patient Navigator Research Program for Minority and Underserved Cancer Patients, 10/27/2005. Available at: http://www.cancer.gov/newscenter/pressreleases/PatientNavigatorGrants. Accessed August 15, 2008.

Office of Management and Budget. Revisions to the Standards for the Classification of Federal Data on Race and Ethnicity Revisions to the Standards for the Classification of Federal Data on Race and Ethnicity Federal Register October 30, 1997. Available at: http://www.whitehouse.gov/omb/fedreg/1997standards.html. Accessed August 15, 2008.

Oppenheimer G. Paradigm lost: race, ethnicity, and the search for a new population taxonomy. Am J Public Health. 2001;91:1049–1055.

Petereit DG, Molloy K, Reiner ML, Helbig P, Cina K, Miner R, Spotted Tail C, Rost C, Conroy P, Roberts CR. Establishing a patient navigator program to reduce cancer disparities in the american Indian communities of Western South Dakota: initial observations and results. Cancer Control. 2008 July;15(3):254–259.

Ponce NA, Hays RD, Cunningham WE. Linguistic disparities in health care access and health status among older adults. J Gen Int Med. 2006;21(7):786–791.

President's Cancer Panel. Facing Cancer in Indian Country: The Yakama Nation and Pacific Northwest Tribes (President's Cancer Panel 2002 Annual Report). Bethesda, MD: National Cancer Institute, 2003.

President's Cancer Panel. Voices of a Broken System: Real People, Real Problems (President's Cancer Panel, Report of the Chairman, 2000–2001). Bethesda, MD: National Cancer Institute, 2001.

President's Cancer Panel. Living Beyond Cancer: Finding a New Balance. 2003–2004, Bethesda MD: National Cancer Institute, 2004.

Rahm AK, Sukhanova A, Ellis J, Mouchawar J. Increasing utilization of cancer genetic counseling services using a patient navigator model. J Genet Couns. 2007;16(2):171–177.

Regenstein M, Mead H, Muessig KE, Huang J. Challenges in language services: identifying and responding to patients' needs. J Immigr Minor Health. June 7, 2008.

Sabin JA, Rivara FP, Greenwald AG. Physician implicit attitudes and stereotypes about race and quality of medical care. Med Care. 2008;46(7):678–685.

Saha S, Arbelaez JJ, Cooper LA. Patient-physician relationships and racial disparities in the quality of health care. Am J Public Health. 2003;93(10):1713–1719.

Schneider EC, Zaslavsky AM, Epstein AM. Racial disparities in the quality of care for enrollees in Medicare managed care. JAMA. 2002;287:1288–1294.

Smedley BD, Stith AY, Nelson AR (eds). Unequal treatment: confronting racial and ethnic disparities in health care. Washington, DC: Institute of Medicine, The National Academies Press, 2003.

Smith WR, Betancourt JR, Wynia MK, Bussey-Jones J, Stone VE, Phillips CO, Fernandez A, Jacobs E, Bowles J. Recommendations for Teaching about Racial and Ethnic Disparities in Health and Health Care. Ann Intern Med. 2007;147:654–665.

Steinberg ML, Fremont A, Khan DC, Huang D, Knapp H, Karaman D, Forge N, Andre K, Chaiken LM, Streeter OE Jr. Lay patient navigator program implementation for equal access to cancer care and clinical trials: essential steps and initial challenges. Cancer. 2006;1;107(11):2669–2677.

Thorpe KE, Howard D. Health insurance and spending among cancer patients. Health Aff (Millwood). 2003 Jan-Jun;Suppl Web Exclusives:W3-189-98.

Urban Institute and Kaiser Commission on Medicaid and the Uninsured. Analysis of the March 2007 Current Population Survey. Available at: http://facts.kff.org/chart.aspx?ch = 365. Accessed August 8, 2008.

U.S. Census Bureau. Racial and Ethnic Classifications Used in Census 2000 and Beyond. 2006. Available at http://www.census.gov/population/www/socdemo/race/racefactcb.html. Accessed 9-17-2008.

USA Today/Kaiser Family Foundation/Harvard School of Public Health National Survey of Households Affected by Cancer, conducted Aug 1-Sept 14, 2006.

Weinick RM, Caglia JM, Friedman E, Flaherty K. Measuring racial and ethnic health care disparities in Massachusetts. Health Aff. 2007;26(5):1293–1302.

Weinrich SP, Boyd MD, et al. Increasing prostate cancer screening in African American men with peer-educator and client-navigator interventions. J Cancer Educ. 1998;13(4):213–219.

Williams DR. The concept of race in health services research. Health Services Res. 1994;29:261.

Chapter 14
Community-Based Approaches to Cancer Disparities

Barbara Gottlieb

I. Introduction

This chapter, while discussing many issues raised throughout this book, focuses on community. Such a perspective allows better understanding of disparities in health outcomes at the group, rather than the individual, level. Chapter 11 of this book addresses policy and advocacy approaches, which invariably involve community action. In this chapter, I use the broad community perspective in first understanding community assets and needs and then applying community-based interventions that appropriately address the full range of structural problems within a conceptual framework. Beginning with an overview of community-level factors that lead to cancer disparities, I then present examples of promising approaches to research and interventions at the community level and conclude with a discussion of the attributes of successful interventions, as well as recommendations for research and an action agenda that will foster structural changes to reduce cancer-related disparities.

II. Community-Level Factors Leading to Cancer Disparities

Community factors are major drivers of health status and outcomes. Community assets, including the human and physical environment, as well as public health, educational, and recreational services, can foster well being. At the same time, features of the environment—including the presence of environmental toxins, discrimination, and violence—can impair the formation of social networks, while inadequate and inappropriate services may undermine health.

As noted throughout this monograph, many studies have linked increased risk of cancer and/or adverse cancer-related outcomes to community-level factors, including environmental elements, social determinants, and inadequate access to health resources. Designing appropriate and effective policy measures,

B. Gottlieb (✉)
Harvard Medical School and Harvard School of Public Health, Boston, MA, USA

H.K. Koh (ed.), *Toward the Elimination of Cancer Disparities*,
DOI 10.1007/978-0-387-89443-0_14, © Springer Science+Business Media, LLC 2009

research, and interventions requires understanding the role of each of these domains and their potential interaction.

What Is Community?

Definitions of community can extend broadly beyond geography and labels of race, ethnicity, or sexual orientation. One definition generated by MacQueen and colleagues (MacQueen et al. 1938) reads "Community is a group of people with diverse characteristics who are linked by social ties, share common perspectives, and engage in joint action in geographical locations or settings." Focusing on domains of identity, Israel and colleagues define community as one of several levels of association, including family and friendship networks, that are "socially constructed dimensions of identity, created and recreated through social interactions." They go on to list features of community: "identification and emotional connection to other members, common symbol systems, shared values and norms, mutual—although not necessarily equal—influence, common interests, and commitment to meeting shared needs." Notably, such communities may transcend geographic borders (Israel et al. 1998).

In their discussion of Community Based Participatory Research (CBPR), Green and Mercer suggest that the definition of community may depend on the purpose of the endeavor. In the case of participatory research, they advocate a broad definition, encompassing "all who will be affected by the research results, including lay residents of a local area, practitioners, service agencies and policymakers" (Green and Mercer 2001). In any case, every program and collaboration must engage in a process to reconcile differences and similarities among its constituents for an appropriate and specific definition of community to emerge.

Physical Attributes of Community: Exposures and Resources

As noted in Chapter 3 and elsewhere, differential exposures to carcinogens can affect community cancer risks and create disparities. Industries with noxious environments tend to be located in poorer countries and, in the United States, within or adjacent to poorer communities. Not surprisingly, rates of certain cancers linked to these environments tend to be higher in these communities. For example, there are numerous reports of high rates of cancers in towns along the petrochemical refining corridor in Louisiana (Wright et al. 1996), Sunnyside, Arizona (associated with aircraft industries) (Nienaber-Clarke and Gerlak 1998), and West Dallas, Texas (associated with a lead smelter and toxic waste dumps) (Robinson 1996). Juxtaposition of poor residential neighborhoods and industry results from lower cost of housing in these areas as well as explicit social policy. Thus, when Maantay studied industrial zones in New York City, she not only found that noxious uses are concentrated in poor and minority industrial neighborhoods but documented the adverse effects of zoning policies. Specifically, they disadvantage poor communities by expanding industrial zones in those neighborhoods while rezoning areas of affluent communities for non-industrial uses (Maantay 2001).

Similarly, Cohen et al. (2003) conducted an ecological study of 107 US cities to determine the relationship between neighborhood deterioration and premature mortality. They found that controlling for race, poverty, education, population change, and health insurance coverage, "boarded-up housing" (an indicator of neighborhood deterioration) was a predictor of all-cause premature mortality due to several conditions, including cancer. The authors postulated that boarded-up housing may be a marker for neighborhoods characterized by fear and social isolation as well as restricted access to health-promoting resources such as fresh fruits, vegetables, low-fat foods, and recreational space. Furthermore, these neighborhoods tend to have an abundance of health-compromising commodities such as tobacco and alcohol, as well as high rates of street violence.

Many of these community disparities can also be linked to socioeconomic status (SES). Residence is highly correlated with social class, the exposures and deprivations of which tend to occur for long periods of an individual's life and impact health. Phillip et al. (1997), for example, describe variation in disease patterns and lifestyle in Britain according to social class. They note disparities at all ages, with lower socioeconomic groups having greater incidence of premature and low-birth weight babies at one end of the lifecourse, and greater incidence of heart disease, stroke, and some cancers later on. Many risk factors cluster in low socioeconomic groups, including lower rates of breastfeeding, higher rates of smoking, physical inactivity, obesity, hypertension, and poor diet (e.g., higher consumption of meats, full cream milk, fats, sugars, preserves, potatoes, and cereals, and lower consumption of fruit, vegetables, and whole grains). The authors point out that nutritional disadvantage continues throughout the lifespan and is related to many factors including expendable income. Households in the top one tenth income brackets spend 18% of their income on food, whereas the bottom one tenth spend a disproportionate 29%. They further point out that while genetic risks for cancer and chronic disease do not cluster according to class, environmental disadvantage will have a greater impact on those who are genetically vulnerable—thereby exerting a disproportional disadvantage on lower socioeconomic groups.

Integrating Environmental Exposures and Social Conditions with Behavior and Genetic Factors

Gastric cancer illustrates the dynamic interaction between environmental exposures, socially constructed behavioral, and individual genetic factors. Behavioral factors, including tobacco and alcohol use and dietary factors, have been found to influence rates of gastric cancer, as have genetic factors. *Helicobacter pylori* (*H. pylori*) infection has also been strongly implicated as a causal factor of gastric cancer. Geographical, socioeconomic, and trends over time in the prevalence of *H. pylori* infection correlate well with variations in mortality from stomach cancer between and within countries. Leon and Davey Smith (2000) explored the relationship between early exposures to substandard living conditions and gastric cancer in adulthood. Calculating death rates from a World Health Organization database, the authors found strong correlation between areas with high rates of infant mortality in the 1920s and current mortality from stomach cancer. They posited that exposure to *H. pylori* during childhood is associated with poor hygiene and substandard living conditions. Controlling for other early factors, and examining potential confounding effects of current circumstances, they concluded that exposure to a poor environment during infancy and childhood is associated with stomach cancer later in life. Although the full pathophysiologic pathways have yet to be elucidated, gastric cancer appears to occur in a vulnerable genetic environment that has been "turned on" by environmental and behavioral exposures. Chapter 3 in this monograph has a more detailed description of gene–environment interactions in cancer.

The concept of "weathering" by Geronimus (2000) and Geronimus et al. (2006) provides a conceptual framework that integrates the impact of environmental exposures over a lifetime on health and well-being with physiologic pathways that mediate illness and disease. According to Geronimus, the factors of poverty that are associated with poor health outcomes include "material hardships, psychosocial conditions of acute and chronic stress, overburdened and disrupted social support and toxic environmental exposures, . . . less access to information, services and technologies, . . . increased tendency to engage in some unhealthy behaviors, [and] depression" (Geronimus 2000). Geronimus points out that there is an apparent dose-response, such that long-term poverty is more devastating than shorter exposures, with a cumulative impact over a lifetime. Using the concept of allostatic load, described by McEwen and Seeman (1999), Seeman et al. (1997), and derived from NHANES III and IV data, Geronimus found that blacks had a higher weathering score than whites for all age strata. Black women consistently had higher scores than black men, while scores for white men and women were similar in all but the oldest age groups. The white–black gap remained statistically significant even when adjusted for income.

This framework therefore connects environmental factors and exposures to stress, including the stress of racism, to physiologic markers that are plausibly related to acute and chronic conditions. To illustrate this point, Geronimus finds that excess deaths between 1980 and 1990 among residents of Harlem, New York attributed to homicide remained stable and even began to decline, while excess deaths attributed to circulatory disease and cancer each doubled for young and middle-aged men. Policy and program interventions to address health disparities must systematically address structural factors. Similarly, program and policy evaluation must account for the cumulative effect of adverse exposures over a lifetime and have realistic expectations for impact and outcome.

Systemic Gaps in Supply and Access to Appropriate Health and Cancer-Related Resources

Racial and other socioeconomic disparities in access to health care and related services are well documented in the literature and elsewhere in this monograph. The physical and emotional burden of cancer and its treatments on the patient and his/her social networks is often more extended and extreme than the burdens associated with other chronic and acute illnesses. Arguably, then, gaps in supply and access to appropriate cancer-related resources can have particularly powerful impact compared to other medical conditions. Disparities exist across the continuum of cancer-related resources: education, needs assessment, screening, prevention, tracking, diagnosis, treatment, and follow-up. Furthermore, these gaps are cumulative. Incremental disparities at each step—particularly with regard to systemic gaps in supply, location, and appropriateness of service design—may magnify the disparities inherited from previous steps in the continuum as illustrated by the following examples.

Knowledge Barriers, Attitudes, and Belief Systems

"Lack of knowledge" has been identified as a major barrier to screening for a variety of cancers. Knowledge barriers to cervical and breast cancer screening among minority, low-income, and non-English speaking women have been particularly well documented by Salazar (1996), Valdina and Cargill (1997), and O'Malley et al. (1997). Knowledge barriers are likely to be greater among ethnic minorities who have less access to mainstream screening information because of language, literacy, and education barriers, as well as belief systems that may require specific information and a culturally informed approach. According to Helman (2000) folk illnesses are rooted in traditional folklore and beliefs, distinct from western scientific models. Cancer, even in modern western societies, retains qualities of a folk illness. As the late Susan Sontag (1989) observed, cancer is a powerful metaphor with strong moral overtones that can dominate the illness experience of individuals, and its interpretation by social groups. Cancer-related services must be cognizant of these metaphoric meanings and their differences between communities.

Fatalism, lack of hope, and ingrained mistrust of research may also affect willingness to participate in treatment, and may explain why rural, non-English speaking, uninsured, immigrant, and American Indian and Alaska Native populations are particularly disadvantaged in the treatment arena. For these reasons, *knowledge* as a barrier to optimal screening is best conceived of at the systems rather than the individual level, as a combination of factors that encompass access to correct information in a culturally, linguistically, and, in the idiom of this chapter, *community*-appropriate manner. Furthermore, this type of barrier is best addressed at the community and systems levels to ensure equal access to treatment.

Barriers to education and screening may be particularly challenging for newer immigrant groups, smaller communities, and groups with non-mainstream belief systems. Such barriers may underlie the increasing mortality rates for cervical cancer among foreign-born women in the United States in recent decades. Women from Asia, South and Central America, and the Caribbean, as well as new immigrants from Europe, have low rates of cervical cancer screening. Using data from the National Health Interview Survey (NHIS), Tsui et al. (2007) found that recent immigrants were twice as likely as established immigrants to have never received a Pap test, whose screening rates were close to US-born women. These differences persisted after adjusting for multiple factors known to influence screening behaviors, including income and education, and were attributed to knowledge barriers. Lee (2000) also explored barriers to cervical cancer screening among Korean American women in New York City using focus groups and found misconceptions about the causes of cervical cancer, structural barriers, including lack of insurance, and time and language barriers. The study identified notions held by individuals that are learned in a cultural context: such as fatalism ("It is God's control. We humans can't do much about it."), embarrassment ("It is Confucian upbringing. It is embarrassing and shameful to show [my] reproductive organ to others."), and lack of familiarity with the notion of preventive services. On the other hand, culturally specific beliefs can be used to advantage in an appropriately designed program. Participants expressed their beliefs in the restorative potential of yin-yang balance, the value of avoiding stress, and placing trust in health professionals.

While it is prudent to avoid generalizing from one cancer to another, across cultural groups and geographic location, and across genders, knowledge about screening and educational beliefs and practices related to cervical cancer may shed light on beliefs and practices regarding other cancers. While there are fewer studies of men's knowledge, attitudes, and perceptions of cancer and cancer screening, in fact, several studies suggest that knowledge barriers operate for men as well. Prostate cancer is the most frequently diagnosed non-dermatologic cancer, and the second greatest cause of cancer deaths among men. Although African American men are at greater risk of developing and dying from prostate cancer than any other group in the United States (Jemal et al. 2008), they are less likely to participate in prostate cancer screening. The ongoing debate about the value of prostate cancer screening certainly impacts these trends (see Chapter 8). Tingen et al. (1998) found that African American men who were not aware of the benefits of early detection were less likely to participate in free prostate cancer screening than those who were.

Qualitative research provides additional insight into knowledge barriers. Linden et al. (2007) conducted focus groups with African American women recruited from churches in Seattle regarding their willingness to participate in breast cancer screening and randomized clinical trials. Salient themes included understanding the elements of the trial, significance of the research topic to the individual and/or the community, the level of trust in the system, preference for "natural treatments" or "religious intervention" over medical treatments, cost-benefit analysis of incentives and barriers, and openness to risk versus a preference for proven treatments. While 80% expressed willingness to participate in the hypothetical trial, they simultaneously emphasized the need for a culturally diverse research staff involved in the development of protocols, recruitment, and procedures to ensure cultural sensitivity and relevance.

Language and Literacy Barriers

Language and literacy barriers are often cited as factors that differentially restrict access to cervical and breast cancer screening for women from Mexico, the Caribbean, Russia, Asia, and India. Language is an obvious potential barrier to education about cancer risks, as well as to the benefits and availability of screening. Population-based studies confirm that women who do not speak English are less likely to receive breast and cervical cancer screening according to guidelines (Jacobs et al. 2005). Using ecological variables derived from the NHIS, Wells and Horm (1998) found that residents of communities with low median education and a high concentration (70–100%) of Hispanic respondents were at risk for never having mammograms. Women residing in areas with high Hispanic concentration, low income, high concentrations of poverty, and high concentrations of recently immigrated respondents were also statistically less likely to have had clinical breast exams or Pap tests. It is noteworthy that in this study, community—rather than individual-level attributes—were associated with underscreening.

Literacy, in addition to language, can be a factor in all health behaviors. Lindau et al. (2002) studied the relationship between health literacy, ethnicity, and cervical cancer screening practices among a cohort of English-speaking adults in ambulatory clinics. Forty percent of participants had low literacy (less than a ninth grade level), including 46% of minority and 15% of white women. Literacy was the only factor independently associated with knowledge related to cervical cancer screening. Although literacy is, arguably, an individual-level factor, it is health systems that fail to identify low literacy individuals and make appropriate adaptations. In the same study, physicians recognized only 20% of those at the lowest literacy levels.

Other Communication Issues

As particularly noted in Chapters 12 and 13 in this book, communication is a key factor that can influence both immediate and long-term interaction with individual providers, the health system as a whole, and long-term health outcomes. Participation in cancer treatment is more complex than other illnesses and requires negotiation and advocacy through multiple systems including insurance, health providers, research institutions, governmental agencies, and charitable organizations. Non-literate, non-English-speaking, and politically and socially vulnerable populations will be disadvantaged in such activities.

Multiple factors are included within the broad category of communication, including information imparted by the provider, responses to patients' questions, and exploration of patients' understanding and possible misconceptions, all of which affect patients' ability to make informed decisions and take appropriate action. The quality of communication can be experienced by a patient as an indicator of respect and concern on the part of the provider (Mandelblat et al. 2003; Liang et al. 2002). Communication can influence women's perceived therapeutic options. In a qualitative study, Kreling et al. (2006) found that women of color reported relatively less communication and information, resulting in lower rates of chemotherapy use because their questions and doubts were not addressed. Ineffective communication can also perpetuate mistaken beliefs and misunderstandings that affect decision making. For example, a study of Veterans revealed the widespread notion that exposure of a lung tumor to air causes the tumor to spread. This belief was more common among African Americans than other groups, and was a major reason why African Americans refused to consider surgery when offered (Margolis et al. 2003).

Quality of communication can influence outcomes such as time to diagnostic resolution as well. Mojica et al. (2007) found that communication influenced follow-up care among Latina immigrant women with breast abnormalities at two public hospitals in Los Angeles, one of which (Hospital A) had a significantly higher inpatient and outpatient volume than the other (Hospital B). Overall, only 60% of cases had reached a diagnostic resolution (either malignant or benign) at six months after detection of an abnormality (56% at Hospital A and 73% at Hospital B). Although neither hospital provided adequate and timely follow-up, it appeared that overburdened systems, as well as larger size and more decentralized layout, may have compromised follow-up in the higher volume hospital. Individual patient-level factors did not appear to account for the differences in follow-up: participants in both groups were poor, had multiple barriers to care, and had many misconceptions about breast cancer. Communication, however, appeared to play a key role: women who were satisfied with how doctors explained their abnormality were most likely to achieve timely diagnostic resolution. A more detailed overview of communication and cancer disparities is within Chapter 12.

Comorbidities

Members of minority populations suffer a greater burden of morbidity from common chronic diseases, including diabetes, renal insufficiency, depression, and cardiovascular disease. Parallel to the way that competing demands might reduce participation in screening, this burden may differentially affect willingness to pursue treatment. Further, strict treatment protocols may exclude individuals with specific comorbidities and/or multiple chronic medications. Minorities are therefore more likely than other patients to be excluded from clinical trials.

Location of Resources

The knowledge base for treating, controlling, and palliating cancers has expanded rapidly in recent decades. Theoretically, these "technologic" solutions should be available to all. Indeed, in the pediatric age group, rates of participation in treatment and clinical trials are high, with less difference between socioeconomic groups and fewer disparities in outcomes. However, among adolescents and adults, barriers to treatment parallel barriers to cancer education and screening. In fact, barriers are magnified because of the complex nature of cancer and its treatment. Because cancer treatment is highly specialized, state-of-the art treatment often involves participation in complex treatment regimens and clinical trials and other research programs, as well as attaining access to the rapidly expanding knowledge base of oncology. These specialized resources are often geographically concentrated in treatment centers. Program resources are finite. Direct service is prioritized over the use of resources for advertisement, outreach, and dissemination of information about treatment programs and research protocols. Primary care providers are typically less involved in cancer care than other specialty care, leaving individual patients and their families to negotiate these complex systems on their own.

Geographic barriers to care are well described for a multitude of health outcomes. Like communication, location is best understood as a composite of factors. In dense urban areas, availability, cost of transportation, parking, familiarity with a site, and, in certain instances, safety of venturing inside certain communities may function as barriers. The vast geography of a country like the United States, with its remote and sparsely populated rural areas, represents an additional challenge to fair and equitable distribution of resources. In their study of prostate cancer disparities, Drake et al. (2006) described the stark urban–rural divide in South Carolina, with high concentrations of poverty, poor health status, and lack of private health insurance in rural areas. In addition, rural areas often lack public health infrastructure, including public health departments and public hospitals, and thus lack channels to disseminate health information to a geographically dispersed population. The authors suggest that this situation, in addition to exposures to potential environmental carcinogens and other possible biologic risks, may contribute to the greater risk that rural African American men face from prostate cancer.

Clinical Trial Participation Rates

Sateren et al. (2002) evaluated the impact of socioeconomic factors on accrual to National Cancer Institute (NCI)-sponsored cancer treatment trials. While accrual rates to cancer clinical trials for all adults are low, there are significant racial and socioeconomic disparities. Black males, Asian American and Hispanic males and females were accrued at lower rates than white counterparts. Accrual rates were statistically significantly higher for those with insurance and Medicare. Geography also played a significant role in accrual, with higher rates in suburban areas and in counties with higher SES measured by income, education level, and employment rates. Supply of clinical oncologists was an additional factor, with higher rates of accrual in locations with more American Society of Clinical Oncologist (ASCO) physicians and ASCO-approved cancer programs. That this same study found no significant racial disparities in the pediatric age group, whose overall accrual rates are significantly higher, suggests that structural factors can be overcome with appropriate policies, systems, advocacy, and provider motivation.

Seidenfeld et al. (2008) found similar disparities in phase 1 trials, in which 90% of participants are self-identified as white and 85% as insured. These findings confirm previous studies that point to the socioeconomic and educational status of phase 1 trial participants. Agrawal et al. (2007) also found that 96% of phase 1 clinical trial participants were insured and 62% were of moderate-high income and high educational attainment.

Summary

Exposure to carcinogens in the physical and biological environment, poor nutrition, physiologic stress (allostatic load), and inadequate access to services and physical and social resources can individually and in combination increase cancer risk and worsen outcomes among members of communities so exposed and deprived. In addition, cancer-related education, prevention, and treatment programs are inadequate in supply, distribution, and accessibility and are often inappropriate in content to address the degree of risk, prevalence, and specific needs of these communities.

III. Promising Approaches to Research and Collaboration

Communities that experience a disproportionate burden of cancer are marginalized and disempowered, largely because they lack both infrastructure and resources. We learn from Geronimus and others that these attributes of community are associated with physiologic processes that are ultimately expressed as health outcomes. Accordingly, McLeroy's ecological model proposes that health promotion programs integrate change at multiple levels, including individual, interpersonal, organizational, community, and public policy (McLeroy et al. 1988). Community-based approaches, whether explicitly employing this model or not, tend to be broad, comprehensive, and extend beyond the medical and public health sectors to effect change in social networks, neighborhoods, churches, and schools (Stokols et al. 1996). Using this ecological model to eliminate cancer disparities in communities requires an integrated approach that includes eliminating exposures that create excess risk; developing appropriate education, outreach, and screening programs; designing effective and responsive systems for follow-up and engagement in care and treatment; and effecting policy changes to promote these activities as well as ameliorate the broader socioeconomic inequalities that provide the context for health inequalities. While it is beyond the scope of this chapter to resolve racism, discrimination, and poverty, it is appropriate to identify interventions that deliberately address these factors through conscious application of principles of equity and social justice and use of strategies that enhance community assets, infrastructure, power, and voice.

Community-Based Participatory Research

Throughout the world, community members, particularly from minority and disadvantaged communities, have begun to advocate for direct involvement as partners in the design of research and intervention projects (Fals-Borda 1987; Macaulay et al. 1998; Holkup et al. 2004). There is ample evidence from social science, nursing, environmental health, and community development that involvement of community members in research and program development can positively contribute to community change (Olden et al. 2001; Duhl 1996; Wing 1996) and growing evidence that community involvement provides certain advantages over traditional approaches in recruitment, retention, and design.

Need for Community-Based Programs

Despite several decades of thoughtful and well-intended community-based programs and interventions, many programs have had only modest impact on behavior change and disease endpoints that they were designed to affect (Merzel and D'Affitti 2003). Researchers and policy makers have therefore been increasingly motivated to involve community members in research design. Green and Mercer (2001), in fact, argue that the push toward dissemination of research findings and establishment of evidence-based guidelines and "best practices" may be misguided. While such research may be well-designed, and scientifically sound from the standpoint of external validity, "best practices" are often derived from controlled trials that may not match the diverse and "real life" communities that experience excess burden of disease. They point out that systematic engagement of community members in research will lead to improved internal validity and greater likelihood of acceptability, applicability, and effectiveness in the specific settings where the research is conducted and where change is needed. Merzel and D'Affitti offer a variety of explanations for this performance gap, including the need to nurture community relationships and develop infrastructure at the initial stages of planning and implementation to uncover knowledge and experience, assure congruity with community needs and values, and utilize networks for dissemination within the community (Merzel and D'Affitti 2003).

This point is echoed in a review of tobacco-related research. Behaviors such as tobacco use are highly specific for age, gender, culture, acculturation, and other socioeconomic indicators that have not been elucidated through traditional research methods (see also Chapter 5 on tobacco use disparities). The National Conference on Tobacco and Health Disparities (NCTHD) convened to review the status of research, identify gaps, and propose an agenda to eliminate tobacco-related disparities (Fagan et al. 2004). More than a hundred of their recommendations focused on high-risk, underserved, and understudied populations. This detailed agenda includes highly specific psychosocial research regarding initiation of smoking, addiction, treatment, identification of cultural norms, and community determinants. The authors point out that the majority of the NCTHD's recommendations focus on the individual rather than on the community. They assert that attention must be paid to "comprehend the complexity of interactions among individual and community factors that influence tobacco use, cessation, and relapse." The authors identified the importance of building networks and infrastructure within communities and developing the tools for conducting community-level research to reach underserved and understudied populations. They emphasized the importance of building community capacity to conduct research so that specific and highly relevant questions could be formulated related to their own populations. The relationships that evolve would then provide channels for carrying out interventions, as well as evaluating and disseminating findings. Community-Based Participatory Research (CBPR) was identified as a potential strategy for enhancing community capacity to conduct research. In addition, governmental agencies and foundations were encouraged to increase the pool of researchers from minority and underrepresented groups from a variety of disciplines to enhance research capacity at the community level. The authors conclude that eliminating disparities will require flexible and creative strategies in research and increased attention to appropriate translation of research findings into policy.

Attributes of Community-Based Participatory Research

Participatory research is not a specific method. It is an approach to research in which community members and other stakeholders transcend the role of subjects and bring their experience and wisdom to the planning, implementation, and analysis stages of research. Participatory research has eclectic roots, drawing heavily on the writings of Freire, who championed the voice of the oppressed and advocated for education as an active process whose ultimate purpose is the positive transformation of the reality in which people live (Freire 2000). Participatory research by definition engages multiple stakeholders in an interactive and collective process that seeks to bring about action, community mobilization, capacity building, and beneficial social change (Koch et al. 2002).

The precise terminology, definition, and practice of participatory research have evolved over the years. In 1995, Green and Mercer wrote that Participatory Action Research (PAR) is (Green et al. 1995):

- Participatory;
- Cooperative, engaging community members in a joint process;
- A co-learning process for researchers and community members;
- A method for systems development and local community capacity building;
- Empowering—participants can increase control over their lives by nurturing community strengths and problem-solving abilities; and
- A way to balance research and action.

Stringer uses slightly different, but complementary language to describe PAR (Stringer, 1999):

- Democratic, enabling participation of all people
- Equitable, acknowledging people's equality of worth
- Liberating, providing freedom from oppressive, debilitating conditions
- Life enhancing, enabling the expression of people's full human potential

Community-Based Participatory Research (CBPR) is a refinement of participatory research in which the partnership is well defined. CBPR is a "collaborative approach to research that equitably involves all partners in the research process and recognizes the unique strengths that each brings. CBPR begins with a research topic of importance to the community, aims to combine knowledge with action to achieve social change, improve health outcomes, and eliminate health disparities" (Kellogg 2001). It has strong roots in community empowerment movements for social change and in asset-based approaches to community organization. Proponents recognize that complex social, economic, and historical issues affect health and that community members have unique experience and expertise related to these factors. CBPR incorporates substantive participation by community members in all stages of research, including design, implementation, analysis, and dissemination.

The Institute of Medicine (IOM) endorses CBPR as a component of public health curricula for its potential role in addressing health disparities (Gebbie et al. 2002). O'Toole et al. endorses CBPR for its potential to improve the health of disenfranchised populations and communities, and asserts the importance of recognizing it as " 'research-plus' that is both methodologically rigorous and that makes unique contributions not possible using other means" (O'Toole et al. 2003).

Israel et al. defined attributes of community-academic partnerships (CAPs) that promote successful CBPR (Israel et al. 1998):

1. Recognize community as a unit of identity.
2. Build on strengths and resources within the community.

3. Facilitate collaborative partnerships in all phases of the research.
4. Integrate knowledge and action for mutual benefit of all partners.
5. Promote a co-learning and empowering process that attends to social inequalities.
6. Involve a cyclical and iterative process.
7. Address health from both positive and ecological perspectives.
8. Disseminate findings and knowledge gained to all partners.

CBPR is particularly suited to test community-based interventions, community-based or targeted translational research, and to describe health outcomes within a community, but it may also be used to generate new knowledge about a specific question or problem. An explicit goal of CBPR is to build the capacity of community members to engage in research and to enhance social networks and infrastructure. Included with the results are, typically, a description and critique of the research process, the engagement of community members, and the process of collaboration. Ultimately, the establishment of solid networks of CBPR sites may provide channels for diffusing interventions for education, screening, early detection, and treatment trials among high risk, underserved target groups.

There is not a single blueprint for CBPR principles and practices, which may require modification in certain communities. For example, Lam et al. (2003) note in their intervention study of community health workers and Pap testing in the Vietnamese American community the cultural pattern of deferring to the authority of senior community leaders and physicians conflicts with the expectation that coalition members "empower" themselves. "We found that the Coalition members were not inclined to struggle with the research staff or one another to seize power and run this project. Instead, they established a one-member, one-vote governance structure in which the research team had one vote. Most Coalition members, already having a sense of their own power, chose to participate by formulating and implementing the project, and allowed the university-based researchers and community-based organizations to engage their complementary capacities to develop content, manage logistics, and evaluate outcomes" (Lan et al. 2003).

Challenges for CBPR

Participatory research is recognized for its potential to yield new knowledge and understanding that is highly relevant and applicable to the participating community. This knowledge can, in turn, provide the basis for effective interventions and improvement in health outcomes. However, for community-based approaches to succeed, community members and researchers must learn to collaborate in an enterprise that is different from traditional research. Commenting on their CAP, Angell et al. acknowledged the challenges to researchers in adapting to authentic partnerships with communities. Researchers must learn

...to be open to novel methods for approaching and assessing participants whose culture and level of trust may be different from those usually studied. It is vital to include underserved and understudied participants in health research, but doing so requires patience, creativity, and a trusting relationship. Researchers need to consistently demonstrate their respect toward participants and to teach them how to tell us about their experience. Community-research partnerships are a way to build a bridge between community experience and academic knowledge, improving our ability to develop interventions that are more effective for more people (Angell et al. 2003).

Research must generate new knowledge, and interventions must be designed and evaluated to reduce and eliminate cancer-related disparities. However, outsider/researcher-directed approaches have generated resistance and mistrust and yielded low rates of participation in many communities. Community members often question "traditional" approaches to experimental design, recruitment, and informed consent. This phenomenon has been studied most extensively among African Americans in the United States. Corbie-Smith et al. (1999) conducted focus groups with African American adults attending medical outpatient and oncology clinics at Atlanta's Grady Hospital. While participants endorsed a variety of reasons for participating in medical research, including obtaining state-of-the-art care and contributing to scientific knowledge, significant mistrust of researchers' motives was apparent. Participants suspected "ulterior motives," including financial reward, rather than purely altruistic motives and desire to advance science, on the part of the researchers. Moreover, participants did not understand the informed consent process, and feared "sign[ing] away" their rights without legal protection. When asked what would enhance participation, participants focused on communication: honest, clear, complete and respectful. It has been noted that many African Americans see the world through the lens of the community rather than the individual and rely on family and social networks to make decisions about participation in treatment and research (Fowler 2006). Corbie-Smith et al. concluded that participation of African Americans in research would be enhanced by inclusion of community members in research design and recruitment and by adapting a communal frame for communication and informed consent.

Pressure from community members has also led to delayed intervention designs rather than traditional control groups so that all participants can benefit from an intervention (Lam et al. 2003; Ammerman et al. 2003). "One in Eight: Women Speaking to Women," a community-based, community-designed cancer education project, for example, challenged the traditional assumption that each recruit requires the same amount of information to be informed and learns at the same rate. Instead, researchers worked closely with community partners to develop a participant-focused recruitment mode that tailored quality and quantity of recruitment contacts to match educational and informational needs, so that each potential participant could make an informed decision about participating. The community recruiters also received extensive training in research design, issues of bias in recruitment, and human subjects regulations and were closely supervised via site visits, feedback from taped assessment interviews, and frequent phone consultation (Angell et al. 2003).

Community-Based Approaches to Cancer

Community-based research encompasses a broad spectrum of research approaches that incorporate some or all of the CBPR principles. These principles have been most widely applied to community-based prevention, education, and screening interventions and are beginning to be applied to treatment. The remainder of this section describes promising interventions that use a collaborative and participatory approach in the context of various issues that appear to influence their success (location, sustainability, targeting, and capacity-building). Selected interventions illustrate the use of these approaches in a broad spectrum of cancer-related programs and a variety of types of collaborations. In evaluating this body of research and interventions, it is important to remember that community engagement and collaboration are complex processes that evolve over time. The sustainability of the collaboration, community self-knowledge, engagement, and empowerment are meaningful indicators of success along with traditionally recognized findings and outcomes (Mincker et al. 2003). For this reason, where possible, descriptions provide details about the processes of community involvement, as well as program design and health and behavioral outcomes.

Location of Interventions

Location can be a critical part of an intervention's success. Is the intervention designed at a national or local level? Where, specifically, is the intervention sited? Answers to these questions are key to determining the potential of a given intervention.

Targeting low-income African American women at high risk of not being screened for breast cancer, Kreuter et al. (2008) compared community settings that are commonly used to disseminate health information. Criteria included accessibility, opportunity, appropriateness, reach, and specificity. Data were gathered over a four-year period from more than 10,000 sites, including beauty salons, neighborhood health centers, churches, social service agencies, health fairs, laundromats, and public libraries. Of these sites, only laundromats were found to provide frequent use (high "reach") and specificity to the target audience.

As we have seen, populations that experience worse cancer outcomes often have less access to "mainstream" channels of health information because of factors including language and educational barriers, and social isolation imposed by place of residence. Community-specific strategies can utilize and strengthen social networks, thereby educating and motivating community members and activating multiple networks to engage participants and disseminate information. For example, Fisher notes that low-income African Americans may be more reliant on and responsive to informal channels, including friends and extended family, and non-health locations such as churches and community centers (Fisher et al. 1992, 1998).

Local community health centers (CHCs) can play a vital role in improving screening rates among vulnerable populations. When vulnerable populations have an identified source of care, it is likely to be a safety net provider such as a community or migrant health center. In 1995, for example, the National Center for Health Statistics (NCHS) surveyed a representative sample of CHC users drawn from a sample of health centers throughout the United States. The survey was designed to be comparable to the NHIS (Regan et al. 1999). At the time, CHCs cared for five million women, with a disproportionate burden of morbidity and mortality from cancer according to a variety of socioeconomic indicators. A significantly higher percentage of CHC women reported appropriate cervical and breast cancer screening than their low-income counterparts from the population-based NHIS. Stratified by race and ethnicity, all in the health center group except Latina women were significantly more likely to receive cervical cancer screening than their counterparts in the low-income group of the NHIS. All racial and ethnic groups of CHC users met or exceeded Healthy People 2000 guidelines for cervical cancer screening (85%) and all but white non-Hispanic women met guidelines for mammography screening. Significantly, black CHC users reported more clinical breast examinations and Pap tests than other groups of women. CHCs are thus considered successful in their breast and cervical cancer screening goals for minority, publicly insured, and uninsured women.

Safety net providers, including CHCs have limited resources and infrastructure compared to providers serving more affluent populations, particularly in relation to the high social and material needs of their clientele. Safety net providers, for example, need inexpensive strategies to improve systems for intensifying outreach and follow-up of women aged 40–79 at risk for underscreening for breast and cervical cancer. A rural Wisconsin CHC conducted a randomized trial comparing a physician reminder letter and telephone reminder to patients to usual care (Lantz et al. 1995). Screening rates were fourfold higher in the intervention group. This relatively low-cost intervention could be easily incorporated into existing systems of resource-poor health centers. This study also found that women who reported difficulty getting released from work to see a doctor were less likely to be screened. Solutions at the policy level must be sought for this barrier.

Targeting people in their own homes can improve the success of local health centers as well. Dietrich et al. (2006) designed a randomized controlled trial to test the effectiveness of a telephone support intervention to increase the rates of breast, cervical, and colorectal cancer screening among minority and low-income women at community and migrant health centers in New York City. All women were given printed guidelines for age-appropriate cancer screening and were randomized to the intervention or usual care. The intervention consisted of a series of telephone calls from a prevention care manager who was trained to address barriers to screening and motivate patients to obtain recommended screenings. Women in the intervention group were more likely to be up-to-date for all three screenings following the intervention. The proportion of women up-to-date for all three types of screenings increased 105%. This intervention can be replicated in diverse settings because it is modest in cost and utilizes non-professional staff who can be recruited from the target community. Further study of these types of intervention is needed to evaluate cost and durability of effect.

Sustainability

Sustainability is a common concern for all health interventions. Community-based interventions provide distinct opportunities for sustainability in that they rely on resources in the form of personnel, buildings, land, and social networks that exist in neighborhoods and faith-based organizations. In addition, they are often designed with explicit objectives of adding needed infrastructure, jobs, and other concrete resources to the community. One successful example is the Garden of Eden (Baker et al. 2006), a community organized and staffed market located in a church in an economically depressed community of St. Louis, Missouri. The project began as a collaboration between faith-based health advocates, lay church members, and academic researchers. Community members noted that information about healthy eating was of limited value without the access to healthy foods. A supermarket was placed in a local church that served low-income African American members. Transportation was provided to and from other churches and senior centers. Health advocates provided information, cooking demonstrations, and recipes in the store and throughout the local community. The pastor at the hosting church commented, "Too many projects come into poor communities and do research and never leave anything behind. We got involved because this effort is different." Produce was priced affordably, allowing enough profit margin that store staff could be paid a livable wage. Program governance was participatory, emphasizing community ownership and sustainability.

Targeting Individuals and Their Social Environment

Individuals encounter health information, establish health-related behaviors, and formulate health-related decisions in the context of their family and social environment. Fowler (2006) interviewed African American women in a variety of settings to determine the processes they use to decide whether or not to obtain a screening mammogram. Five social processes were mentioned with equal frequency: experiences with health systems and providers, personal religious beliefs and supports, fears and fatalistic beliefs about breast cancer, care giving responsibilities, and the opinions of significant others.

Using Traditional Community Networks and Organizing Strategies

Social networks are important across many cultures. A multi-site case study was carried out to determine how American Indian and Alaska Native (AI/AN) tribal programs implemented National Breast and Cervical Cancer Early Detection Program (NBC-CEDP) comprehensive screening guidelines in their target areas (see also Chapters 6, 9, and 11 on this topic) (Orians et al. 2004). Participatory research was used to identify key strategies employed by successful programs. All targeted the social and cultural environment and included the following: (1) reinforcing the social fabric of the community by honoring women, particularly elders, use local languages, local images, and personal testimonies; (2) using personalized contact, and exploiting the valued social role that word-of-mouth plays in Native communities; (3) having health providers use any contact to educate AI/AN people about cancer screening and early detection, given that preventive medicine visits are not the norm; (4) involving community members, particularly cancer survivors, in advisory committees; (5) utilizing local media to disseminate information; (6) making use of the AI/AN gift-giving tradition by providing non-monetary incentives for participation; and (7) continually evaluating and improving strategies and approaches.

Community-based interventions often use traditional community organizing strategies for educating communities and bringing about behavior change, including mobilizing leaders, enhancing social networks, media, and multiple simultaneous activities. Neighbors for a Smoke Free North Side (Fisher et al. 1998) used a community organizing approach to promote smoking cessation among African Americans. This controlled, quasi-experimental designed study was an academic-community partnership that involved community members in planning and implementing the program elements. The intervention involved multiple sectors of the community and created multiple levels of program infrastructure, from local neighborhoods to a citywide planning council. The project generated an array of activities, including health fairs, billboards, written promotional materials, smoking cessation classes, a youth choir "gospelfest" featuring anti-smoking songs, and informal activities such as presentations at neighborhood and church meetings. Tobacco use declined from 34 to 27% in program neighborhoods compared to a 1% decline in the control neighborhoods (34–33%). Smoking prevalence declined in all demographic sub-samples. The decrease was greatest (40–27%) among those who had "heard of the program." There was a significant decline among women of childbearing age. Despite the fact that the project areas were predominantly African American and that the program specifically targeted African

Americans, the decline in smoking was significantly higher among whites in the program area (40–24%) compared to African Americans (33–28%), suggesting the need for further targeting and intensifying the intervention. Acknowledging the limitations of the quasi-experimental design, the authors attribute the apparent success of their program to the fact that it was a locally designed and locally implemented program. They contrast their experience to the more limited success of locally implemented but nationally designed programs such as COMMIT (COMMIT Research Group 1995a,b).

Churches as Sites for Health-Related Activities

Extensive literature supports the value of churches as sites for health-related activities, both because of their role in providing social networks and social support and because of the potential role that religious participation and spirituality play in promoting health and healthful behaviors. In their literature review of health programs in faith-based organizations, DeHaven et al. (2004) found that one half focused on primary prevention, with general health maintenance, cardiovascular health, and cancer together comprising the remaining half. Programs were generally successful in promoting health, including cholesterol, blood, pressure, and weight checks, disease management, and mammograms and breast self exams. Paskett et al. (1999) examined the relationship between several indicators of religious belief and participation in cancer screening in a cohort of 290 primarily African American women. In their study, church attendance, rather than specific religious beliefs, was the only religious variable related to cancer screening frequency, supporting the notion of religious affiliation as a health-related activity. Other studies suggest that churches may provide a social network through which information and other factors that motivate health-related behaviors can be disseminated. Weinrich et al. (1998), for example, surveyed African American men who attended an educational program on prostate cancer at their church. They found that having a member of the congregation who had been diagnosed with cancer was a significant cue to participation in the educational program.

Aaron et al. (2003) also examined the relationship between church participation and health care practices among adults in an urban African American community. They found that 37% of community residents attended church at least once a month and that church attendance was associated with dental visits and blood pressure measurement. Church attendance was also positively associated, though not statistically significant, with mammography use and Pap testing. However, there were significant, interactions between church participation, insurance status, and comorbidity. For example, among uninsured women, church attendance more than doubled the likelihood of Pap testing—making church attendance almost as important as having a regular source of care. Furthermore, for women with two or more comorbid health conditions, church participation nearly doubled the likelihood of having a Pap test, similar to the effect of having a regular source of care, but had no effect on those with fewer than two comorbid conditions. In this study, church participation had a particularly positive impact on more vulnerable populations, including the uninsured and those with multiple chronic illnesses. The authors conclude that churches represent an important partner in the safety net and that collaborating with churches might strengthen public health programs targeting low-income populations. Because of their potential importance, DeHaven encourages faith-based programs to formally evaluate their impact and disseminate their findings (DeHaven et al. 2004). However, to the extent that church participation is not universal (37–52%, Taylor et al. 2000), interventions should not rely exclusively on churches.

Besides encouraging cancer screening, churches are also effective sites for primary prevention activities (Derose et al. 2000). The Black Churches United for Better Health project (Campbell et al. 1999) was designed to increase fruit and vegetable consumption as a strategy for decreasing cancer risk among rural African American church members in an area of North Carolina with excess cancer-related morbidity and mortality compared to the state as a whole. Fifty churches were matched and randomly assigned to intervention or delayed intervention. Community input was obtained through all phases of the project, and an ecological framework, targeting individual knowledge and behavior, group messaging, and establishing new social norms guided the development of project activities. Each church had a team of congregation members who guided local implementation. The 20-month project utilized informal leaders—church members who were identified as "natural helpers"—to attend bimonthly trainings on social support and stages of change. Community coalitions including churches, grocery store owners, community leaders, and farmers enacted multiple activities including classes, gospelfests, health education from the pulpit, bulletin board notices, and pamphlet distribution. At the two-year follow-up point, the intervention group consumed 0.85 more servings of fruits and vegetables than the control group, a statistically significant difference and greater than the expected increase of 0.5 servings. Noting the durability of behavior change, the authors point out that churches may represent not only an effective location for an intervention, but a potential avenue to institutionalize and maintain behavior change among regular church attendees.

Other projects suggest that churches can be successful sites for recruitment as well, which can, in turn, affect health outcomes. The Detroit Education and Early Detection (DEED) (Powell et al. 1997) study recruited African American men into a study of prostate cancer through churches and compared recruitment and outcomes with men who were seen through standard channels in a urology setting. Education, testing, and follow-up related to prostate cancer was provided to 1105 age-eligible African American men, and results and outcomes for study participants compared to those of African American and white men who presented to the urological clinic during the same time period. Despite the fact that the DEED population was older than the comparison group, it had lower average and median PSA. Of those who ultimately had malignancies, the screened group had significantly fewer late stage tumors. Of those diagnosed with cancer, 65% of DEED men, compared to 35% of African American clinic patients had organ-confined disease, and recurrence rates for the DEED population was less than one-third the rate for African American clinic patients. This study successfully recruited African American men for prostate screening, identified early stage disease, and seems to have had an impact on recurrence rates. This type of community-based screening has the potential to narrow the gap in prostate cancer outcomes for African American men.

Identifying Key Community Leaders

Effective community organizing strategies identify key individuals to serve as leaders and brokers in order to introduce a health program into a community. Religious leaders are key opinion leaders in many communities. Markens et al. (2002) interviewed pastors of black churches in Los Angeles to identify characteristics of pastors willing to engage in health-related activities as part of the Los Angeles Mammography Promotion in Churches Program, funded by the NCI. Pastors who were the most committed to the program had a holistic approach to their ministry, valuing physical along with spiritual well-being. Many were aware of the potential power of the church to influence community members and hoped to contribute to the overall health of the community. As one respondent stated, "If you don't help keep people alive, you're not going to have a congregation." Pastors were also motivated to connect their congregations with broader sectors of society and were pleased to acknowledge the concern and interest of "outsiders." Enthusiastic pastors tended to have multiple secular commitments, larger congregations, and limited resources. At the same time, some pastors were wary of participating in a research study. One respondent stated, "As black people, we've been researched and researched and researched. And people just get tired of it. And that's what my folk heard. ...We don't need nobody to come in here and research us."

Many of the positive sentiments expressed in Los Angeles were echoed in Ammerman's study of pastors and lay leaders who participated in the PRAISE! Project, a 5-year randomized trial, funded by the NCI to identify barriers to healthy eating and develop a culturally sensitive behavior change intervention in rural North Carolina. The project, which used a CBPR approach, was designed as a church-based intervention, and heavily relied on pastors and lay leaders as role models and early adopters of behavior change. Church leaders chose to participate because of interest in cancer prevention and general concern for the health of their congregations. Respondents endorsed the importance of communication, cultural sensitivity, and support. They described research as a form of giving back to the community. Leaders' and community members' expectations were met (Ammerman et al. 2003; Corbie-Smith et al. 2003). Community members expressed high levels of trust, perceived benefit, and satisfaction with the research process, and low perceived burden. The congregations reached through this intervention had limited resources and previously limited exposure to health promotion interventions.

Relationship Building

Derose et al. (2000) describe another aspect of community organizing in the Los Angeles mammography promotion program: relationship-building. To engage churches as collaborators in the program, researchers developed relationships with church and other community leaders for 10 months prior to recruitment. A variety of efforts including group and individual meetings, breakfasts, and close follow-up with individual pastors was required to build the trust that ultimately allowed researchers and church personnel to collaborate. Pastors and church members were intimately involved in the early phases of implementation, including outreach to eligible women. Despite initial mistrust on the part of some of the project's ministers, many aspects of the program succeeded. Thirty churches were randomized to test the effectiveness of telephone counseling to promote adherence to mammography screening recommendations, allowing researchers to recruit 1443 eligible women. Peer counselors were recruited and hired from the churches. The intervention included educational and behavioral goals. Peer counselors provided telephone information regarding mammography screening, identifying barriers, discussing personal risk factors, and encouraging contact with medical providers to schedule mammograms. After one year, women who were non-adherent at baseline who were randomized to the intervention group demonstrated significant improvement in mammography screening (Duan et al. 2000).

Targeting Interventions to Specific Community Needs

Community-based interventions have the potential to deliver interventions that are highly specific to the cultural, linguistic, and health needs of their populations. Many interventions successfully use lay health workers, recruited from the target population, to provide outreach and education. In a Vietnamese American community in Santa Clara County, California, for example, a coalition of community-based organizations collaborated with an academic researcher to design and implement a randomized trial to increase knowledge of cervical cancer and Pap testing (Lam et al. 2003). In this intervention, 400 Vietnamese American women were randomized to a media campaign alone ("media only" group) and a media campaign combined with lay health worker outreach ("health worker" group). The media campaign consisted of television and radio broadcasts, advertisement in Vietnamese newspapers, posters, and an information booklet distributed at medical and other community facilities. Health workers, recruited from the target population, held informational meetings to educate Vietnamese women about HPV, Pap tests, and cervical cancer, using flip charts and oral presentations. Although both arms of the intervention were associated with increased knowledge, knowledge increased more in the media plus health-worker group. This intervention seemed to be particularly effective in addressing widespread misconceptions, such as the belief that women who have not had penetrating intercourse or who are postmenopausal do not need Pap tests. The intervention also had a positive effect on behavior, with significant improvement in adherence to Pap testing guidelines in the health worker group, as well as increased expressed intention to get a Pap test. The authors conclude that using health workers replicates familiar cultural patterns of obtaining health information through intimate social networks.

In a similar study, Navarro et al. (1998) trained female Latina cancer survivors in the rural Southwest to provide education and motivation for Latina women to participate in breast cancer screening. This intervention resulted in increased knowledge of breast cancer screening among Latina women, and increased participation in breast self exam, clinical breast exam, and mammography (Hansen et al. 2005).

Another study supporting the effectiveness of concrete social support from a community member comes from Tingen et al. (1998) who conducted an intervention study to determine predictors of participation in a free prostate cancer screening program. The researchers selected 1522 primarily African American men aged 40–70 from community sites including churches, barbershops, industries, housing projects, and car dealerships. The study then compared four educational interventions: (1) traditional prostate cancer education, (2) traditional method supplemented by personal testimony by a peer educator on the importance of prostate cancer screening, (3) traditional education supplemented by a "client navigator" who assisted the participant in negotiating the health care system—via transportation, written reminders, and phone calls—to participate in screening, and (4) a combination of traditional, peer educator, and client navigator. Multivariate regression analysis determined that men who received the client navigator and the combination interventions were twice as likely to participate in prostate cancer screening than men who received the traditional intervention. This apparent "dose-response" also supports the potential for synergy between program elements and the need for interventions that are intensive among individuals and populations that experience multiple barriers.

Health worker interventions are not uniformly successful, however. In designing such interventions it is important to ascertain that the role is consistent with the cultural scripts and expectations of the community and that the intervention has sufficient reach and intensity. Campbell et al. (2004), for example, conducted a randomized trial to compare the effectiveness of a tailored print and a video intervention and a lay health advisor to increase colorectal cancer screening among 587 African Americans who were members of 12 rural North Carolina churches. The Wellness for African Americans Through Churches Project (WATCH) found that the print and video information significantly improved fruit and vegetable consumption, recreational physical activity, and increased fecal occult blood testing. The health advisor intervention, however, was not found to be effective. Authors concluded that the intervention did not reach the target population, nor did it deliver its message with sufficient intensity.

Building Capacity Through Collaboration and Coordination

Collaboration and coordination appear to be particularly effective ways to address problems in supply and distribution of resources (Probst et al. 2004), and the success of partnerships for prevention and other behavioral research has increased interest in applying this model to treatment. One striking example is the Massey Cancer Center at Virginia Commonwealth University, which collaborated with rural hospitals and providers to enhance cancer care. Oncologists at Massey provided clinical consultation at the hospitals, as well as education and telephone consultation to primary care physicians. Coordination of systems resulted in reduced cost and improved quality of care for rural breast cancer patients compared with baseline measures (Desch et al. 1999).

Focusing on CAPs, the NCI's Cancer Disparities Research Partnership (CDRP) program has funded six sites across the United States to reduce cancer disparities through a variety of strategies, including treatment trials. Rogers and Petereit (2005) describe one such partnership serving three tribes in western South Dakota. Collaborators, partners, and stakeholders include two academic medical institutions, several hospitals, the Department of Veterans Affairs, multiple tribal councils, and an array of community organizations. Collaborators faced a wide array of challenges in the early stage of the partnership: geographic distances, transportation, multiple health and federal bureaucracies, and multiple institutional review boards. At the same time, the authors affirm the importance of cultural consciousness in building effective collaborations, noting that "[p]erhaps the most fundamental obstacle to this project is the historical reality of relationships between the Lakota and non-Native American (white) populations over the past century and a half." They observe that many Native Americans in western South Dakota have had experiences or heard stories that led them to doubt their welcome in Rapid City and that "building trust" is therefore an essential component of their activities. "Trust," they continue, "requires openness, honesty, culturally appropriate messages, culturally integrated staff, services that people can appreciate, long-term commitments, consistency, patience, and time."

Infrastructure: Community-Academic Partnerships

An expanding evidence base suggests that encouraging community participation and increasing social capital are important components of strategies for reducing health disparities in a variety of communities (Cheadle et al. 2001). Recognizing the potential role of community participation, federal agencies and private foundations have encouraged the creation of CAPs (Institute of Medicine 2005). CAPs stress collaboration between community-based groups, academic partners, and public health agencies. Although CAPs are typically convened to address health disparities, they take an assets approach, beginning with an inventory of all resources. Unlike single-focused research projects and interventions, they focus broadly on an array of social determinants. Their time frame is long, typically beginning with a planning period during which diverse stakeholders are brought together and initial relationships are established, and which extend far into the future (Gasewood et al. 2006).

Community-academic partnerships can deepen a community's ability to recognize and utilize its own assets and garner resources through relationships and networks with outside institutions. By participating in CAP activities, community members develop leadership skills and the ability to participate substantively in research, community development, and policy activities. The Deep South Network for Cancer Control (DSNCC), for example, is a partnership involving public health agencies in Mississippi and Alabama, several academic institutions, and a variety of community agencies. The network's mission is to eliminate cancer disparities between African Americans in the two states through community-based interventions and research. The DSNCC trains community members in CBPR, trains community health advocates, and provides funds for research and interventions. The trust and capacity that have been built is reflected in the marked success the DSNCC has had in overcoming barriers to recruiting increasing numbers of African Americans to cancer screening and treatment trials (Partridge et al. 2005).

Addressing Social Determinants Through Partnerships

Broad collaborations with a long-term perspective can address some of the social determinants that underlie health disparities. There are many examples of such collaborations, including Poder es Salud/Power is Health, a community-based participatory prevention research project funded by the Centers for Disease Control and Prevention to reduce health disparities in African American and Latino communities in Multnomah County, Oregon (Farquhar et al. 2005). The project's name embodies the project's fundamental principle that community health and community empowerment are inextricably linked. Poder es Salud uses participatory methods to capture the voice of the community and to provide culturally specific programs for African American and Latino communities. Community health workers are carefully chosen for training in leadership, advocacy, community organizing, health promotion, and disease prevention. The community has identified priority health issues, including diabetes, cardiovascular disease, and cancer screenings. Popular education activities such as socio-dramas and learning games engage community members and activate their knowledge and understanding. These activities are carried out alongside CBPR, community assessments, and organizing. Such collaborations illustrate the extended processes that are required to build community capacity and address social determinants of health by enhancing ties among individuals and community groups, engaging a broad array of partners and building an enduring partnership with an academic institution. Metrics of evaluation must recognize that the work is iterative, slow and deliberate, and may not have tangible outcomes for a very long time.

Similarly, in New York, the Northern Manhattan Environmental Justice Partnership is a broad coalition of community groups and individuals and academic institutions formed to fight exposures to home-based and environmental hazards and neighborhood deterioration through community organizing, education, research, and political advocacy (Prakash 2008). Formed in 1997 to address the disproportionate burden of cancer, respiratory, and other chronic diseases born by Harlem and surrounding communities (Srinivasan et al. 2003), this partnership has been recognized as an example of the potential of CAPs to build community capacity. A series of trainings between 1999–2004 taught participants of a variety of ages, education, and literacy levels the science of environmental hazards and related political and regulatory issues. Trainees have themselves become leaders in the environmental justice movement, the efforts of which have led to legislation to protect children from home hazards, changes in bus routes and traffic patterns, and other concrete improvements in the community. The impact on cancer rates will take more time to measure.

Johns Hopkins' Urban Health Initiative is a broad collaboration initiated by an academic institution to "marshal the resources of the university and external groups to improve the health and well-being of the residents of East Baltimore and to promote evidence-based interventions to solve urban health problems nationwide" (Fox et al. 2004). East Baltimore residents suffer from disproportionately high rates of preventable morbidity and mortality from cancer, chronic diseases, HIV, substance abuse, low birth weight, violence, and sexually transmitted diseases. Consistent with a broad understanding of health, including the importance of infrastructure, the institute has identified three major goals: (1) strengthen research and learning; (2) reduce disparities in health and health care for East Baltimore residents; and (3) promote economic growth in East Baltimore. A broad cross-sector collaboration of community members; city officials, university staff, and faculty engaged in an extensive planning process. In keeping with an underlying commitment to align health objectives with social determinants, the planning process culminated in the formation of two categories of working groups: disease-oriented groups and community action groups, which focused on tasks such as economic revitalization, employment, the environment, and communication.

Summary

A new and valuable knowledge base is emerging from many promising examples of interventions that address barriers and engage vulnerable populations in needed services. In addition, there are models of community participation in the design and implementation of research and intervention, collaborations among providers, and partnerships between communities and academic institutions that address social determinants and hold promise to eliminate cancer-related disparities. In the next section, specific needs and gaps are discussed that must be addressed to bring community-based solutions to the next level.

IV. Recommendations

While there are many examples of successful community-based health interventions, many do not achieve their desired endpoints. The degree of behavior change is often modest and short-lived. The effectiveness of even the most successful programs may be attenuated in translation and replication. What is needed to allow communities to deliver on their potential to contribute to behavioral change, health, and well-being? In the next section, we will discuss approaches to developing the knowledge base that will be needed to eliminate cancer-related disparities. These approaches attempt to answer a variety of questions, including the following: What kinds of data support the development of effective interventions? Who should be involved in designing programs? What is known, and what do we need to know about designing and evaluating effective programs? Where should interventions take place? Are we fully incorporating the voice of community? How can the knowledge gap be closed? What are the target levels of interventions: Individuals? Communities? Systems? What policies will foster effective community-level programs?

Importance of Local Data

Nationally representative data sets often fail to collect data relevant to vulnerable populations that would be helpful in guiding policy and program development. Cancer-related behaviors, such as tobacco use, for example, are strongly influenced by culture and other community factors. National data sets, such as the Current Population Survey, fail to disaggregate data by country of origin within broad categories such as Hispanic or Asian/Pacific Islanders, or distinguish between foreign- and US-born members of the same ethnic group. In contrast, data drawn from specific locations and sub-populations reveal significant heterogeneity and patterns of difference within these broad categories (Baluja et al. 1998). Highly specific descriptive data, including length of residence in the United States, languages spoken, and age at time of immigration are needed to guide program development and target interventions at the community level.

Several studies have exemplified important differences that emerge when data are appropriately disaggregated. For example, relatively low smoking prevalence of large urban areas can mask markedly higher rates in specific communities (Northridge et al. 1998). Shah et al. (2006) compared findings from a population-based health survey conducted in six Chicago communities with corresponding data from the city as a whole. They found statistically significant differences between communities, and between the communities and the city as a whole for conditions such as hypertension, depression, asthma, and diabetes; health behaviors such as smoking and physical activity; and indicators of access to care, including insurance status and having a mammogram in the past year.

For some programs, even more specific and targeted data are needed. For example, CHCs need denominator data and adequate information systems in order to design and monitor effective surveillance and tracking programs. Moreover, creative approaches to local data can be used as leverage in the public arena. The Garden of Eden project (Baker et al. 2006) discussed above used data from a 6-month audit of food stores within a specified geographic area, measuring mean availability of fruits and vegetables. Maps of audit findings were overlaid on maps of income and racial composition and illustrated the stark findings that availability of fruits and vegetables was positively correlated with income. Race paralleled class disparities. Predominantly white areas had greater supply and selections than predominantly African American or mixed race areas. This data confirmed impressions held by community members and helped to justify the need for a produce market in the under-supplied areas. The NCTHD (Fagan et al. 2004) report on tobacco use echoed the need for highly specific data, studies of small populations, and differences within small groups in order to understand individual- and community-level factors and their complex interactions.

Measuring Relevant Constructs

Multiple streams of evidence point to the fact that racism, and the experience of racial discrimination, is responsible for many of the health disparities initially ascribed to an inaccurate notion of biological race. Guthrie et al. (2002) provide an excellent example of a detailed study of smoking behavior of adolescent African American girls. They found that experience of high levels of discrimination is common and is a risk factor for smoking. Although the study was in a small convenience sample, the findings may suggest one pathway in Geronimus' concept of weathering (Geronimus 2000; Geronimus et al. 2006), such that racial discrimination leads to tobacco use, which, in turn, has multiple health consequences. Moreover, constructs such as the experience of racism are crucial to guide program and policy interventions.

Community-Specific, Validated Tools

Besides community-based and collaborative approaches to research and appropriate data fields at the appropriate level, community-appropriate tools are required as well. To compare community-specific findings to national data sets and appropriately matched counterparts, survey instruments must be validated and calibrated to the specific community in question. In certain instances it might even be necessary to design tools for a specific community. For example, in addition to the usual challenges required for developing a questionnaire, designing the Breast Health Behavior Questionnaire (BHBQ) to measure breast health behavior among Hispanic women required extensive testing of psychometric properties in English and Spanish versions, with particular attention to Spanish idioms and literacy level (Wells et al. 2001). The result was a tool that can be used for "needs assessment, asset mapping, diagnosing and structuring of health teaching, counseling, promoting self-care, and evaluating self-care."

Linking Health to Community Voice, Community Empowerment

As the role of social determinants in health and health disparities has become increasingly clear, the link between community capacity and community empowerment and the health of the community has been recognized as a necessary, core strategy for reducing health disparities. Certain universal principles underlie this approach, particularly recognition of community assets and the need to enhance material and other resources within the community, honor and enhance the knowledge and leadership of community members, build from the inside-out rather than the outside-in (Kretzmann and McKnight 1993), and build collaborations and partnerships intentionally, with full respect for the contribution of community partners (http://depts.washington.edu/ccph/principles.html#principles. Accessed 7/29/2008). However, beyond these broad principles, historical, cultural, geographic, local, and other community-specific factors should influence the priorities and processes for community empowerment and capacity building.

New and existing partnerships and collaborations must also allow time for the exploration and expression of core community values and beliefs. For example, Chino and DeBruyn (2000) contend that Western models that are "linear, static, time-oriented" may not reflect the values and perspectives of indigenous communities. They contend that indigenous people must acknowledge and heal the wounds caused by colonization, historical trauma, and racism before entering into the first steps of a Western-defined planning process. They further assert that for Native and non-Native partners to collaborate, there must be a participatory process that allows for "mutual learning... without the potential for abuses and exploitation and [that] repair(s) lines of trust between non-indigenous researchers and tribal communities." They go on to describe a process for program design and community development that has been used successfully to address a variety of health issues, including cancer, partner violence, and health disparities. The four steps parallel the life course: (1) building relationships (infancy and childhood)—focusing on establishing open communication and identifying common ground and goals; (2) building skills (adolescence)—honoring the concept of mastery and allowing participants to develop interpersonal and practical skills; (3) working together (adulthood)—"interdependence"—integrating the tradition of community and reinforcing the notion that groups are stronger when they solve problems together; and (4) promoting commitment (elders)—encouraging participants to examine their responsibility and give back to community and family as advocates and mentors. The authors note that this approach is readily embraced by indigenous people because it is "deeply embedded in history and context...goes beyond the surface structure of cultural competence to the deeper structure of the cultural, historical, social and environmental forces that shape health behaviors among indigenous people." Every community has fundamental values and philosophies that must be expressed in evolving partnerships and collaborations. To shortchange the expression of such values risks trust and perhaps the viability of the partnership.

Flaskerud critically reviews two approaches to inclusion of women and ethnic and racial minorities in research and offers a framework for improving participation of these underserved groups (Flaskerud and Nyamathi 2000). The cultural responsiveness approach (Sue et al. 1991) focuses on the similarity between the researcher and the participants in language, gender, and ethnicity. Similarity engenders greater participation. In contrast, the resource provision perspective focuses on providing economic and social resources to empower community members to participate in research (Flaskerud and Winslow 1998). Flaskerud contends that the latter is the operative construct. She argues that it is the lack of resources rather than contrasting values and attitudes that keep marginalized, low-income women, and people of color from participating in research. While not negating the importance of language and cultural barriers nor the importance of research being culturally responsive, Flaskerud concludes that participants must be provided with financial support, skills, and knowledge and that research budgets must anticipate these costs. While Flaskerud's review focuses on participation in research, her conclusions are relevant to screening, prevention, and treatment as well.

Identifying Key Targets in Eliminating Cancer-Related Disparities

As noted, all aspects of cancer-related activities, including education, screening, prevention, treatment, and follow-up, reflect and contribute to cancer-related disparities. Understanding the relative contribution of each in order to identify sentinel indicators and key targets for intervention is critical. However, unlike other conditions for which there are disparities, cancer is not a single entity. It is likely that key targets will differ according to type of cancer, gender, race/ethnicity, geographic location, and the myriad definitions of community. In addition to identifying gaps and effective interventions in the important domains of cancer activities, attention should ideally be paid to identifying key leverage points. However, in the absence of this information, interventions should err on the side of inclusiveness, and even redundancy, to avoid excluding populations and inadvertently furthering disparities.

Education, prevention, and screening have a predictable, yet hypothetical impact on cancer disparities. In contrast, disparities related to treatment are concrete at least to the extent that treatment involves individuals who have, in fact, been diagnosed with cancers. In the interest of justice and equity, it is therefore appropriate to devote specific and immediate efforts and attention to reducing disparities related to treatment. These would include the following: (1) increasing community, patient, and provider knowledge; (2) developing broad public campaigns on the availability and effectiveness of cancer treatments; (3) enhancing the knowledge and role of safety net and other primary care providers in facilitating involvement of underserved populations in treatment; (4) enhancing capacity to serve underserved cancer patients; (5) developing the role of case managers, advocates, and patient navigators to connect and maintain patients' ability to engage in treatment; (6) developing treatment consortia to span geographically underserved areas; (7) providing cancer treatment programs, including those engaging in clinical trials, with adequate resources for outreach to underserved communities; (8) examining barriers to participation in cancer treatment, including clinical trials that are particularly relevant to underserved communities; and (9) developing interventions to address these barriers. These interventions might include re-examination of exclusion criteria from clinical trials, culturally sensitive recruitment, consent and retention procedures, and accessible location of treatment facilities.

Changing Public Policy Focus

Public policy must recognize its powerful role in establishing norms and effecting behavior change. Health outcomes are expressed at the individual and even smaller biological levels—as in the expression of genes, cellular behavior, and sub-cellular chemical reactions. However, public policy has the ability to generate change and effect improvement in these health outcomes through its capacity to communicate to large numbers of people and reframe norms, and through its ability to prioritize and shift resources. In this vast spectrum, community is where policy and biology meet. Resources are distributed (or not) among communities. Educational messages, knowledge, and norms are filtered—interpreted and diffused—through communities. For communities to deliver on their potential to eliminate cancer disparities, public policy must recognize and facilitate this pivotal role of communities.

To begin with, public policy must recognize the reality that health disparities reflect societal problems that cannot be addressed solely through the health sector. It is unrealistic, and potentially damaging to public confidence, to expect the health sector to eliminate violence, infant mortality, or disparities in cancer on its own. Rather, social policies must address broad social determinants of health—specifically, housing, environment, employment, education, and protection of vulnerable populations such as children, elders, and immigrants, as well as the poor and the sick. With such policies in place, the health sector will be able to contribute its unique and crucial role in eliminating disparities more effectively.

We also need to recognize that safety net providers must receive adequate resources to care for the most vulnerable members of society. This includes resources to maintain programs already known to be effective, as well as resources to develop and evaluate improvements and new programs to serve their communities. As new programs are found to be effective, resources must expand to disseminate, scale-up, and replicate promising programs.

Public policy must further support a research agenda that recognizes the importance of community engagement in integrating new knowledge into research and program development. Funding allocation must recognize the complexity of CAPs, including the time required to establish trust, the training needs, and the changes in all aspects of the research process—hypothesis generation, recruitment, consent, design, and dissemination—that will take place as a function of community participation. In all research endeavors at the community level, moreover, adequate resources must be provided for program evaluation to guide local implementation, replication, and translation. In addition, public policy governing funding must be willing to re-examine its approach to "best practices," valuing, instead, where appropriate, internal validity arrangement and learning to capture and translate broad lessons from highly effective specific interventions (Green and Mercer 2001). Furthermore, explicit policies are critical to ensure that data from studies are accessible to a variety of audiences and users, including user-friendly presentation of data and appropriate training. For that reason, public policy must support the provision of resources for appropriate data collection to inform community-based programs, including maintenance of the infrastructure and support for data collection that elucidates social determinants and health disparities.

Public policy must also support cross-sector, multi-disciplinary research collaborations. As we have seen, engagement of diverse community members and stakeholders is a promising step in generating innovative interventions and research processes. The research questions and hypotheses that arise will require the involvement of multi-disciplinary expertise to uncover the pathways that connect the community environment to biological outcomes, and to design local and policy-level solutions. Srinivasan et al. (2003) point the need for research to "identify mechanisms by which the built environment adversely and positively impacts health and to develop appropriate interventions to reduce or eliminate harmful health effects." In particular, they emphasize the dearth of studies on the benefits of aspects of the "built environment" as the basis for policy changes to benefit public health and quality of life. The authors call for multi-disciplinary collaboration to identify the measures and indicators for sustainable communities, coordination among federal and non-federal agencies to promote such research, community participation in this research, and development of "multi-level techniques of measurement in order to assess the impact of the built environment, accounting for individual, community and systemic variables, including biological factors, socioeconomic factors, and neighborhood and physical environment variables." Finally, we will need methods to translate research findings into policy and programs at the community level to improve public health. CBPR and other collaborative approaches are appropriate strategies to implement this ambitious research agenda.

Coordinating Systems and Building Infrastructure

Whatever the specific strategy used, the education, knowledge, and belief systems that function as barriers to participation in screening, follow-up and, ultimately, treatment must be addressed through multiple, coordinated, and mutually reinforcing channels. Providers must be knowledgeable about these barriers and address them in the clinical encounter. Health care systems must be attentive to these issues and devise monitored and responsive quality improvement systems for tracking and follow-up. Community-based strategies must reach out to individuals at high risk of not being screened to provide appropriate information and motivation, based on community-specific data, and then provide assistance in navigating screening, follow-up, and treatment. To the extent that high-risk individuals and communities, by definition, experience multiple barriers to appropriate care, systems must have some degree of redundancy. Ideally, this approach will allow clinical and community-based systems to function in a coordinated manner, providing a consistent message, reliable and timely access to education, screening resources, and care, and will allow these systems to respond to the specific challenges we have seen in urban and rural areas.

Structural Changes

In addition to all the recommendations discussed above, eliminating cancer-related disparities entirely will require additional resources and infrastructure. It is beyond the scope of this chapter to discuss social policies and strategies to create structural changes that will provide the bases for improving health status, such as safe and health-promoting physical environments, employment and economic opportunities, appropriate and high-quality educational opportunities across the lifespan, and political voice and empowerment at local and national levels. It is, however, relevant to be cognizant of these structural factors, and be attentive to building infrastructure in these domains when designing health-related research, systems change, and interventions.

Looking Critically at Community-Based Programs

It is appropriate to conclude this discussion with a critique of community-based programs themselves. As we have seen, despite their promise, a performance gap remains, as do many unanswered questions about the design, implementation, and evaluation of community-based programs. Here it is helpful to think in terms of two fundamental questions discussed at greater length in Merzel's critical review of community-based programs (Merzel and D'Affitti 2003).

What Are the Most Effective Strategies for Engaging Communities?

Community-based programs employ a variety of techniques to engage communities. Critically assessing the actual engagement that is accomplished, as well as how the voice of communities is incorporated into the various stages of the program, is essential. As Merzel points out: "Few projects have been able to fully apply key principles of community-based health promotion, which emphasize facilitating community capacity and readiness to mobilize and establishing true partnerships in which researchers and communities share decision-making and resources" (Merzel and D'Affitti 2003).

To what Extent Is the Ecological Model Actually Implemented?

Although the ecological model offers a useful framework for designing interventions, few programs actually implement and integrate interventions at all levels. Activities and program measures tend to be focused on individual-level behaviors and indicators, at least partially, because these indicators are more easily defined. Merzel recommends that programs should fully reflect the ecological framework and attempt to influence not only individual risk but community-level factors and the normative social environment. Similarly, evaluation should go beyond individual behavior change and measure impact on community organizations, social norms, and social policy. She reminds us that interventions may not be able to change individual behavior substantially without changing the broader social environment (Merzel and D'Affitti 2003).

This brings us to a set of recommendations to enhance the potential of community-based programs. We must:

- improve the metrics of evaluation as well as the resources devoted to this important activity;
- improve the application of the ecological framework to learn how efforts at all levels can be mutually reinforcing;
- critically evaluate the expected outcomes of interventions at each level of the ecological framework to ensure that outcomes are appropriate for each level;
- expand the practical and theoretical understanding of community-based interventions, particularly with regard to scale, intensity, and duration;
- explicitly incorporate policy-level objectives and measures;

- improve the knowledge base of translation and replication so that successful programs can be brought to scale where appropriate; and
- establish realistic expectations for what community-based programs can and cannot accomplish.

V. Conclusion

Community-based programs can reach populations, including those thought of as "vulnerable" and "inaccessible," by exploiting social networks such as family, neighborhood, religious, and other key affiliations. Community-based programs can address the social context in which health choices and other health behaviors occur and take place in the real environments in which people live, providing reliable evidence of how programs and policies can influence health behaviors, and, ultimately, health. These programs can provide an opportunity to build community capacity and civic engagement and incite empowering social change. Implemented in a favorable policy environment, with appropriate resources and expectations, and synergy across all layers of the ecological model, community-based programs can deliver on their promise and potential to be a powerful tool in the fight against cancer and other health disparities.

References

Aaron KF, Levine D, Burstin HR. African American church participation and health care practices. J Gen Intern Med, Nov 2003;18(11):908–913.

Agrawal M, Grady C, Fairclough DL, Meropol NJ, Maynard K, Emanuel EJ. Patients' decision-making process regarding participation in phase 1 oncology research. J Clin Oncol, 2007;25(5):548–554.

Ammerman A, Corbie-Smith G, St George DM, Washington C, Weathers B, Jackson-Christian B. Research expectations among African American church leaders in the PRAISE! Project: A randomized trial guided by community-based participatory research. ASPH, Oct 2003;93(10):1720–1727.

Angell KL, Kreshka MA, McCoy R, Donnelly P, et al. Psychosocial intervention for rural women with breast cancer. JGIM, July 2003;(18)7:499–507.

Baker EA, Kelly C, Barnidge E, Strayhorn J, Schootman M, Struthers J, Griffith D. The Garden of Eden: acknowledging the impact of race and class in efforts to decrease obesity rates. AJPH, July 2006;96(7):1170–1174.

Baluja KF, Park J, Myers D. Inclusion of immigrant status in smoking prevalence statistics. AJPH, April 2003;93(4):642–646.

Campbell MK, Demark-Wahnefried W, Symons M, Kalsbeek WD et al. Fruit and vegetable consumption and prevention of cancer: The Black Churches United for Better Health Project. AJPH, Sept 1999;89(9):1390–1396.

Campbell MK, James A, Hudson MA, Carr C, Jackson E, Oates V, Demissie S, Farrel D, Tessaro I. Improving multiple behaviors for colorectal cancer prevention among African American church members. Health Psych, Sept 2004;23(5):492–502.

Cheadle A, Wagner E, Walls M, et al. The effect of neighborhood-based community organizing: results from the Seattle Minority Youth Health Project. Health Serv Res, 2001;36:671–677.

Chino M, DeBruyn L. Building true capacity: indigenous models for indigenous communities. AJPH, Apr 2006;96(4):596–599.

Cohen DA, Mason K, Bedimo A, Scribner R, Basolo V, Farley TA. Neighborhood physical conditions and health. AJPH, 2003;(93)3:267–471.

COMMIT Research Group. Community intervention trial for smoking cessation (COMMIT): I. Cohort results from a four-year community intervention. AJPH, 1995a;85:183–192.

COMMIT Research Group. Community intervention trial for smoking cessation (COMMIT): II. Changes in adult cigarette smoking prevalence. AJPH, 1995b;85:193–200.

Corbie-Smith G, Ammerman AS, Katz ML, St George DMM, Blumenthal C, et al. Trust, benefit, satisfaction and burden, a randomized controlled trial to reduce cancer risk through African-American churches. J Gen Int Med, 2003;18:531–541.

Corbie-Smith G, Thomas SB, Williams MV, Moody-Ayers S. Attitudes and beliefs of African Americans toward participation in medical research. J Gen Intern Meds, Sept 1999;14(9):537–546.

DeHaven MJ, Hunter IB, Wilder L, Walton JW, Berry J. Health programs in faith-based organizations: Are they effective? ASPH, Jun 2004;94(6):1030–1036.

Derose KP, Hawes-Dawson J, Fox SA, Maldonado N, Tatum A, Kington R. Dealing will diversity: recruiting churches and women for a randomized trial of mammography promotion. Health Educ Behav, Oct 2000;27(5):632–648.

Desch CE, Grasso MA, McCue MJ et al. A rural cancer outreach program lowers patient care costs and benefits both the rural hospitals and sponsoring academic medical center. J Rural Health, 1999;15:157–167.

Dietrich AJ, Tobin JN, Cassells A, Robinson CM et al. Telephone care management to improve cancer screening among low-income women: a randomized controlled trial. Ann Int Med, 18 Apr 2006;144(8):563–571.

Drake BE, Keane TE, Mosley CM, Adams SA et al. Prostate cancer disparities in South Carolina: early detection, special programs and descriptive epidemiology. JSC Med Assoc, Aug 2006;102(7):241–249.

Duan H, Fox SA, Derose KP, Carson S. Maintaining mammography adherence through telephone counseling in a church-based trial. AJPH, Sept 2000;90(9):1468–1471.

Duhl LJ. An ecohistory of health: the role of "healthy cities." Am J Health Prom, 1996;10:258–261.

Fagan P, King G, Lawrence D, Petrucci SA et al. Eliminating tobacco-related health disparities: directions for future research. AJPH, Feb 2004;94(2):211–217.

Fals-Borda O. The application of participatory action-research in Latin America. Int Sociol, 1987;2:329–247.

Farquhar SA, Michael YL, Wiggins N. Building on leadership and social capital to create change I 2 urban communities. AJPH, Apr 2005;95(4):596–601.

Fisher E, Auslander W, Sussman L, Owens N, Jackson-Thompson J. Community organization and health promotion in minority neighborhoods. Ethn Dis, 1992;2:252–272.

Fisher EB, Auslander WF, Munro JF, Arfken CL, Ross C, Owens NW. Neighbors for a smoke free North Side: evaluation of a community organization approach to promoting smoking cessation among African Americans AJPH, Nov 1998;88(11):1658–1663.

Flaskerud JH, Nyamathi A. Attaining gender and ethnic diversity in health intervention research: cultural responsiveness versus resource provision. Adv Nurs Sci, Jun 2000;22(4):1–15.

Flaskerud JH, Winslow BJ. Conceptualizing vulnerable populations' health-related research. Nurs Res, 1998;47(2):69–78.

Fowler BA. Social processes used by African American women in making decisions about mammography screening. J Nurs Scholarsh, Sept 2006;38(3):247–254.

Fox CE, Morford TG, Fine A, Gibbons MC. The Johns Hopkins Urban Health Institute: A collaborative response to urban health issues. Acad Med, Dec 2004 79(12):1169–1174.

Freire, P. Pedagogy of the oppressed. New York: Continuum International Publishing Group, 2000: p. 183.

Gasewood JD, Rollins LK, Galazka SS. Beyond the horizon: the role of academic health centers in improving the health of rural communities. Acad Med, Sept 2006;81(9):793–797.

Gebbie K, Rosenstock L, Hernandez LM. Who Will Keep the Public Health? Educating public health professionals for the 12th Century. Washington, DC: Institutes of Medicine, National Academy of Sciences, 2002.

Geronimus AT, Hicken M, Keene D, Bound J. "Weathering" and age patterns of allostatic load scores among blacks and whites in the United States. AJPH, May 2006;96(5):826–833.

Geronimus AT. To mitigate, resist, or undo: addressing structural influences on the health of urban populations. AJPH, Jun 2000;90(6):867–872.

Green LW, George MA, Frankish CJ, Herbert CJ, Bowie WR, O'Neil M. Study of Participatory Research in Health Promotion: Review and Recommendations for the Development of Participatory Research in Health Promotion in Canada. Ottawa: Royal Society of Canada, 1995

Green LW, Mercer SL. Can public health researchers and agencies reconcile the push from funding bodies and the pull from communities? ASPH, Dec 2001;91(12):1926–1929.

Guthrie BJ, Young AM, Williams DR, Boyd CJ, Kintner EK. African American girls' smoking habits and day-to-day experiences with racial discrimination. Nurs Res, May/Jun 2002;51(3):183–190.

Hansen LK, Feigl P, Modiano MR, Lopez JA et al. An educational program to increase cervical and breast cancer screening in Hispanic women: a Southwest Oncology Group study. Cancer Nurs, Jan/Feb 2005;28(1):47–53.

Helman CG. Culture, Health and Illness, 4th ed. London: Hodder Headline Group, 2000. p. 88.

Holkup PA, Tripp-Reimer T, Salois EM, Weinert C. Community-based participatory research: an approach to intervention research with a Native American Community. Adv Nurs Sci, July/Aug/Sept 2004;27(3):162–175.

Institute of Medicine. Quality Through Collaboration: The Future of Rural Health Care. Washington, DC, National Academies Press, 2005.

Israel BA, Schulz AJ, Parker EA, Becker AB. Review of community-based research: assessing partnership approaches to improve public health. Annual Review of Public Health, 1998;19:173–302.

Jacobs EA, Karavolos K, Rathouz PJ, Ferris TG, Powell LH. Limited English proficiency and breast and cervical cancer screening in a multiethnic population. AJPH, Aug 2005;95(8):1410–1416.

Jemal A, Siegel R, Ward E, Hao Y, Xu J, Murray T, Thun MJ. Cancer statistics, 2008. CA Cancer J Clin 2008;58:71–96.

Kellogg WK. Community Health Scholars Program, 2001 (quoted in Hartwig K, Calleson D, Williams M). Developing and sustaining community-based participatory research partnerships: a skill-building curriculum, 2006. Accessed February 16, 2009, http://depts.washington.edu/ccph/cbpr/append/dappend.php

Koch T, Selim P, Kralik D. Enhancing lives through the development of a community-based participatory research program. J Clin Nurs, January 2002;(11)1:109–117.

Kreling B, Figueiredo MI, Sheppard VL, Mandelblatt JS. A qualitative study of factors affecting chemotherapy use in older women with breast cancer: barriers, promoters, and implications for intervention. Psychooncology, Apr 2006;15(12):1065–1076.

Kretzmann JP, McKnight JL. Building Communities from the Inside Out: A Path Toward Finding and Mobilizing a Community's Assets. Evanston, IL: Institute for Policy Research, 1993.

Kreuter MW, Alcaraz CI, Pfeiffer D, Christopher K. Using dissemination research to identify optimal community settings for tailored breast cancer information kiosks. J Pub Health Manage Pract, Mar/Apr 2008;14(2):160–169.

Lam TK, McPhee SJ, Mock J, Wong C et al. Encouraging Vietnamese-American women to obtain Pap tests through lay health worker outreach and media education. J Gen Intern Med, 2003;18:516–524.

Lantz PM, Stencil D, Lippert MAT, Beversdorf S, Jaros L, Remington PL. Breast and cervical cancer screening in a low-income managed care sample: the efficacy of physician letters and phone calls. AJPH, June 1995;85(6):834–836.

Lee MC. Knowledge, barriers and motivators related to cervical cancer screening among Korean-American women: A focus group approach. Cancer Nurs, June 2000;23(3):168–175.

Leon DA, Davey SG. Infant mortality, stomach cancer, stroke, and coronary heart disease: ecological analysis. BMJ, 24 June 2000;320(7251):1705–1706.

Liang W, Burnett CB, Rowland JH, Meropol NJ, et al. Communication between physicians and older women with localized breast cancer: Implications for treatment and patient satisfaction. J Clin Oncol, Feb 2002;120(4):1008–1016.

Lindau ST, Tomori C, Lyons T, Langseth L, Bennett CL, Garcia P. The association of health literacy with cervical cancer prevention knowledge and health behaviors in a multiethnic cohort of women. Am J Obstet Gynecol, May 2002;186(5):938–243.

Linden HM, Reisch LM, Hart A, Harrington MA, Nakano C, et al. Attitudes toward participation in breast cancer randomized clinical trials in the African American Community: a focus group study. Cancer Nurs, July/Aug 2007;30(4):261–269.

Maantay J. Zoning, equity and public health. AJPH, July 2001;91(7):1033–1041.

Macaulay AC, Delormier T, McComber AM, et al. Participatory research with native community of Kahnawake creates innovative Cod eof Research Ethics. Can J Pub Health, 1998;89:105–108.

MacQueen KM, et al. What is community? An evidence-based definition for participatory public health. AJPH, 2001;91:1929–1938.

Mandelblat JS, Edge SB, Meropol NJ, Senie R. Predictors of long-term outcomes in older breast cancer survivors: Perceptions versus patterns of care. J Clin Oncol, Mar 2003;21(5):855–863.

Margolis ML, Christie JD, Sylvestri GA, Kaiser L, et al. Racial differences pertaining to a belief about lung cancer surgery: Results of a multi-center survey. Ann Intern Med, October 2003;139(7):558–563.

Markens S, Fox SA, Taub B, Gilbert ML. Told of Black churches in health promotion programs: lessons from the Los Angeles Mammography Promotion in Churches Program. ASPH, May 2002;92(5):805–810.

McEwen BS, Seeman T. Protective and damaging effects of mediators of stress: elaborating and testing the concepts of allostasis and allostatic load. Ann NY Acad Sci, 1999;896:30–47.

McLeroy KR, Bibeau D, Steckler A, Glanz K. An ecological perspective on health promotion programs. Health Educ Q, 1988;15(4):351–377.

Merzel C, D'Affitti J. Reconsidering community-based health promotion: Promise, performance, and potential. AJPH, Apr 2003;93(4):557–574.

Mincker M, Blackwell AG, Thompson M, Tamir H. Community-based participatory research: Implications for public health funding. AJPH, Aug 2003;93(8):1210–1213.

Mojica CM, Roshan B, Ninez AP, Boscardin WJ. Latinas with abnormal breast findings: patient predictors of timely diagnostic resolution. J Women's Health 2007;16(10):1468–1477.

Navarro AM, Senn KL, McNicholas LJ, Kaplan FM, Roppe B, Campo MC. Por La Vida model intervention enhances use of cancer screening tests among Latinas. Am J Prev Med, 1998;15(1):32–41.

Nienaber-Clarke J, Gerlak A. Environmental racism in southern Arizona: the reality behind the rhetoric. In: Camacho DE, ed. Environmental Injustices, Political Struggles: Race, Class and the Environment. Durham, NC: Duke University Press, 1998, pp. 82–100.

Northridge ME, Morabia A, Ganz ML, et al. Contribution of smoking to excess mortality in Harlem. Am J Epidemiol, 1998;147:250–258.

O'Malley AS, Mandelblatt J, Gold K, Cagney KA, Kerner J. Continuity of care and the use of breast and cervical cancer screening services in a multiethnic community. Arch Intern Med, 1997;157(13):1462–1470.

O'Toole TP, Aaron KF, Chin MH, Horowitz C, Tyson F. Community-based participatory research, opportunities, challenges, and the need for a common language. J Gen Intern Med, July 2003;18:592–594.

Olden K, Guthrie J, Newton S. A bold new direction for environmental health research. AJPH, 2001;91:1964–1967.

Orians CE, Erb J, Kenyon KL, Lantz PM, et al. Public education strategies for delivering breast and cervical cancer screening in American Indian and Alaska Native populations. J Pub Health Manage Pract, Jan/Feb 2004;10(1):46–53.

Partridge EE, Fouad MN, Hinton AW, et al. The Deep South Network for Cancer Control: eliminating cancer disparities through community-academic collaboration. Fam Comm Health, 2005;28:6–19.

Paskett ED, Case LD, Tatum C, Velez R, Wilson A. Religiosity and cancer screening. J Relig Health, Mar 1999;38(1):39–52.

Phillip W, James T, Nelson M, Ralph A, Leather S. Socioeconomic determinants of health: the contribution of nutrition to inequalities in health. BMJ, 24 May 1997;314(7093):1545–1549.

Powell IS, Heilbrun L, Littrup PL, Franklin A, et al. Outcome of African American men screened for prostate cancer: The Detroit Education and Early Detection Study. J Urol, 1997:158(1):146–149.

Prakash S. "Taking action in Northern Manhattan." Environmental Health Perspectives Feb 2005. FindArticles.com. 14 May 2008 http://findarticles.com/p/articles/mi_m0CYP/is_2_113/ai_n15625847

Probst JC, Moore CG, Glover SH, Samuels ME. Person and place: the compounding effects of race/ethnicity and rurality on health. AJPH, 2004;94:1695–1703.

Regan J, Lefkowitz B, Gaston MH. Cancer screening among community health center women: eliminating the gaps. J Ambul Care Manage, Oct 1999;22(4):45–52.

Robinson R. West Dallas versus the lead smelter. In: Bullard R, Ed., Unequal protection: Environmental justice and communities of color. San Francisco, CA: Sierra Bluc Books, 1996, pp. 92–109.

Rogers D, Petereit DG. Cancer disparities research partnership in Lakota Country: clinical trials, patient services, and community education for the Oglala, Rosebud, and Cheyenne River Sioux tribes. AJPH, Dec 2005;95(12):2129–2132.

Salazar MK. Hispanic women's beliefs about breast cancer and mammography. Cancer Nurs, 1996;19(6):437–446.

Sateren WB, Trimble EL, Abrams J. How sociodemographics, presence of oncology specialists and hospital cancer programs affect accrual to cancer treatment trials. J. Clin Oncol, 2002;(20):2109–2117.

Seeman TE, Singer BH, Rowe JW, Horowitz RI, McEwen BS. Price of adaptation-allostatic load and its health consequences. Arch Intern Med, 1997;157:2259–2268.

Seidenfeld J, Horstmann E, Emanuel EJ, Grady C. Participants in phase 1 oncology research trials: are they vulnerable? Arch Int Med, Jan 14 2008;168(1):16–20.

Shah AM, Whitman S, Silva A. Variations in the health conditions of 6 Chicago community areas: A case for local level data. ASP, Aug 2006;96(8):1485–1491.

Sontag S. Illness as Metaphor and AIDS and Its Metaphor. New York: Picador USA, 1989.

Srinivasan S, O'Fallon LR, Dearry A. Creating healthy communities, healthy homes, healthy people: initiating a research agenda on the built environment and public health. AJPH, Sept 2003;93(9):1446–1450.

Stokols D. Translating social ecological theory into guidelines for community health promotion. Am J Health Promot, 1996;10:282–298.

Stringer ET. Action Research (2nd Ed.) Thousand Oaks, CA. Sage Publications, 1999.

Sue S, Fujino DC, Hu L, Takeuchi DT, Zane NWS. Community mental health services for ethnic groups: a test of the cultural responsiveness hypothesis. J Consult Clin Psychol, 1991;59:533–540.

Taylor RJ, Ellison CG, Chatters LM, Levin JS, Lincoln KD. Mental health services in faith communities: the role of clergy in black churches. Soc Work, 2000;45:73–87.

Tingen MS, Weinrich SP, Heydt DD, Boyd MD, Weinrich MC. Perceived benefits: a predictor of participation in prostate cancer screening. Cancer Nurs, Oct 1998;21(5):349–357.

Tsui J, Mona S, Trevor T, Dey A, Richardson L. Cervical cancer screening among foreign-born women by birthplace and duration in the United States. J Women's Health, 2007;16(10):1447–1457.

Valdina A, Cargill LC. Access and barriers to mammography in New England community health centers. J Fam Pract, 1997;45(3):243–249.

Weinrich S, Holdford D, Boyd M, Greanga D, et al. Prostate cancer education in African American churches. Publ Health Nurs, Jun 1998;15(3):188–195.

Wells BL, Horm JW. Targeting the underserved for breast and cervical cancer screening: the utility of ecological analysis using the National Health Interview Survey. AJPH, Oct 1998;88(10):1484–1489.

Wells JNB, Bush HA, Marshall D. Psychometric evaluation of Breast Health Behavior Questionnaire: SPANISH VERSION. Cancer Nurs, Aug 2001;24(4):320–327.

Wing S, Grant G, Green M, Stewart C. Community based environmental justice: southeast Halifax environmental reawakening. Environ Urban, 1996;8:129–140.

Wright B, Bryant P, Bullard R. Coping with poisons in Cancer Alley. In: Bullard R, ed. Unequal Protection: Environmental Justice and Communities of Color. San Francisco, CA: Sierra Club Books, 1996, pp. 110–129.

Index

Printed in the United States
152570LV00001B/34/P